BIOLOGICAL BASES OF PSYCHIATRIC DISORDERS

BIOLOGICAL BASES OF PSYCHIATRIC DISORDERS

Alan Frazer, Ph.D.
Veterans Administration Hospital and
Departments of Psychiatry and Pharmacology
University of Pennsylvania School of Medicine
Philadelphia, PA

and

Andrew Winokur, M.D., Ph.D.
Departments of Psychiatry and Pharmacology
University of Pennsylvania School of Medicine
Philadelphia, PA

SP
SP Books Division of
SPECTRUM PUBLICATIONS, INC.
New York • London

SPECTRUM PUBLICATIONS, INC.
175-20 Wexford Terrace, Jamaica, N.Y. 11432

Library of Congress Cataloging in Publication Data

Main entry under title:

Biological bases of psychiatric disorders.

    Bibliography: p.
    Includes index.
    1. Mental illness--Physiological aspects.
I. Frazer, Alan. II. Winokur, Andrew. [DNLM:
1. Neurophysiology. 2. Psychophysiology.
3. Mental disorders WM100 B6143]
RC455.4.B5B56   616.8'9'071   77-413
ISBN 0-89335-011-7

Contents

Contributors

AARON T. BECK, M.D.
Department of Psychiatry
University of Pennsylvania
School of Medicine
Philadelphia, Pa.

ALEXANDER L. BECKMAN, Ph.D.
Department of Physiology
University of Pennsylvania
School of Medicine
Philadelphia, Pa.

ROBERT CANCRO, M.D.
Department of Psychiatry
New York University School of Medicine
New York, N.Y.

ALAN FRAZER, Ph.D.
Veterans Administration Hospital
Departments of Pharmacology and Psychiatry
University of Pennsylvania
School of Medicine
Philadelphia, Pa.

RUTH L. GREENBERG, B.A.
Department of Psychiatry
University of Pennsylvania
School of Medicine
Philadelphia, Pa.

RAQUEL GUR, Ph.D.
Department of Psychiatry
University of Pennsylvania
School of Medicine
Philadelphia, Pa.

RUBEN C. GUR, Ph.D.
Department of Psychology
University of Pennsylvania
Philadelphia, Pa.

JERRE LEVY, Ph.D.
Department of Psychology
University of Pennsylvania
Philadelphia, Pa.

CONTRIBUTORS

JOSEPH LIPINSKY, M.D.
Harvard Medical School
Psychiatric Research Laboratories
Massachusetts General Hospital
Boston, Mass.

STEVEN MATHYSSE, Ph.D.
Harvard Medical School
Psychiatric Research Laboratories
Massachusetts General Hospital
Boston, Mass.

WILLIAM T. McKINNEY, JR., M.D.
Department of Psychiatry
Director, Wisconsin Psychiatry Research Institute
University of Wisconsin
Medical School
Madison, Wisconsin

JULIAN MENDLEWICZ, M.D., Ph.D.
Institut de Psychiatrie
Universite Libre de Bruxelles
Bruxelles, Belgium

HELEN L. MORRISON, M.D.
Wisconsin Psychiatric Research Institute
Department of Psychiatry
Center for Health Sciences
University of Wisconsin
Madison, Wisconsin

RUSSEL E. POLAND, B.A.
Department of Pharmacology
UCLA School of Medicine
Los Angeles, California

T. ALAN RAMSEY, M.D.
Veterans Administration Hospital
Department of Psychiatry
University of Pennsylvania
School of Medicine
Philadelphia, Pa.

KARL RICKELS, M.D.
Departments of Psychiatry and Pharmacology
University of Pennsylvania
School of Medicine
Philadelphia, Pa.

ROBERT T. RUBIN, M.D., Ph.D.
Department of Psychiatry
UCLA School of Medicine
Harbor General Hospital Campus
Torrance, California

PETER STERLING, Ph.D.
Department of Anatomy
University of Pennsylvania
School of Medicine
Philadelphia, Pa.

JAMES L. STINNETT, M.D.
Department of Psychiatry
University of Pennsylvania
School of Medicine
Philadelphia, Pa.

ANDREW WINOKUR, M.D., Ph.D.
Departments of Psychiatry & Pharmacology
University of Pennsylvania
School of Medicine
Philadelphia, Pa.

Foreword

THE BRAIN is the organ of behavior. Everything we do, everything we feel, everything we think is the result of the physiological activity of the brain. More than that, the brain is plastic. It records all experience as some set of complex and as yet unknown changes within its own biological structure. This plasticity, of course, is what accounts for the great influence of past experience in the control of behavior and makes learning such an important determinant of what the higher organism is. Yet the basic biological properties of the brain are given by heredity and appear in the course of maturation and development. Thus both heredity and environment determine the biological properties of the brain, and as a result, the behavior and the mind of man.

Nowhere is this relation between brain and behavior more dramatically illustrated than in the domain of the behavior disorders, particularly the psychiatric disorders. Our scientific knowledge is so primitive that we cannot yet detail the mechanisms that have gone awry in schizophrenia, manic-depressive psychosis, depression, *anxiety and other neurotic manifestations, or psychosomatic disorders. Nevertheless, enormous strides have been made in the last 25 years in our understanding of the basic principles of neurobiology and in the growth of our empirical knowledge of the action of behavior-altering or psychotropic drugs. Thus we are on the threshold of understanding the mechanisms underlying many psychiatric disorders and have the possibility of developing the basis for their cure.*

For this reason alone, this book is an important introduction for the next generation of neurobiologists and neuropsychiatrists. But it is more than that. It is an invitation to an exciting intellectual venture into the most intricate organ of the body and into the most complex and most important problem facing modern medicine: the mind and its disorders.

The book does a remarkable job illustrating the fruitful partnership of basic science and clinical investigations in not only solving practical problems, but in framing fundamental questions that will advance basic knowledge. For this reason, the book is eminently suitable for: 1) college students with an interest in behavioral biology, neurobiology, and physiological psychology; 2) graduate students in anatomy, neurobiology, pharmacology, physiology, and psychology; 3) medical students interested in neurology, psychiatry, and psychosomatic medicine; and 4) residents in psychiatry and neurology.

The book is an interdisciplinary one, written as it is by contributors from anatomy, biology, pharmacology, physiology, psychology and psychiatry. It deals with the modern anatomical concept of the brain as a complex network, with highly differentiated ultrastructure, providing a physical substrate for a variety of chemical processes and physiological interactions. Thus the neuro-anatomy becomes important. The function of this network is to process information in myriads of local neuronal circuits, and transmit this information via propagated nerve impulses along axions to multiple loci in the brain. Thus, the neurophysiology becomes important. In both the local circuits and the longer pathways, the critical action takes place in the synapses, due to the release of neurotransmitter substances such as dopamine, norepinephrine, serotonin, and acetylcholine. Thus, the neurochemistry of the brain becomes important. Furthermore, it turns out that it is on these neurotransmitter mechanisms that many of the potent psychotropic drugs such as chlorpromazine, imipramine, iproniazid, and lithium, meprobamate, diazepam, and chlordiazepoxide act. Thus the pharmacology of the brain becomes important.

The book goes on to summarize what is known of the genetic factors in the etiology of psychiatric disorders, at the very least a strong predisposing factor. But until the genetic mechanism is determined, its influence can only be suggestive of the role of the inherited biological determinants of psychosis.

In a similar way, more and more is being revealed of the neuroendocrine mechanisms that may underlie psychosis. We know that the brain controls the activity of the endocrine glands. Neuro-secretory cells in the hypothalamus of the brain act upon the anterior pituitary gland via a special portal circulation. In this way, the activity of the thyroid, adrenal medulla, adrenal cortex, pancreas, and gonads are controlled by environmental influences, such as psychological stress, acting on the brain. Thus the way is pointed toward an under-standing of the mechanisms underlying psychosomatic disorders, and more generally, toward the biological mechanisms which may participate in the precipitation of psychiatric disorders.

How well we understand how these mechanisms work depends a great deal on our conception of the organization of the brain as a neurological system. For example, we know the brain is a bilateral system, but we are now learning that it is far from symmetrical, with language function predominating in the left hemisphere of right-handed people and spatial perception pre-dominating in the right hemisphere. So despite the fact that it is evident that the brain is a vastly interconnected network, there is still specialization of function in its various subdivisons.

On the basis of this fundamental biological background, the book then deals with substantive issues in the major behavior disorders: schizophrenia, manic-depressive psychosis, depression, opiate addiction, and alcoholism. It is obvious from this treatment that much is yet to be learned, particularly at the behavioral level in the diagnosis and specification of the behavior disorders them-selves. At the biological level, too, much is yet to be learned, but the outlines of the basic mechanisms are beginning to appear at an accelerating pace. The biological ground is getting firmer, and one might even hope that progress in our biological knowledge of the behavior disorders will help us sort and clarify the diagnostic categories themselves. Furthermore, there is hope that biological progress will lead to insights about the role of the environment, particularly early life experences, as well as identification of genetic influences. Thus there is hope that we may indeed be able to control genetic as well as environmental factors.

The broad outline of exciting possibilities is being drawn.

The reader is invited to join the basic science and clinical investigators represented in the authorship of these chapters and embark upon a creative intellectual adventure that will map the mind of man in his brain and find the cure of his most devastating and perplexing disorders.

Eliot Stellar
Philadelphia, Pennsylvania
1977

BIOLOGICAL BASES OF PSYCHIATRIC DISORDERS

Part I

Pre-clinical Neurosciences

THIS SECTION *consists of chapters reviewing important concepts of neuroanatomy, neurophysiology and neuro-chemistry. A working familiarity with these disciplines is an important prerequisite to understanding the biological mechanisms of behavior and behavioral disorders. It should be pointed out, however, that the traditional distinctions between "basic science" and "clinical" issues frequently prove to be artificial. In many cases, fundamental biological principles and relevant clinical problems involve a high degree of overlap and integration. In fact, the most creative and fruitful research efforts often arise from the collaborative efforts of investigators representing a variety of disciplines who are united by their interest in a specific problem.*

The chapter on neuroanatomy provides a brief orientation to the organization of the brain and to some of the important structures of the central nervous system. The complex connections of neuronal networks is emphasized, and the implications of such intricate interconnections is stressed. It appears that studies utilizing sophisticated techniques to explore the implications of neuronal organization may extend our understanding of the structural aspects of brain function and behavior. This subject is developed further in Chapter 8, which describes clinical studies of brain organization and behavior.

The manner in which messages, in the form of neuronal impulses, are initiated and carried throughout the central nervous system is described in Chapter 2. Basic concepts such as the structure of the neuron and the roles of monovalent and divalent cations in impulse conduction and neurosecretion are reviewed. Since behavior is based upon transmission of messages in the central nervous system and thus involves complex integration of sensory input and effector responses, the mechanisms underlying such a communication system must have enormous behavioral significance.

An understanding of such mechanisms is furthered by the extensive description of the chemical process of communication between pre- and postsynaptic neurons provided in Chapter 3. The metabolic pathways of the catecholamines and indolealkylamines are described, since the neurotransmitters included in these categories are currently thought to be most involved in behavioral disorders and in psychotropic drug effects. Among all the steps associated with the transfer of information in the central nervous system, the neuro-transmission process seems most amenable to alteration and manipulation by drugs, and for this reason is of particular relevance to many of the subjects discussed later in the book.

The basic neural mechanisms involved in the control of behavior are far from fully understood. Nevertheless, attempts to explore the biological aspects of psychiatric disorders must be closely tied to our most extensive knowledge of these basic neural mechanisms. Future developments in clinical areas may well be determined by technological and theoretical advances in the preclinical neuro-science disciplines.

Chapter 1

Principles of Central Nervous System Organization

Peter Sterling

This book is about mental illness and drugs that are used to treat it. We begin with a chapter on the brain because the ways in which one views mental illness and clinical neuro-psychopharmacology rests heavily on one's conception of how the brain works.

Consider, for example, the automobile engine. It is a device in which an explosion of gasoline pushes a piston that turns a drive shaft. Certain complexities must be added to convert this simple causal chain into a workable engine. The explosion in each cylinder must be correctly timed, requiring a "distributor." The fuel mixture must be regulated (carburetor), and also its flow rate (accelerator).

A mechanic confronted with a broken car is confident that with patience he can find the unique source of the difficulty and fix it—by setting the timing, readjusting the carburetor, and so on. His confidence rests on the assumption that each part has a single well-defined function. If, however, the mechanic thought that each part had different functions at different times and that it was difficult to predict which one was important at any given moment, he would not be so confident about making a diagnosis. Furthermore, he would want to be highly conscious of the possibility that altering a certain part might improve one of its functions but cause the

A

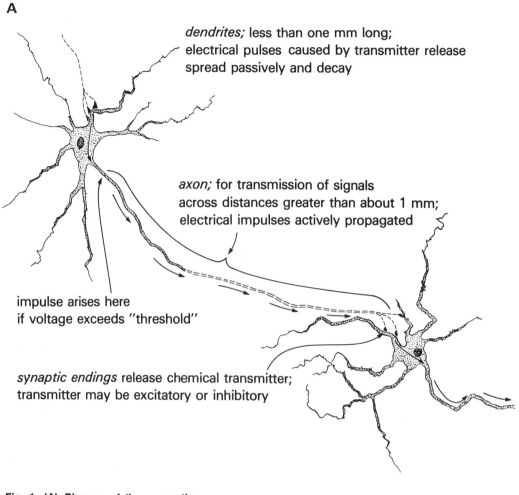

dendrites; less than one mm long;
electrical pulses caused by transmitter release
spread passively and decay

axon; for transmission of signals
across distances greater than about 1 mm;
electrical impulses actively propagated

impulse arises here
if voltage exceeds "threshold"

synaptic endings release chemical transmitter;
transmitter may be excitatory or inhibitory

Fig. 1. (A) Diagram of the connections between 2 neurons.

deterioration of others.

In this chapter, we shall first describe the brain in the way it has been thought to work for at least a century, as a machine made of serially linked functional "centers." Later, we shall point out some of the difficulties with this conception that have been appreciated increasingly over the last decade or so. Finally, we shall redescribe the brain, emphasizing the extraordinary degree to which its parts are interconnected. This description will suggest that to understand the brain one might more usefully approach it as an ecologist than as a mechanic.

Machinery of the brain: The building blocks

The brain is made up of countless billions of nerve cells, or "neurons," each of which is basically a receiver and a transmitter of information (Fig. 1). A neuron receives information from other nerve cells by their contacts, called "syn-

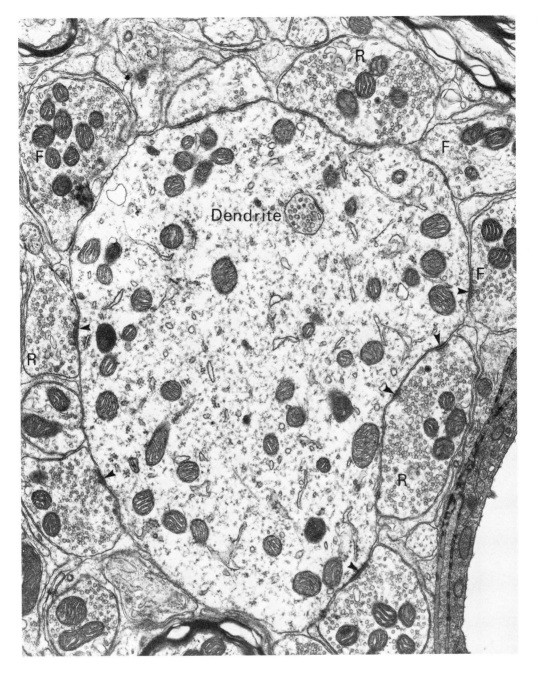

apses," on its short side branches (dendrites) and on its cell body. When active, these synaptic contacts release small packets of chemical "transmitter" substance that tend either to turn the cell on, to excite it, or to turn it off, to inhibit it. This excitatory process is a flow of electrical current into the cell; the inhibitory process is a short-circuiting of that current flow. If the total amount of excitation exceeds the total amount of

Fig. 1. (B) Cross-section through a dendrite magnified 30,000 times in the electron microscope. The dendrite's external surface is studded with 10 synapses. These contain clusters of vesicles, either round (R) or flat (F), whose contents are released onto the dendrite (arrowheads). It is known that in some cases round vesicles are excitatory and flat vesicles are inhibitory. Photograph courtesy of Dr. R.F. Spencer.

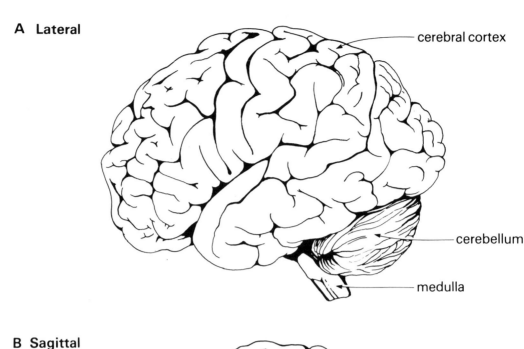

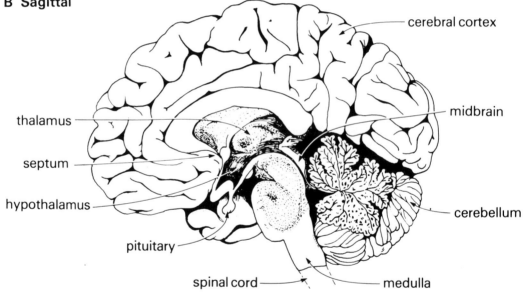

Fig. 2 (A) Diagram of the human brain. Lateral or "side" view of the left hemisphere. (B) Sagittal view of the right hemisphere. Brain has been divided front-to-back to show internal structure.

inhibition, the cell reaches a "threshold" and sends an electrical impulse down its main branch, the axon. At the end of the axon, the nerve impulse causes release of a "transmitter" that excites or inhibits the next cell. The following two chapters will describe in more detail the mechanisms underlying the nerve impulse and the actions of neural transmitter substances.

From this description, one might conceive of the neuron as a device something like an electromechanical relay controlling a telegraph key. On this premise, when there is enough excitatory current, and not too much inhibitory short-circuiting, the key closes and a message is relayed down the axon to the next station. Particular kinds of information are thought to be transmitted along particular lines. For example, "pain" is transmitted by activating "pain" receptors in the skin that transmit to "pain" neurons in the spinal cord, while "touch" is transmitted by activation of a different chain of neurons.

Concepts of the whole brain: assembly of building blocks into chains of functional centers

We return now to the whole brain and consider how its pieces are supposed to be related. Fig. 2 shows two drawings of the human brain. Viewed from the outside (Fig. 2A), the brain appears primarily as a furrowed mass. This tissue is the cerebral cortex that, in man, hides the rest of the brain. Fig. 2B is a view in which the brain is split down the middle from front to back. This reveals the spinal cord, brain stem (medulla and midbrain), cerebellum, diencephalon (thalamus and hypothalamus), and forebrain (cerebral cortex and subcortical structures, the "basal ganglia"). This view also shows that there are several cavities termed "ventricles" within the brain. These contain cerebrospinal fluid (CSF) that is continuously secreted from special ventricular blood vessels (termed "choroid plexus") at the rate of about a liter per day. The CSF percolates through the ventricular system, and escapes from several openings in the brain at the level of the medulla. The CSF is sequestered by a membranous sac (the "meninges") that encases the brain and spinal cord. As a consequence, the whole central nervous system is actually suspended in a fluid medium much as is the embryo in the amniotic fluid.

Invariably, the first question asked about the gross structures, such as the forebrain and the cerebellum is, "What do they do?". It is a reasonable question, particularly in view of our experience with the common sorts of machines in which specific parts have unambiguously defined functions. The usual answer is that each piece contains "centers" that carry out particular functions. The brain is considered as an assembly of "centers" arranged in hierarchical fashion. The spinal cord and brain stem are considered to contain "lower" ("reflex") centers, the automatic machinery for controlling basic bodily functions, such as posture, breathing, heart rate and blood pressure. The cerebral cortex is supposed to contain "higher" centers for conducting "higher" functions such as sensation, perception, thought, language and "voluntary" movement. All information arriving at the central nervous system enters two parallel, linear paths: one is a reflex path toward motor neurons, which arise in the spinal cord and innervate skeletal muscle, and the second is a pathway that ascends toward the higher centers.

Several examples are shown in Figs. 3 and 4. In the first, a stimulus activates a sensory neuron specialized to detect "pain." This neuron sends information into the reflex chain that quickly removes the body from the stimulus. Simultaneously, the information enters the pathway leading toward the cerebral cortex. Centers along the path to the cortex, the thalamus, for example, are considered primarily as "relay" stations that modify very little the information arriving at the cortex.

For visual stimuli (Fig. 4), there is also a separate pair of "lower" and "higher" pathways quite parallel to those

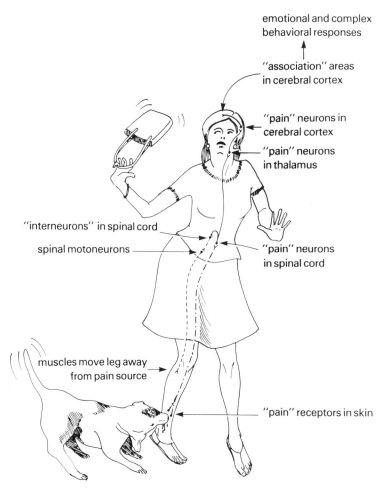

emotional and complex
behavioral responses

"association" areas
in cerebral cortex

"pain" neurons in
cerebral cortex

"pain" neurons
in thalamus

"interneurons" in spinal cord

spinal motoneurons

"pain" neurons
in spinal cord

muscles move leg away
from pain source

"pain" receptors in skin

Fig. 3.   Two pathways for "pain" information entering the nervous system, one for "automatic," or "reflex" control, and the other for "higher" centers.

for pain. Visual information enters the reflex paths in the midbrain that control the pupil size, blinking and automatic orientation of the head and eyes toward the stimulus. The same information enters the relay system through the thalamus to the cortex. Both thalamus and cortex are subdivided so that particular parts of thalamus are associated with particular cortical regions. Thus, the parallel, private lines are maintained.

The cortex itself is subdivided into centers, again arranged in serial array. Visual information arriving from the thalamus in the "primary" visual cortex is then relayed to the visual "association" cortex. If the visual information is written language, it is supposed to be relayed to a region called Wernicke's area where the visual patterns are "recognized" as words. The relay proceeds from there to Broca's area where the words are assembled into grammatical language, and from there to the motor cortex which controls, by means of instructions to lower centers, the articulatory organs (either mouth and vocal cords for speaking, or hands for writing).

It is also supposed that there are distinct brain centers for emotion and for

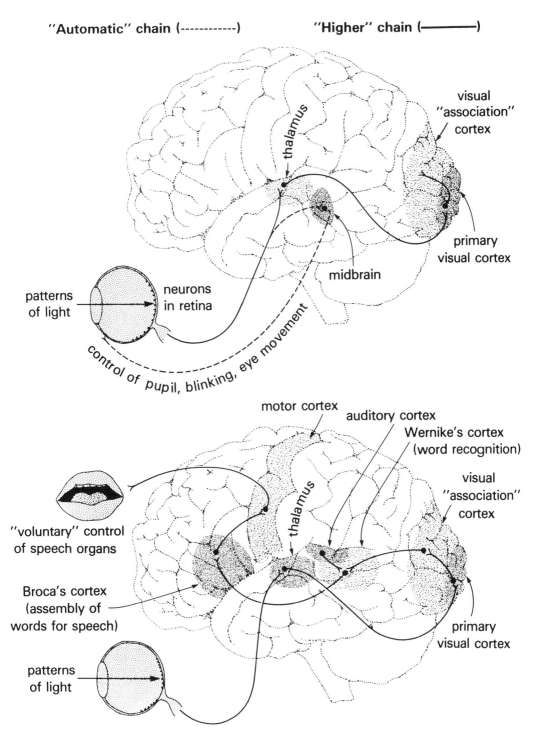

"Automatic" chain (-----------)   "Higher" chain (—————)

visual "association" cortex

thalamus

primary visual cortex

midbrain

patterns of light   neurons in retina

control of pupil, blinking, eye movement

motor cortex   auditory cortex   Wernike's cortex (word recognition)

visual "association" cortex

thalamus

"voluntary" control of speech organs

Broca's cortex (assembly of words for speech)

primary visual cortex

patterns of light

Fig. 4. "Automatic" and "higher" pathways for vision. Location of functionally distinct regions of the cortex were mapped by electrical stimulation in awake humans. Drawing based on the work of Penfield.

"motivated" behavior, such as feeding, drinking, fighting and sexual behavior. These centers are supposed to be located in the hypothalamus (Fig. 2B) and to be "modulated" by information relayed from ascending sensory systems, by hormones, and also by complex pathways descending from the cerebral cortex. The set of centers and pathways involved in emotion and "motivated" behavior has been termed the "limbic system" (Fig. 9B).

The plan we have just sketched portrays the brain as a machine built with chains of simple elements that are linked in linear, causal sequences, not different in principle from such familiar machines as the gasoline engine. Like these machines, the brain also contains numerous organs and systems that are important modifying mechanisms, but, nevertheless, are separate from the primary causal chain. The cerebellum, for example, has been viewed as a timing organ, analogous to a distributor, for ensuring that muscular contractions occur with the correct timing, so that the body does not "run rough." The "ascending reticular activating system" is a pathway ascending from the spinal cord and brain stem to the cerebral cortex. It has been described as a general regulator of cortical activity and thus of consciousness—something like a volume control or accelerator. In the past few years, other systems have been discovered that ascend from the brain stem to diencephalon, basal ganglia and cortex. These systems, recognized because their chemical transmitters (called "catecholamines") can be induced to fluoresce brilliantly, have been considered by some as regulators of "mood" (see Chapter 3).

Experimental basis for the concept of functional centers

This concept of the brain as an assembly of parallel, serially-linked functional centers rests on two kinds of experiments. One can either produce a "lesion" in a particular structure, i.e., destroy it, and observe which capacities are lost, or one can stimulate electrically a particular structure and observe which behaviors are evoked. The missing or evoked behaviors are then attributed to the structure that was destroyed or stimulated. For example, when all of the brain above the midbrain is destroyed in a cat, the animal can still carry out most of its basic life functions. It can breathe, swallow, stand and walk; it maintains adequate blood pressure, heart rate, and so on. The animal does not, however, find food by itself nor respond with appropriate emotion or behavior to sensory stimuli. It is this kind of experiment that localizes the basic functions in the spinal cord and brain stem and the "higher" functions in the cerebral cortex.

The concept of the "pain pathway" from skin to the cerebral cortex arises from experiments in which pain can be abolished by destroying particular structures along the pathway to the cortex and from others in which pain can be evoked by stimulating these structures electrically.

The parceling of the cerebral cortex rests on similar experiments. Fig. 4 shows the cortex mapped by electrical stimulation in awake human subjects. Stimulation of the "motor" cortex leads to specific body movements: "somatosensory" cortex stimulation produces tingling sensations; "visual" cortex stimulation—flashes of light; "auditory" cortex stimulation—a buzzing. Stimulation of the "interpretive" cortex sometimes evokes a vivid experience that seems to be a memory, elicited from a stored stream of consciousness. Wilder Penfield, who performed these experiments, states that as the electrode is moved from the purely "sensory" to the "interpretive" areas,

"There is no longer a sound, but a voice, no longes a rumbling, but music. Visual flashes ... give way to a scene, or the sudden appearance of a familiar person."

In the case of the serially connected language centers illustrated in Fig. 4, the reason for considering Wernicke's area as a "word recognition center" is that its destruction is accompanied by a loss of comprehension of written and spoken language. The patient's speech remains fluent and rhythmic, but it is devoid of meaning. Broca's area is considered a "grammar center" because its destruction is accompanied by a loss in fluency. The patient can comprehend language and can speak, but only haltingly and with an enormous effort.

The pathways and centers subsumed by the term "limbic system" have also been assigned their functions on the basis of behavioral changes associated with stimulation and ablation. The amygdala, for example, has been considered a center for violent or aggressive behavior because such behavior is evoked by electrical stimulation and amygdalar destruction is followed by placidity. The septum has been regarded as a "pleasure center" since animals will work hard to be permitted to deliver stimuli through electrodes implanted in this region ("self-stimulation"), and human subjects have reported a variety of pleasurable sensations during septal stimulation. A "hunger center" has been described in the lateral hypothalamus because stimulation there causes an animal to eat and destruction results temporarily in a failure to eat. This by no means exhausts the list of centers in the limbic system—there are centers for satiety, drinking, sex, etc., all discovered by lesion or stimulation.

The brain's other organs and systems are assigned functions on similar grounds. When the cerebellum is removed, there is a deterioration of posture and movement. Balance is poor and movements are shaky. The cerebellum is, therefore, considered a "preventer" of tremor, or, in more positive terms, a "smoother" of movement. Electrical stimulation of the ascending reticular activating system is followed by behavioral activation and its destruction—by somnolence. Similarly, catecholamine and indolealkylamine systems have been considered to be mood regulators because mood changes are induced by drugs that alter the functional activity of these systems.

Problems with the concept of brain "centers"

At this point, it would appear that the brain is not so mysterious after all. Although the number of neurons is vast and the number and variety of centers great, the neurons themselves seem to be relatively simple. The experiments described above ostensibly provide some basic ideas of what the various parts of the brain do, and apparently confirm the concept of private relay lines and "centers."

Nevertheless, there are difficulties with the concept of "centers." One is that the results of ablation and stimulation experiments are invariably more complex and contradictory than are often described in popular accounts. If the brain really worked as a linear machine, one would anticipate that destruction of the same part in different brains would lead to highly predictable changes in function. Thus, it should be possible, for example, to relieve pain by interrupting the "pain pathway" at any point on its way to the cerebral cortex (Fig. 3) and to obtain the same result in different individuals. Astonishingly enough, what appear to be the same lesions in different animals or people, frequently produce very different results. Interruption of the "pain pathway" may relieve the pain, or it may not; furthermore, pain may return in even more intense form.

Certain ablation experiments call sharply into question the time-honored distinction between "higher" and "lower" centers. For instance, if the "primary" visual cortex (Fig. 4) is removed from a cat, there is very little detectable loss in the animal's ability to recognize and discriminate visual stimuli. If, however, the visual part of the midbrain (formerly supposed to be a "lower" reflex center) is destroyed, the most profound visual losses ensue, including loss of the ability to discriminate visual patterns.

Another difficulty is that even when behavioral losses are dramatic and repeatable, as for example in the syndromes that follow destruction of Wernicke's and Broca's areas, it is usually impossible to define precisely what is lost. Each attempt at an exact formulation invariably turns up contradictions. For example, Broca's area cannot *really* be a "grammar center" because a patient with Broca's syndrome *can* produce grammatical speech. When asked about the weather, he can reply, "Weather . . . overcast," haltingly, but with the basic grammatical structure intact. Similarly, in Wernicke's syndrome, it is not really the recognition of *words* that is lost—for they come tumbling out—it is their *meaning* that is lost. However, if one retreats and calls Broca's area a "fluency center" and Wernicke's area a "meaning center," one is reduced to merely redescribing the syndromes without clarifying how language is really organized in the brain.

In many situations, a dramatic effect of ablation may be shown to depend on the context in which the organism is operating. If the motor cortex of one hemisphere is removed in a monkey, the arm on the opposite side of the body hangs limply. The animal will not use it to reach for food or groom itself, and the arm appears to be paralyzed. It might be concluded that the motor cortex is responsible for voluntary movement.

However, if the normal arm is restrained, the animal will immediately begin to use the "paralyzed" arm for feeding and grooming. This observation indicates how difficult it is to pin down either what is meant by "voluntary" or "paralyzed," or what is really lost when the motor cortex is removed. At the very least, it indicates that there must be other parts of the brain that share the responsibility for "voluntary" movement. Indeed, one can find other regions of the brain that, when destroyed, also cause the arm to hang limply and to be used only when the "good" arm is restrained.

This example illustrates a very general feature of the brain that has only recently begun to be fully appreciated: responsibility for virtually every function or behavior is widely shared. Aggressive behavior, originally associated with the amygdala, is now known to be evoked by stimulation of certain regions of the hypothalamus, midbrain, and even the cerebellum. Similarly, feeding and drinking behavior, formerly thought to originate in the hypothalamus, have been evoked from many points in the brain, again including the cerebellum. It has also proved possible to evoke pleasure-seeking behavior, originally associated with a septo-hypothalamic "center" from many, widespread points.

As multiple centers were discovered for each function, the simplest way to salvage the general concept of "centers" was to consider them as arranged in linear, hierarchical series. In the case of aggressive behavior, for example, the series would be: amygdala → hypothalamus → midbrain → spinal cord. This salvage operation founders on another feature of neural organization, which also has only recently been appreciated: each region of the brain participates in *multiple* functions.

The cerebellum, formerly thought of as a center for controlling posture and movement, is now known to be involved as well with feeding, grooming, aggressive behavior, attention-emotional arousal, and control of blood pressure. The amygdala is concerned not merely with aggressive behavior but also with sexual behavior, feeding, drinking, blood pressure, and secretion of many different hormones. The frontal lobe in humans has long been known to be involved in both intellectual and emotional spheres —and debate has raged for years as to which of these functions was primary in the hierarchy and which secondary.

The multiple functions represented within each structure are not randomly distributed but arranged in ways that contribute to the necessary coordination between systems. Thus, the part of the cerebellum that contributes to the maintenance of an upright posture by skeletal muscle also contributes to sustaining a pattern of blood vessel constriction appropriate to such a posture. Similarly, the regions of the amygdala and hypothalamus from which particular behaviors are evoked contribute to muscular, blood flow, and hormonal patterns that must accompany the behavior. In retrospect this is not astonishing; one would not want the cerebellum to give a command, "Stand!" without also providing adequate blood pressure to the head—otherwise fainting would result. Nevertheless, to see the cerebellum as contributing to control of blood pressure, hormonal patterns, attention, and "motivated" behaviors is quite different from seeing it as a purely "motor" center.

There seems to be a major paradox. On one hand, we have seen that the brain is made of discrete units connected in specific ways. On the other hand, the difficulties with the linear, hierarchical conception of the brain now appear overwhelming. Destruction of the same region in different animals of the same species does not invariably produce the same loss in function. Furthermore, the functions are hard to define and often depend on the immediate or historical context. Each function seems to be multiply represented in the brain and

each structure is apparently involved in multiple functions. Finally, it is no longer so obvious that some structures are "high" and others "low." How did we arrive at such a paradox and what is the way out?

One must realize that the apparent congruence between the original linear machine concept of the brain and the physiological observations was to some extent a consequence of an experimental design that favored discovering only simple kinds of functional localization and that tended to exaggerate it. In the left half of Fig. 5, for example, ablation of area C_2 will cause a total loss of function in the chain $A_2 \rightarrow B_2 \rightarrow C_2$. It would be entirely correct in a system connected in this way to attribute the observed behavioral deficits to the loss of that chain. In such a system, ablation would be a powerful experimental tool. Suppose, however, that the system were arranged as on the right in Fig. 5, with the same number of neurons and synapses but with more widely distributed connections. In this instance, the behavioral deficit following ablation of C_2 could not properly be attributed to the loss of $A_2 \rightarrow B_2 \rightarrow C_2$ but to partial losses in all of the chains converging on C_2. In this case, ablation would be less useful as an investigative method for it would not point directly to the role of any single chain. This model, as we shall see, approaches more closely the actual patterns of connection that exist in the brain.

Use of the ablation method on a system with such widely distributed connections often leads directly into a logical trap. Recall the joke in which a man trains a flea to jump on command. He removes the flea's legs, one at a time, commanding "Jump!" after each detachment. The flea responds with successively weaker jumps. When the last leg has been detached and the flea no longer responds to the command, the man concludes that a flea with no legs cannot hear. He has "localized" the center for

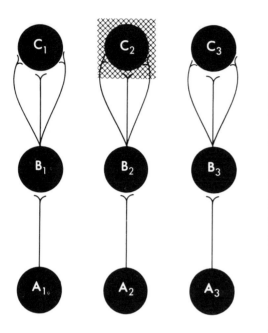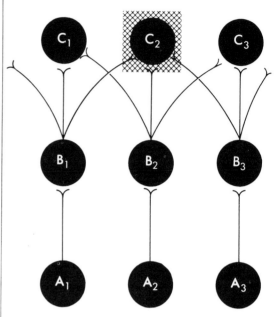

Fig. 5. Diagrams to illustrate the effects of removal of a higher "center" (C_2). On the left, the whole chain $A_2 \rightarrow C_2$ is lost. On the right, there are partial losses in all 3 chains, but not a total loss in any one.

hearing in the last remaining leg. This is what scientists tend to do when they remove a piece of brain (e.g., motor cortex), find a defect (loss of voluntary movement), and attribute it to a "center" (for "willed movement") in the missing piece. The more dramatically the behavior is altered following a lesion or stimulation, the more strongly the observers may believe that a "center" exists. The logical fallacy is obvious but is usually discovered only in retrospect after the effects of context (such as restraining the arm) and the roles of other structures have been searched for.

Another reason that the ablation-stimulation approach and the linear model lead to a paradox is that the observations tend to be selected to fit our own conceptual categories rather than the inherent categories of the brain. It seems very unlikely, for example, that the brain's language system actually uses

such categories as "word recognition," "grammar," or "meaning," even though we analyze language in this way. Partial resolution of the paradox may come as we attempt to discover the brain's natural categories.

The visual system offers a concrete illustration of what is meant by natural categories. In the 1940s and 1950s scientists imagined that the visual image striking the retina was "displayed" in the visual cortex by an array of neurons that were either "on" or "off," a display that in most important respects is analogous to the formation of an image from light and dark dots on a T.V. screen. It was discovered, however, that most neurons in the primary visual cortex do not fire many impulses when small spots of light are presented to the eye. Instead, they fire vigorously upon the presentation of straight lines or edges of particular orientation and length

(Fig. 6). This suggests that one of the *brain's* ways of initially analyzing a visual image is to signal the presence in the image of lines and edges. Therefore, lines and edges form a natural category for the brain that we could not have anticipated from our non-biological engineering experience.

A *different view of the brain: Redefinition of the building blocks*

The essence of the model of the neuron shown in Fig. 1 is that information flows in only one direction within and between nerve cells. Dendrites receive information, conduct it to the cell body, and from there down the axon, where it passes without further modification to the dendrites of the next cell. Electron microscope studies of neurons in many different parts of the brain have shown that the model in Fig. 1 is far too simple.

It was discovered, for example, that axons, in some cases, terminate not only on dendrites (axo-dendritic synapses), but also on the synapses made by other axons (axo-axonic synapses). This means that the message "relayed" from a neuron is not immutable once it has left the cell body but is modified at its destination. What cell A "relays" to cell B depends on what cell C has to say (Fig. 7A).

Another recent discovery is that dendrites, formerly thought merely to be receivers, also *transmit* information to other neurons by means of synaptic contacts (dendro-dendritic synapses). This means that a neuron responds not only to its own axonal inputs, but also to axonal inputs to the dendrites of neighboring neurons. In some cases, the synaptic contacts between dendrites are reciprocal (Fig. 7B). The dendrite of cell A is turned on by the dendrite of cell B, but it also turns off the dendrite of cell B. In this instance, the neurons are not passive receivers but modify their own inputs. In essence, they tell

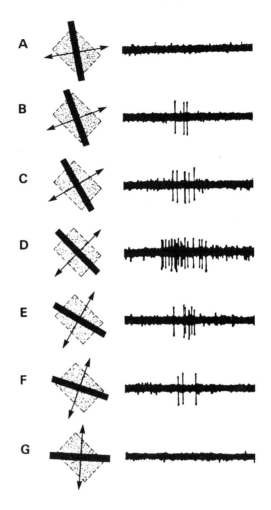

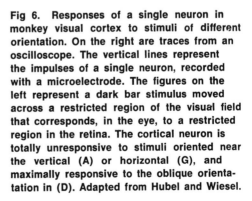

Fig 6.   Responses of a single neuron in monkey visual cortex to stimuli of different orientation. On the right are traces from an oscilloscope. The vertical lines represent the impulses of a single neuron, recorded with a microelectrode. The figures on the left represent a dark bar stimulus moved across a restricted region of the visual field that corresponds, in the eye, to a restricted region in the retina. The cortical neuron is totally unresponsive to stimuli oriented near the vertical (A) or horizontal (G), and maximally responsive to the oblique orientation in (D). Adapted from Hubel and Wiesel.

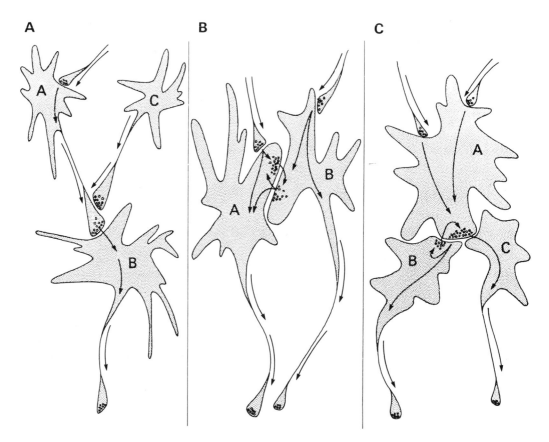

Fig. 7. Some types of neural connections discovered with the electron microscope. (A) Axo-axonic contact from cell C to A. (B) Dendro-dendritic contact from cell A to cell B and reciprocally from B to A. (C) "Dyadic" contact from cell A to both B and C. Reciprocal contact from cell B to A also influences cell C. Arrows indicate functionally significant directions of current flow in the cells.

their informant what they are willing to hear. A more complex variant of this arrangement has been discovered in the retina involving three types of cells. Cell type A contacts dendrites of type B and C and also receives a reciprocal contact from B. Here, type B not only tells A what it wants to hear, but also modifies the message that A transmits to C (Fig. 7C).

Many of these complicated synaptic interactions do not require nerve impulses to be conducted from the cell body but only local depolarization to cause release of transmitter. As a consequence, each complex of interacting synapses, such as illustrated in Fig. 7, may act as an indepedent analytic element, quite apart from what is occurring in other, more distant regions of the neurons in question. A single neuron, whose dendritic branches are involved in many of these complexes, may not be the most basic functional unit after all, for the neuron may participate simultaneously in many different functions. The important unit in such cases is probably the network made up of a particular set of these synaptic complexes which are carrying out a particular operation.

A simple analogy in electricity would be a network of resistors and capacitors that operate to filter out signals at certain frequencies and pass others. In analyzing such a circuit, one tries to determine that it is a *filter* one is looking at and not to be distracted by the properties of individual resistors and capacitors. Similarly, in the brain it may often be important to understand the specific *process* accomplished by a network of synaptic complexes rather than the all-or-none impulses given off by a single neuron. This is not to deny that particular neurons within the network carry out specific functions. It is rather to emphasize that the degree of interconnectedness is so great, that to try to assign a function to a single neuron may be to miss the point. Let us reexamine the "division of labor" between regions of the brain where we shall see the same principle in operation.

The whole brain as a network

There are methods of studying the brain that do not emphasize localization of particular functions, but rather, the interconnectedness of various regions. With these methods, one does not ask directly about a structure, "What does it do?" Instead, one asks, "What are all the sources of information flowing into it and to what parts of the brain does this structure transmit?" This is a powerful way of asking what a structure is concerned with. If it receives both auditory and visual information, we can be certain that it has something to do with both of these senses, even though destroying it may not produce noticeable behavioral defects. In this respect, this method is more sensitive than the ablation technique.

When the brain is studied in this manner, one finds that most structures are so elaborately interconnected that the simple linear chains of neurons simply disappear. Recall the concept of the visual system as two separate, linear paths, a lower reflex chain and higher cortical chain (Fig. 4). Compare this to the connections that have actually been described (Fig. 8A). First, note that there is not a single, vaguely defined "association area" at the end of the pathway, but nine distinct regions of the cortex, each of which contains a representation of the visual world. Second (Fig. 8A), notice that the path from eye to midbrain is not separate from the "higher" pathway, but makes connections via a different part of the thalamus with all the cortical visual areas. Thus, the cortex does not deal with visual information arriving along a single linear chain, but is informed by a whole series of parallel pathways. Third (Fig. 8B), note that the connections between successive cortical stations (V_1–V_9) are also not arranged as a simple, linear series, but rather as a *cascade* of forward connections. V_9 does not merely receive the output of V_8 but also the outputs of all the earlier stages. Finally (Fig. 8C), notice that each of the cortical regions feeds back to earlier structures on the pathway—again not in a simple, serial manner, but as a cascade that includes cortical areas, thalamus and midbrain.

When all the components are assembled (as in Fig. 8C), the original, separate chains, though still present, are hardly recognizable. Should one consider the midbrain a "lower center" because it receives information from the eye and projects to the cerebral cortex, or a "higher center" because it is thoroughly informed by all of the visual cortical areas? Electrical recordings from single neurons in the visual midbrain show that the cells are quite as sophis-

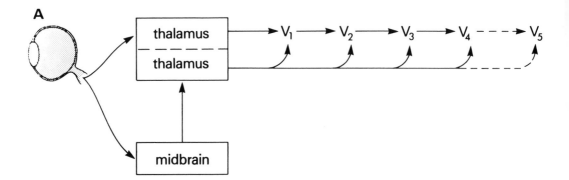

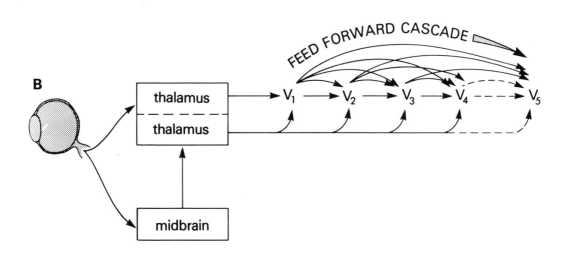

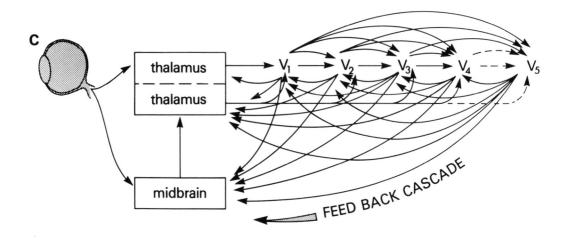

ticated as many in the visual cortex and more closely reflect the activity of the cortex than the activity of the retina itself.

A recent study on the visual capacity of humans, following ablation of the "primary" visual cortex, provides a dramatic example of how one's conception of the machine circumscribes one's observations. Neurologists holding the linear conception of the brain have long believed that ablation of the primary visual cortex in humans leads to "blindness." Indeed, if one shines a figure on a screen, a patient with such brain damage will vigorously deny "seeing" it. Recently, however, some British neuropsychologists, acting on their understanding of the visual system as a network, took a giant step in the examination of such a patient. They insisted that he try to point to where he thought the figure might be and urged him to "guess" whether the figure was an "X" or an "O." The patient pointed accurately and "guessed" correctly on this and other tests. Thus, although he has abnormal vision because part of the visual network has been destroyed, there is some sense in which he *does* "see" even though the nature of this vision is hard to describe.

Clearly, the brain is a machine, one of whose main principles is the interconnectedness of its parts. This is true both at the level of single neurons (Fig. 7), and at the level of gross structures (Fig. 8). Each region can be found at the end of many processes and also at the beginning of many others. This is why no one lesion produces a single, simple defect, and why it is so hard to agree on the defects that accompany lesions.

It is now possible to appreciate by a glance at the connections of the frontal lobe why there have been arguments about whether intellectual or emotional processes were primary in that region. Fig. 9A shows that the frontal lobe receives information from structures that

Fig. 8. Diagram of the connections in the visual system. (A) Note that there are at least 9 distinct visual areas in the cortex (V$_1$-V$_9$). These are fed directly *via* one part of the thalamus and indirectly by the midbrain *via* another part of the thalamus. (B) Note that areas V$_1$-V$_9$ are not linked in a simple series, but in a cascade of "forward" connections. (C) Note that V$_1$-V$_9$ form a cascade of "feedback" connections with thalamus and midbrain.

A. Neocortical cascades to the frontal lobe

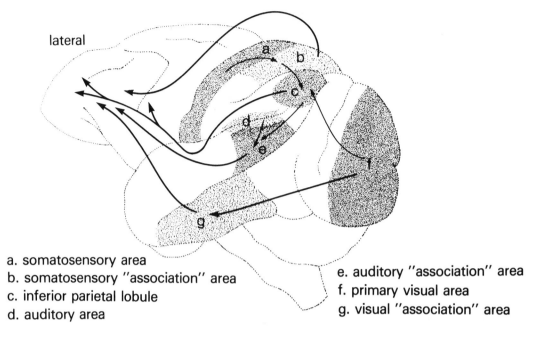

a. somatosensory area
b. somatosensory "association" area
c. inferior parietal lobule
d. auditory area

e. auditory "association" area
f. primary visual area
g. visual "association" area

B. Limbic cascades to the frontal lobe

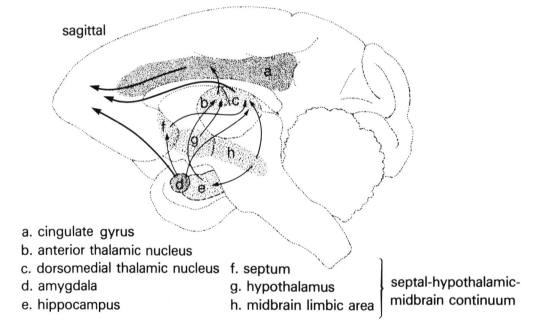

a. cingulate gyrus
b. anterior thalamic nucleus
c. dorsomedial thalamic nucleus
d. amygdala
e. hippocampus

f. septum
g. hypothalamus
h. midbrain limbic area

septal-hypothalamic-midbrain continuum

Fig. 9 Diagram of some connections of the frontal cortex. Cascades arrive in the frontal lobe from neocortical systems which analyze the "outer" world (A), and also from the limbic system that analyzes the "inner" world (B). The results are transmitted back to both neocortex (C) and to limbic structures (D), again by means of cascades. Many connections have been omitted for the sake of clarity.

C. Frontal lobe cascades to the neocortical system

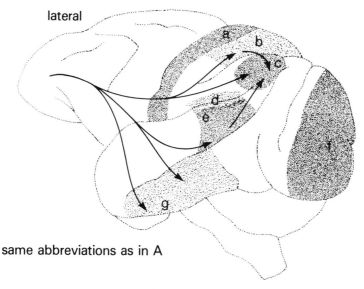

same abbreviations as in A

D. Frontal lobe cascades to the limbic system

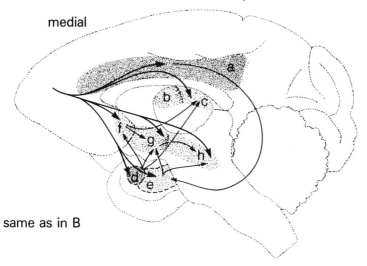

same as in B

carry out complex perceptual and ideational processes concerning the "outside world." These connections are arranged, as with the visual system, in cascade fashion, from the visual, auditory and somatosensory systems. The frontal lobe also projects *back* to these regions, again in a complex cascade (Fig. 9C). The frontal lobe also receives multiple connections from structures representing the internal states of the body, and the

emotions (Fig. 9B). These structures, termed the limbic system, are themselves highly interconnected, and, again, receive a cascade of connections *from* the frontal lobe (Fig. 9D).

Thus, the frontal lobe belongs neither solely to the "higher" functions of thought and analysis, nor solely to the more "primitive" functions—the emotions. Rather, it is one of the pivotal points in the brain between thought and emotion. The frontal lobe is in a perfect position to influence emotions by thought and also to focus and reinforce thoughts by emotion.

Conclusion

We have seen that the destruction of each region of the brain produces behavioral changes that at first glance appear to be quite specific and describable in simple terms. If it were not for hindsight, it would be easy to believe that the brain is organized in linear chains of functional "centers." We recognize now, however, that when one carefully analyzes behavior following brain lesions, it is impossible to find a single lesion that destroys a single "category" of behavior, and that the categories such as "seeing," which at first seem simple, are complex. This is the lesson of "blind" sight described earlier. We can now appreciate that this is so because the neurons are not organized as linear chains but as carefully intermeshed networks. Perhaps it is now clear why the brain must be approached not as a mechanic would approach a car, but as an ecologist approaches the environment, looking not for "centers," but for processes and their interconnections.

Selected References

Bateson, G.: *Steps Toward an Ecology of Mind.* Ballantine Books, New York, 1972.

Carpenter, M.B., *Human Neuroanatomy*, 7th ed. Williams and Wilkins Co., Baltimore, 1976.

Hess, W.R.: *The Functional Organization of the Diencephalon.* Grune and Stratton, New York, 1957.

Hubel, D.H., and Wiesel, T.N. Receptive fields and functional architecture of monkey striate cortex. *J. Physiol.* 195:215-243, 1968.

Kuffler, S.W., and Nicholls, J.G.: *From Neuron to Brain.* Sinauer Associates, Inc., Sunderland, Mass., 1976.

MacLean, P.D.: The Hypothalamus and Emotional Behavior. In W. Haymaker, E. Anderson, and W.J.H. Nauta, eds. *The Hypothalamus*, Charles C. Thomas, Springfield, Ill. 1969, pp. 659-678.

Nauta, W.J.H.: The problem of the frontal lobe: a reinterpretation. *J. Psychiat. Res.* 8:167-187, 1971.

Papez, J.W.: A proposed mechanism of emotion. *Arch. Neurol. Psychiat.* 38:725-743, 1937.

Penfield, W. and Rasmussen, T.: *The Cerebral Cortex of Man. A Clinical Study of Localization of Function.* Macmillan, New York, 1950.

Chapter 2

Principles of Neurophysiology

Andrew Winokur
and Alexander L. Beckman

Introduction

The central nervous system (CNS) serves as the major information processing system of the body: collecting data (in the form of sensory input) about conditions in the external and internal environment, and producing a multitude of physiological and behavioral re- sponses. Our attempt to understand the biological bases of behavior must surely incorporate the study of the elements of CNS function, i.e., the transmission of messages among its cellular units. This chapter will consist of a discussion of basic mechanisms involved in the initiation, propagation and transmission of impulses in the central nervous system. A thorough understanding of these topics is crucial to a more general understanding of the physiological processes underlying normal as well as disordered behavior.

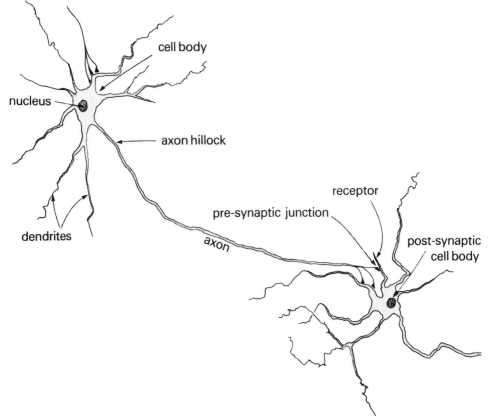

Fig. 1   Schematic representation of the characteristic features of a neuron.

Overview of Neuronal Function

Brain tissue is made up of two types of cells, *glial* and *neuronal*. Glial cells surround the axonal portion of neurons, serving to insulate the axon and improve conduction of the nerve impulse. In addition, glial cells are thought to be involved in other functions, including the metabolic activity of neurons and the long-term storage of information.

The neuron is, for our purposes, the most important component of brain tissue, since it is the neuron that provides conduction of signals throughout the central nervous system, as well as to and from the periphery. The neuron comprises the basic unit for initiation and conduction of the action potential, which is the basic "message unit" of the nervous system. A schematic structure of a neuron showing the cell body, dendrites, and the axon is depicted in Fig. 1.

The cell body contains the nucleus, which regulates the DNA to RNA transcription processes. The cytoplasm of the cell body contains ribosomes which are involved in protein synthesis. Moreover, the endoplasmic reticulum within the cytoplasm plays a role in the packaging of proteins called neurotransmitters that are secreted by the active neuron.

Several processes extend from the cell body, the longest of which is the *axon*; more highly branched processes which are usually shorter than the axon are called *dendrites*. The dendrites increase the receptive area of a given neuron to signals from the axons of other neurons. Axons can make functional contact (form a "synapse") with the cell body or with the axon of the target neuron as well. Action potentials reaching the terminal of the axon produce an effect on the postsynaptic neuron (the next neuron in the chain) by releasing a chemical substance referred to as a *neurotransmitter*. The neurotransmitter diffuses across the gap separating the terminal from the postsynaptic cell (i.e., the synaptic cleft) and combines with a specialized portion of the membrane of the postsynaptic cell, the *receptor*. This topic is discussed in more detail in the following chapter. The transmitter-receptor interaction results in a local flow of current across the membrane, that alters the latter's resting electrical potential. This current flow is conducted by the dendrites and the cell body in a *decremental* manner, which means that the strength of the current diminishes with increasing distance from its site of origin. At any instant, a number of dendrites of a given neuron may be in the process of being activated, resulting in the flow of electrical current toward the cell body, while the cell body itself may be receiving direct stimulation from the axons of other neurons. The cell body integrates (i.e., *algebraically sums*) the total current flow. If the current flow exceeds the *threshold* value, an *action potential* is generated at the junction of the cell body and the axon (the axon hillock) that is propagated along the length of the axon. Action potentials travel down the axon in a non-decremental manner, i.e., with a constant amplitude. The mechanism underlying this process will be discussed in more detail later in this chapter.

The terminal portion of the axon, the *presynaptic junction*, is itself a specialized structure that contains characteristic bodies, called synaptic vesicles. Neurotransmitter agents of a given type are stored in the synaptic vesicles, ready to be released when the terminal is rapidly depolarized by an incoming action potential. As noted, the synaptic cleft, which separates the pre- and postsynaptic membranes, is extremely small, generally 200 to 500 angstroms. The synaptic junction can be demonstrated by electron microscopic techniques.

The presynaptic region, in combination with the adjoining postsynaptic membrane area, can also be isolated by centrifuging brain homogenate preparations at progressively greater rates (differential centrifugation) and then separating subcellular organelles by centrifuging them on a gradient comprised of material of varying densities (density gradient separation). During the isolation process, the pre- and postsynaptic material rounds up and forms a *synaptosome* (Fig. 2). The synaptosome is comprised of pre- and postsynaptic membrane, synaptic vesicles and mitochondria, and can remain functionally active for a number of hours in an *in vitro* incubation system. Thus, it has been possible to utilize synaptosomal preparations to study the synthesis, uptake and release of various neurotransmitters.

The receptor area of the postsynaptic membrane appears thickened, when viewed through an electron microscope, and is characterized by a high protein content. The synaptic junction conducts action potentials in only one direction, from the presynaptic to the postsynaptic neuron.

Resting Membrane Potential

Prior to discussing the events associated with the firing of an action potential, it is necessary to describe the basal condition that underlies the excitable properties of a neuron, namely the existence of a resting *membrane potential*.

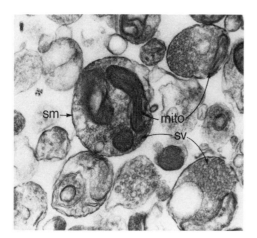

Fig. 2. Electron micrograph of a synaptosomal preparation (X 31,300). Note the mitochondria and characteristic synaptic vesicles contained within the mitochondria. (Kindly supplied by Dr. R. Davis, University of Pennsylvania.)

Fig. 3. Representation of the concept of pores in the neuronal membrane. It is believed that pores containing a negative charge allow the passage of positively charged ions (e.g., Na+ and K+), while positively charged pores permit the passage of negative ions (e.g., Cl-). From Eyzaguirre and Fidone (1975). Used by permission.

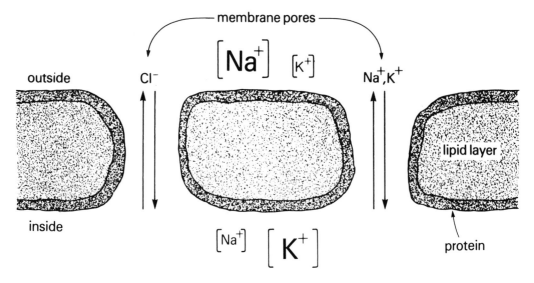

A membrane potential refers to an electromotive force established as a result of the separation of charged particles (ions) across the membrane. The formation of this potential is based, in part, upon the physical properties of the neuronal membrane which is a semipermeable structure containing numerous minute *pores* that allow the passage of ions (Fig. 3). The ability of an ion to pass through a membrane pore is related to the diameter of the hydrated sphere formed by the ion and the water molecules that immediately surround it. The diameter of the hydrated potassium ion is smaller than that of the sodium ion and, as a consequence, the resting membrane is approximately 100 times more permeable to potassium ions than it is to sodium.

Information concerning the relationship between the movement of ions across the neuronal membrane and the excitable properties of neuronal tissue was obtained primarily through a brilliant series of experiments on the giant axon of the squid, conducted by a number of investigators, notably Hodgkin, Huxley and Katz. The general methodology of these experiments involved placing the axon in an incubation medium which maintained the preparation in a biochemically and physiologically active state for a number of hours (Fig. 4). The large diameter of the axon (about 1mm) permitted electrodes to be introduced with-

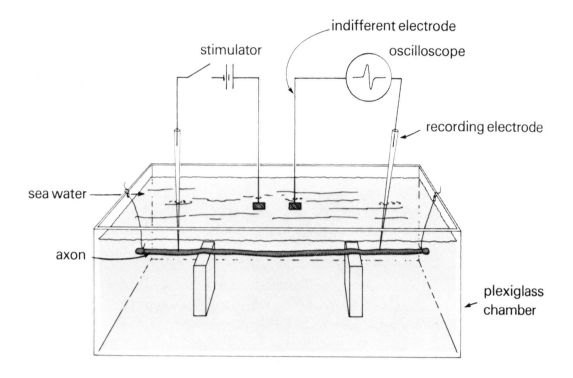

Fig. 4. Schematic representation of a squid giant axon isolated in a perfusion medium. Currents can be passed through a stimulating electrode, while electrical activity can be monitored by means of a recording electrode attached to an oscilloscope. An axon isolated in this manner can maintain its excitable properties for a number of hours.

in the axon, that made it possible to measure the electrical potential (the voltage) across the membrane. Using this *in vitro* preparation, the ionic events underlying the resting membrane potential and the action potential were determined by observing the effects of changes in internal or external ionic concentrations on these potentials. The passive electrical characteristics of the axon and also the manner in which the action potential is propagated along the axon were determined using multiple recording electrodes spaced along the length of the isolated axon.

Measurement of the electrical potential across the membrane of the squid giant axon, as well as across the mem-

brane of numerous other types of neurons, has shown that the inside of the axon is negative (in the range of –60 to –90 mv) with respect to the outside. This voltage is produced by the tendency of charged particles (ions) to flow across the membrane.

As mentioned above, the resting membrane has a very low permeability to sodium ions. The high extracellular and low intracellular concentration of sodium provides a strong chemical driving force for moving it into the axon. However, the impermeability of the resting membrane to this ion blocks its inward flux and little sodium crosses the membrane during the resting state. This phenomenon is important because it means that

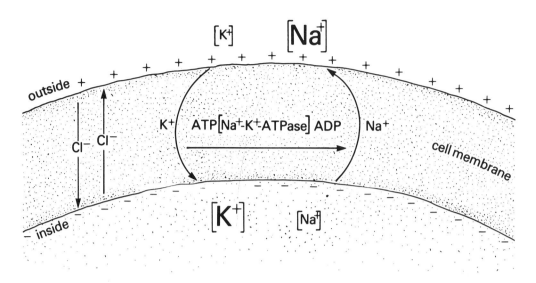

the resting membrane potential does not depend upon sodium, since ions must be free to flow in order for a voltage to be produced. Potassium ions are also separated into unequal concentrations across the membrane, in this case with higher concentration inside compared to outside. The high internal concentration provides a driving force for moving potassium out of the axon. Because the resting membrane is permeable to potassium, potassium ions move across the membrane and accumulate just outside the membrane. This accumulation of positively charged particles produces an electrical field that retards the further movement of potassium ions down their concentration gradient into this area. At equilibrium (i.e., electrochemical equilibrium of potassium), the electrical force just opposes the driving force produced by the potassium concentration difference. This electrical force, measured as a voltage across the membrane, is known as the *resting membrane potential*. The separation of charged particles across the cell membrane is a critical factor in establishing the excitable properties of the neuron. Both the maintenance of the resting membrane potential and the firing of an action potential (to be discussed later)

depend upon properties of the membrane, which control the passage of ions through the membrane and are probably related to the configuration of the membrane pores.

It has proven useful to express the relationship between the membrane potential and the distribution of ions across the cell membrane in terms of an equation generally referred to as the Goldman equation:

$$E_m = -58 \ln \frac{P_K[K]i + P_{Na}[Na]i + P_{Cl}[Cl]_0}{P_K[K]_0 + P_{Na}[Na]_0 + P_{Cl}[Cl]_i}$$

where E_m represents the voltage across the membrane,
58 is a calculated constant,[*]
P is the permeability constant for a given ion,
$(i)_0$ is the ionic concentration outside the membrane,
and $(i)_i$ is the concentration of the ion within the cell.

The Goldman equation describes the contribution of the constituent ions to

---

[*]The value of 58 is derived from the constant $\frac{RT}{nF}$. See Katz (1966) for the derivation of these terms.

Fig. 5. Schematic representation of the sodium-potassium pump. Sodium is pumped out of the cell against both an electrical (positive charge outside the cell) and chemical (high [Na+] outside the cell) gradient. K+ passes into the cell in conjunction with the outward flux of Na+. Energy for this process is provided by the breakdown of ATP by the enzyme Na+, K+-activated ATPase.

the membrane potential. For example, as described previously, the membrane is virtually impermeable to the passage of sodium during the resting state. Thus, P_{Na} is essentially zero, and sodium drops out of the equation. E_m for the resting membrane is, therefore, proportional to the relative concentrations and permeability characteristics of potassium and chloride ions. Intracellular and extracellular ion replacement studies indicate that potassium is of more importance to the maintenance of the resting membrane potential than is chloride.

An important mechanism involved in the maintenance of sodium and potassium concentrations across the neural membrane is the *sodium-potassium pump*. Sodium is pumped out of the cell against both an electrical gradient (i.e., positive charge outside the cell) and a chemical gradient (high sodium concentration outside the cell) (Fig. 5). The active (i.e., energy requiring) transport of sodium out of the cell is coupled to the transport of potassium into the cell. Energy for the pump is provided by the breakdown of the high-energy compound, adenosine triphosphate (ATP), and the administration of metabolic inhibitors, such as cyanide, can block this process. The rate at which sodium is

pumped out of the cell depends upon its internal concentration and the external concentration of potassium. During the resting state, when the internal sodium level is low, the pump shows relatively little activity. However, the increased internal concentration of sodium that occurs during the firing of an action potential results in enhanced activity of the pump.

The existence of an enzyme related to the sodium-potassium pump mechanism has been demonstrated. This enzyme, located in the cell membrane, causes the hydrolysis of ATP. It is activated not only by magnesium ions but also by potassium and sodium ions. This enzyme is referred to as the sodium, potassium-activated ATPase. It has been demonstrated that, under normal conditions, potassium ions activate the enzyme at an extracellular site, whereas the site for sodium ion activation is inside the cell. Such locations are consistent with the notion that this enzyme catalyzes the transport of sodium ions back into the cell. In a variety of tissues with different rates of sodium ion transport, an excellent correlation exists between the activity of the sodium, potassium-activated ATPase and sodium-potassium pump activity. Moreover, drugs such as ouabain (a cardiac glycoside), which are known to retard the efflux of sodium from nerve and muscle cells, have been shown to inhibit this enzyme.

Contributions of the sodium-potassium pump to the physiological activity of neurons have been well demonstrated. For example, depolarizing the resting membrane potential leads to an influx of sodium ions, while potassium tends to move out of the cell. With pharmacological inhibition of the pump, repeated depolarization of a neuron can result in a decrease of the sodium and potassium gradients across the membrane. As a consequence of this effect, the cell loses its excitability. To cite a common analogy, the situation is similar to a battery losing its charge. However, the sodium-potassium pump serves to restore the concentration gradients by pumping sodium out of the cell in exchange for potassium. Thus, the gradients are re-established and the excitable properties of the cell are preserved. In other words, as a result of the action of the sodium-potassium pump, the battery is re-charged.

The ionic movements associated with neuronal activation are frequently discussed in terms of the passive properties of the neuron. However, a more accurate description of neuronal activity involves a complex combination of passive and active mechanisms.

Action Potential

Initiation of an Action Potential

The forces described in the previous section tended to maintain the membrane potential at the resting level. However, when depolarizing currents decrease the membrane potential sufficiently, a transient alteration in the properties of the membrane ensues that creates an *action potential*.

The generation of an action potential is associated with the inward flux of sodium ions. The role of sodium in carrying the action potential has been demonstrated by a technique commonly referred to as the voltage clamp, in which electrical current is passed into the cell through an indwelling micropipette in order to counterbalance the effects of ionic flow (current) across the cell membrane. The injected current is precisely controlled in terms of direction (inward or outward) and magnitude so that the membrane voltage remains constant. Monitoring the direction and magnitude of the injected current reveals the direction and magnitude of the ionic current that the voltage clamp is opposing. With this technique, it is possible to maintain ("clamp") the axon at a desired potential and study the ionic currents resulting from this alteration from the resting state.

Experiments using the voltage clamp have shown that an action potential is associated with three distinct current flows: First, a brief outward surge of current, reflecting release of the charge on the membrane; next, an inward flux of sodium ions; and finally, a longer lasting outward flow of current, which is related to the outward flux of potassium ions. With depolarization of the membrane potential to the threshold level for generating an action potential, some unidentified property of the membrane changes and sodium permeability increases dramatically. The enormous driving force resulting from the combined effects of the sodium concentration and the resting E_m (high concentration of sodium ions outside the membrane, low concentration inside; membrane positively charged outside,

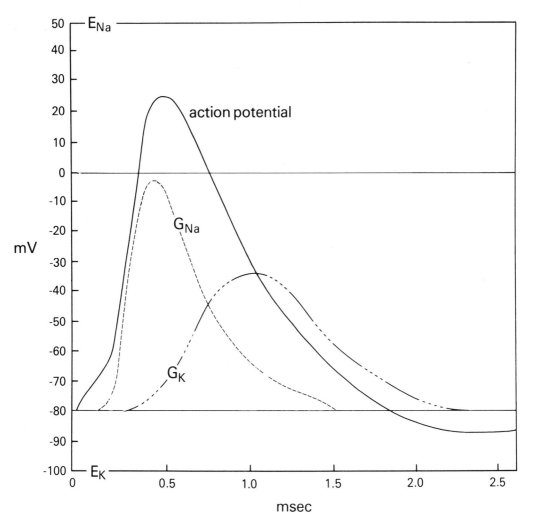

Fig. 6. Representation of data obtained from voltage clamp studies. An action potential is associated with an initial increase in sodium conduction (G_{Na}). Shortly thereafter, potassium conductance (G_{K}) increases, and this event is associated with the process of repolarization. This representation is based upon the work of Hodgkin and Huxley (1952). Adapted from Eyzaguirre and Fidone (1975). Used by permission.

negatively charged inside) moves sodium ions rapidly across the membrane into the interior of the axon.

Data obtained from voltage-clamp studies have demonstrated that the influx of sodium ions (the sodium current) produces the rising phase of the action potential. As sodium ions enter the axon, the polarity of the membrane decreases toward zero and overshoots to a potential of about +30 mv. Thus, the polarity briefly reverses during the action potential (Fig. 6). However, sodium permeability abruptly ceases before sodium ions reach electrochemical equilibrium. As in the case of increased sodium permeability, its decrease has also been demonstrated to be voltage dependent.

The mechanism that relates membrane voltage to changes in sodium permeability is, as yet, unknown but may well involve effects on the patency of membrane pores.

The Goldman equation illustrates the relationship of sodium permeability to the action potential. With a large increase in membrane permeability to sodium, $P^{(Na)o}/_{(Na)i}$ becomes very large, and overshadows the other terms in the equation. Thus, E_m is primarily dependent on sodium flux during the initial phase (the rising portion) of an action potential.

Even as the action potential is reaching its peak, the process of *repolarization,* which works to restore the resting potential, has already begun. Repolarization is produced by the outward movement of potassium ions. This represents the third stage of current flow, the movement of potassium ions out of the axon. This outward flux reaches its peak following the restoration of resting levels of sodium permeability. The outward flow of potassium drives the membrane voltage back to resting levels, transiently hyperpolarizing the membrane. In the course of this repolarization process, the neuron is first absolutely then relatively refractory to responding to another stimulus with a second action potential. During the absolute refractory phase, a neuron is incapable of generating an action potential, even in response to a very large depolarizing input. While the relative refractory phase is in process, the threshold for initiating an action potential can be reached with supranormal depolarizing currents.

Propagation of the Action Potential

As indicated previously, the action potential is produced by the transient, rapid influx of sodium. From that point, the impulse is rapidly transmitted down the axon to the nerve ending. One of the notable features of this conduction process is that there is no loss of signal strength along the entire length of the axon. This occurs because the impulse is carried by a wave of depolarization that results in the continuous reproduction of the action potential along the length of the axon (Fig. 7). At each point, an action potential of the same strength is generated. This is understandable since, at each point, the movement of charged ions underlying the firing of an action potential reduplicates the events that initially occurred at the site of origin.

For an unmyelinated axon, the spread of the action potential, as described above, can best be thought of in terms of a series of depolarizing currents leading to action potentials occurring in minute steps down the length of the axon. As portrayed in Fig. 7, at a given instant, the action potential will be present at one locus, with the polarity across the membrane reversed from the resting state (i.e., positively charged inside the membrane with respect to the outside). Just ahead of the action potential, the depolarizing current will be tending to reverse the membrane potential, while behind the action potential, a wave of repolarization restores the resting potential. The rate at which an impulse travels down an unmyelinated axon is proportional to the diameter of the axon.

There are drawbacks to having the rate of conduction of an impulse depend upon the size of the axon. For example, small organs that have finally controlled functions, such as the retina of the eye, require thousands of axons to be contained in a very small space. The problem of how to speed impulse conduction is solved by the presence of a lipoprotein material, called *myelin,* that surrounds axons. Myelin forms an insulating sheath which is punctuated at regular intervals by gaps called *Nodes of Ranvier* (Fig. 7). The presence of this sheath serves to confine the flow of depolarizing current along the interior of the axon, there-

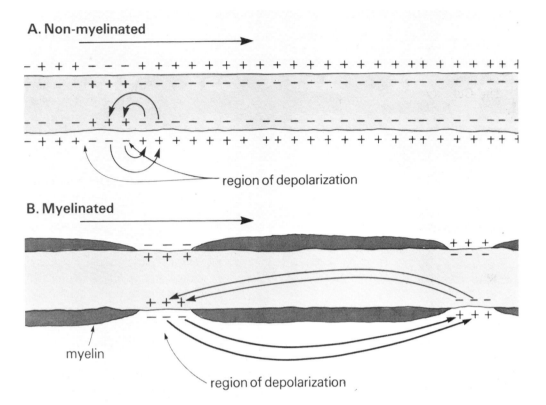

A. Non-myelinated

region of depolarization

B. Myelinated

myelin

region of depolarization

Fig. 7. Impulses traveling down a non-myelinated and myelinated axon. Conduction down a non-myelinated axon occurs by depolarization in minute steps, and is relatively slow. Impulses conducted along a myelinated axon jump rapidly across the high-resistance myelinated regions, with depolarizations occurring only at the non-myelinated Nodes of Ranvier.

by reducing the loss of current strength due to leakage through the membrane. Electrical resistance across the myelinated portion of the membrane is considerably higher than at the unmyelinated nodes. As a consequence of this, current flowing from the patch of activated membrane (site of the action potential) cross the membrane at the Nodes of Ranvier. Consequently, action potentials are only generated at the Nodes and the impulse is propagated in a series of jumps, resulting in rapid conduction.

Effect of the Action Potential on the Presynaptic Nerve Ending

When an action potential reaches the nerve terminal, it triggers a series of events that result in the release of neurotransmitter from the presynaptic neuron. It is not fully understood how an electrical process (the action potential) is coupled to a chemical process (secretion

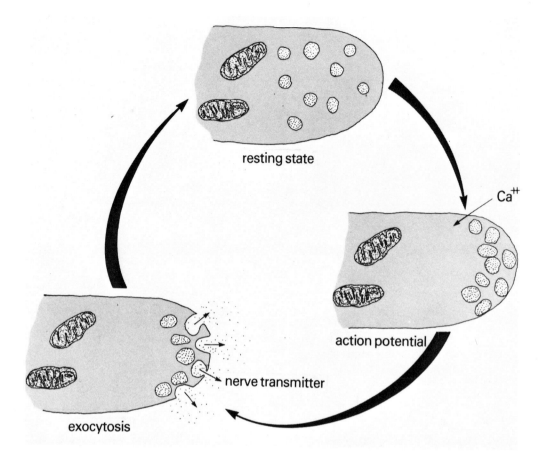

resting state

Ca⁺⁺

action potential

nerve transmitter

exocytosis

of a neurotransmitter agent). However, the following model is useful to approximate this aspect of nerve function.

Depolarization of the nerve terminal region results in an altered alignment of the synaptic vesicles (Fig. 8). Some of these appear to fuse with the presynaptic membrane and release their contents into the synaptic cleft (Chapter 3). According to this theory, the supply of synaptic vesicles has to be replenished as the vesicles become fused with the presynaptic membrane. This could represent an important regulatory step in the neurosecretion process.

Calcium, an agent ubiquitously involved in excitation-secretion processes, is necessary for the release of neurotransmitter. The mechanisms underlying the effects of calcium are not fully understood. However, a considerable amount

of data indicates that removal of calcium from the external perfusion solution causes a profound decrease in the release of neurotransmitter in response to an action potential. It appears that calcium enters a depolarized nerve terminal as a result of increased permeability. Once inside the nerve terminal, calcium may interact with some subcellular membrane structures in order to increase the likelihood of neurotransmitter release. One theory holds that calcium binds to synaptic vesicles, resulting in fusion of the synaptic vesicles with the membrane lining. Subsequently, the contents of the vesicles are released into the synaptic cleft by a process called *exocytosis*.

Magnesium, another divalent cation, has also been shown to alter neurotransmitter release, apparently exerting opposite effects to those produced by

Fig. 8. A theory of the release of neuro-transmitter substances. In the resting state, vesicles are scattered within the nerve terminal. Depolarization produces an influx of Ca++ causing vesicles to fuse with the membrane lining. Neurotransmitter is then released by the process of exocytosis.

calcium. Thus, high concentrations of magnesium in the external perfusion solution (or removal of calcium) causes a loss of neurotransmitter release in response to an action potential. The effects of high magnesium concentration can be counter-balanced by increasing the calcium level. The ratio of calcium to magnesium ions, as well as the presence of the individual cations alone, seem to influence the release of neurotransmitter. It is not clear why magnesium produces opposite effects to those seen with calcium. The roles of divalent cations in the release of neurotransmitter is an area requiring further investigation.

Some additional discussion of the action of calcium in neuronal processes is in order because it is important to emphasize the involvement of the divalent cations (such as calcium and mag-

nesium) in various aspects of impulse initiation, conduction, and neurotransmitter release. It is often the case that attention is focused primarily upon the role of the monovalent cations (sodium and potassium) in carrying the current for the action potential. While the latter are clearly vital to these activities, the divalent cations also play a sensitive and critical role in many of the control processes of neuronal function. For example, data obtained from a variety of studies point to calcium being involved in the stabilization of membranes and in the regulation of membrane permeability. Calcium is able to bind avidly to axonal (and many other) membranes. The ability of calcium to bind with negatively charged membrane sites appears to be the basis for its membrane stabilizing effect, resulting in low permeability of the membrane to other cations. There is some evidence suggesting that the increase in membrane permeability associated with depolarization is regulated by the release of calcium from its membrane binding sites, although this has not yet been directly demonstrated. In the absence of calcium, the sodium inward current is increased, the membrane potential is lowered and the axon becomes more excitable (more readily stimulated to threshold). An apparent competition between sodium and calcium for entry into the cell is further supported by the finding that decreased external sodium concentration leads to an increased inward flux of calcium.

As a result of extensive basic research, considerable information has been obtained about the varied and important roles of calcium in neuronal activity. The importance of such findings for understanding the biological aspects of psychiatric disorders or the mechanism of action of the psychotropic drugs has not been well explored and awaits further investigation.

Neurotransmission

The neurotransmitter substance released from the nerve terminal upon activation of the neuron serves to carry a "message" to the next neuron in the chain. To do this, the neurotransmitter must first interact with what has been termed the receptor portion of the postsynaptic cell membrane. Activation of the postsynaptic receptor by the neurotransmitter results in either depolarization or hyperpolarization of the membrane, depending upon several factors, including the specific neurotransmitter involved and the type of receptor.

As noted, a given neuron may receive thousands of inputs from other axons, with the contact occurring most commonly at the dendrites and cell body. An axon impinging upon another neuron can exert an excitatory or an inhibitory influence through the action of its neurotransmitter upon the receptor sites of the postsynaptic neuron. Activation of the receptor site might result in *depolarization* of the neuron (the membrane potential becomes less negative) or *hyperpolarization* (the membrane potential becomes more negative), depending upon the membrane process controlled by the receptor. A depolarizing current, termed an excitatory postsynaptic potential (EPSP), is produced by increased sodium conduction whose time course is related to the duration of the action of the neurotransmitter and to the passive electrical properties of the postsynaptic membrane. As these depolarizing currents raise the potential toward threshold, they make the neuron more excitable to subsequent stimuli. Conversely, a hyperpolarizing current, termed an inhibitory postsynaptic potential (IPSP), is produced by an increased conductance of potassium and chloride. Hyperpolarizing currents drive the membrane potential in a more negative direction, and the neuron will be less likely to fire in response to subsequent excitatory stimuli.

It is important to emphasize that inhibition of a neuron produced by a neurotransmitter does not necessarily imply inhibition of behavior. It is possible to produce behavorial activation either by stimulating an excitatory neuron or by suppressing an inhibitory neuron. For example, removal of the influence of an inhibitory neuron might allow the expression of a given behavior. Conversely, excitation of a different neuron might stimulate an inhibitory input that suppresses the given behavior. Thus, the behavorial output for a neural network (See Chapter 1) is a function of the sum of the excitatory and inhibitory processes working in concert to regulate the behavior associated with that network.

For example, the cerebral cortex generally exerts an inhibitory influence on other brain structures. Drugs that inhibit cortical function may produce an excitatory effect on CNS activity. To cite a well-known instance of this phenomenon, alcohol exerts an inhibitory effect on the central nervous system. A moderate dose will initially inhibit the cerebral cortex, resulting in a release of cortical inhibition on other brain structures. The consequence of this effect is the familiar excitation and lack of behavioral inhibitions associated with the early stages of alcohol intoxication (see Chapter 16).

The effects upon neuronal activity of a number of chemicals generally regarded as neurotransmitter agents in the central nervous system have been studied by means of the technique of micro-iontophoresis. It involves the use of fine multi-barrelled glass micropipettes to administer tiny amounts of these chemicals to actively firing neurons and study their effects upon neuronal activity.

Norepinephrine and serotonin both exert predominantly inhibitory effects while acetylcholine, another CNS neurotransmitter, generally has an excitatory action.

A number of other chemicals endogenous to the central nervous system have also been shown to affect neuronal activity. The amino acids, glutamic acid and aspartic acid cause excitation, while inhibition is produced by glycine and gamma-aminobutyric acid (GABA). In addition to these amino acids, other substances affecting neuronal activity include histamine, a polypeptide called substance P, and the hypothalamic releasing hormones, thyrotropin releasing hormone and luteinizing hormone releasing hormone (see Chapter 4). The evidence suggests that a number of these compounds may act as neurotransmitters in the CNS. Since the list of accepted neurotransmitter agents may expand substantially in the near future, it will be a considerable challenge to understand the patterns of interactions among the various neurotransmitters acting in the central nervous system.

Plasticity in Neuronal Circuits

Throughout this chapter, the central nervous system has been portrayed as a very simple system in order to emphasize some of the factors involved in the initiation and transmission of impulses. However, it is appropriate to address some comments to the issue of complexity in neural systems.

In Chapter 1, it is pointed out that the interconnectedness of neurons should not be thought of in terms of a simple linear relay model (like a telegraph system), but should more accurately be conceived in terms of complex networks. There are several factors that illustrate the enormous complexity of such networks. First, any single neuron may receive synaptic input from tens of thousands of other neurons. These influences

may be expressed at the dendritic tree, the cell body, or directly at the nerve terminal.

Despite the complexity introduced by such factors, one could assert that the system in question is still basically a simple, perhaps even rigid one. Accordingly, the neural regulation of behavior would be based upon the patterns of neuronal interconnections, i.e., the "wiring diagrams" for such systems. However, a number of investigators have raised objections to viewing neuronal function in this manner. For example, Kandel (1970) has posed the question: "How does one reconcile the known malleability of behavior with a preprogrammed and rigidly 'wired' nervous system?"

A response to this involves the concept of *plasticity*, which asserts that neuronal connections may be rigidly determined, but the functional effectiveness of neuronal systems can be influenced or modified by experience. An example of such a phenomenon, referred to as *post-tetanic potentiation*, is the observation that stimulation of certain neuronal pathways results in a greater responsiveness of these neurons to subsequent stimuli. In other systems, an opposite phenomenon, *post-tetanic inhibition*, has been observed. In this case, prior stimulation of neurons results in a decrease in synaptic responsiveness to subsequent stimulation.

Additional information has been obtained about the characteristics of plasticity in neuronal circuits. For example, plastic changes have been observed in some systems after low frequency stimulation. In other networks, one stimulus frequency results in depression of activity, while another frequency produces facilitation. In the case of post-tetanic potentiation, the mechanism underlying this response appears to be an increased amount of neurotransmitter agent released per action potential. It is possible that the increased permeability to calcium, associated with multiple depolarizations, may produce this enhancement of neurotransmitter release.

The concept of plasticity emphasizes the relationship between the activity of neuronal systems and the functional consequences of that activity. A number of investigators, such as Kandel, are currently exploring these types of interactions by studying the "wiring diagrams" of simple organisms. For example the abdominal ganglion of the *Aplysia* contains only about 1,800 cells. In this species, the neural circuits regulating various behaviors can be studied in great detail, and the effects of physiological stimulation of these circuits can be observed. Such techniques are providing information about the effects of experience on subsequent physiological and behavioral responsiveness. Studies of this type may help to elucidate the neural mechanisms related to learning and memory.

Conclusion

In this chapter, we have attempted to highlight the important features of the initiation and propagation of impulses in the central nervous system. At the moment, it is not known whether the factors discussed here actually play a significant role in disorders such as depression or schizophrenia. It is clear, however, that since behavioral responses derive from the basic mechanisms of brain function, our concepts of the biology of behavior must incorporate these basic mechanisms. An appreciation of neurophysiological mechanisms can point to factors of potential importance in experimental and clinical studies of behavior as well as in understanding sites of psychotropic drug actions. Thus, such factors as the sodium pump, the role of calcium and magnesium in the release of neurotransmitters, and the receptor response to neurotransmitter activation should all be considered in studies of the biology of behavior. The effects of psychotropic drugs on such neurophysiological mechanisms represent an important area for future investigations. Thus, an increased awareness of the basic mechanisms of neural activity opens the way to more relevant clinical studies of the biological aspects of psychiatric disorders.

Selected References

Cooper, J.R., Bloom, F.E., and Roth, R.H.: *The Biochemical Basis of Neuropharmacology*. Oxford University Press, New York, 1974.

Eyzaguirre, C. and Thidone, S.J.: *Physiology of the Nervous System*. Second Edition. Year Book Medical Publishers, Inc., Chicago, 1975.

Hodgkin, A.L. and Huxley, A.F.: Currents carried by sodium and potassium ions through the membrane of the giant axon of *Loligo*. *J. Physiol*. (London) 116: 449-472, 1952.

Hodgkin, A.L. and Huxley, A.F.: The components of membrane conductance in the giant axon of *Loligo*. *J. Physiol*. (London) 116:473-496, 1952.

Hodgkin, A.L. and Huxley, A.F.: The dual effect of membrane potential on sodium conductance in the giant axon of Loligo. *J. Physiol*. (London) 116:497-506, 1952.

Huxley, A.L.: *The Conductance of the Nervous Impulse*. Charles C. Thomas, Springfield, 1964.

Kandel, E.R.: Nerve cells and behavior. *Scientific American* 223:57-70, 1970.

Katz, B.: *Nerve, Muscle and Synapse*. McGraw Hill Book Company, New York, 1966.

Rubin, R.P.: *Calcium and The Secretory Process*. Plenum Press, New York, 1974.

Chapter 3

Neurochemistry of Central Monoamine Neurons

Alan Frazer

The chemical substances thought to mediate the process of synaptic transmission in the central nervous system (CNS) have been the object of extensive research. This is probably due to the fact that most drugs modify neuronal activity by altering synaptic transmission rather than neuronal conduction. Local anesthetics are the only major class of drugs used in clinical medicine which inhibit the conduction process. However, psychotropic drugs have a variety of effects on the process of synaptic transmission (Chapter 10), and these effects

have been postulated to produce their clinical efficacy.

In this chapter, the distribution and metabolism of those substances considered to be neurohumoral agents in the CNS will be reviewed. Particular attention will be given to the catecholamines, norepinephrine (NE) and dopamine (DA), and to the indolealkylamine 5-hydroxytryptamine (serotonin), since the neuronal systems that they subserve are thought to be particularly important with regard to psychotropic drug effects. An understanding of these substances will form the framework for much of what is discussed in other chapters. For example, alcohol and narcotic drugs may produce some of their behavioral effects by modifying the activity of these mono-amine-containing neurons in brain. Furthermore, the schizophrenias and the affective disorders have been postulated to arise due to abnormal functioning of these neurons.

Criteria that must be fulfilled for a substance to be qualified as a transmitter agent have been established in the peripheral nervous systems; whether the same criteria should be applied with regard to the central nervous system is debatable though, in view of the complex morphology of the CNS. Generally speaking, what seems important for a putative transmitter agent is that it be present where it is presumed to act; that some mechanism be available for synthesis and/or storage of the transmitter

agent within the neuron; that the transmitter be released from the neuron upon appropriate stimuli; that some mechanism be available to terminate the action of the transmitter at its receptor; and that the suspected transmitter be able to produce the same electrophysiological actions as the natural neurohumoral substance.

With these ideas in mind, we can review the distribution and metabolism of some of the monoamine transmitter substances in the brain. While specific differences in metabolism will be noted, certain general principles will emerge. These similarities between the different transmitter systems far outweigh the specific differences and are important to remember.

Catecholamines and Indolealkylamines

Chemistry

The term "catecholamine" refers to all organic compounds containing a catechol nucleus (a benzene ring with two adjacent hydroxyl substituents) and an amine group (Fig. 1). The three catecholamines usually considered of greatest physiological importance are DA, NE, and epinephrine (E) (Fig. 1).

Due to the amine constituent of the catecholamines, which serves as a proton acceptor at the physiological pH, these compounds exist as positively charged molecules in the body. Also, the hydroxy groups on the benzene ring make these compounds more soluble in water than in oils (lipids). One important consequence of this is that catecholamines do not readily pass through the lipid containing blood-brain barrier from the plasma into most regions of the brain. The impermeability of the blood-brain barrier to catecholamines has made it difficult to investigate the direct action of these agents on the CNS and to study

their metabolism in the brain. To circumvent this problem, the catecholamines have been injected directly into the cerebrospinal fluid (CSF), by being administered into either the lateral ventricles or the cisterna magna. The amines are removed from these spaces and taken up by cells in the brain. While questions remain as to the extent and specificity of the uptake of amines from these subarachnoid spaces, considerable use has been made of this technique to study amine metabolism in the CNS.

Serotonin belongs to the class of chemicals termed "indolealkylamines." As shown in Fig. 2, these compounds have an alkylamine in covalent linkage with a carbon atom in an indole nucleus. As in the case with catecholamines, indolealkylamines, such as serotonin, exist as positively charged molecules at pH 7.4. They are subject, therefore, to the same distribution barriers as the catecholamines.

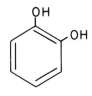

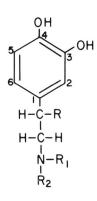

COMPOUND	R	R_1	R_2
Dopamine	H	H	H
Norepinephrine	OH	H	H
Epinephrine	OH	H	CH_3

Fig. 1. The chemical structure of catechol and different catecholamines.

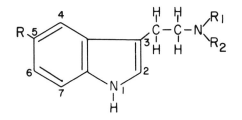

COMPOUND	R	R_1	R_2
Tryptamine	H	H	H
Serotonin	OH	H	H
Dimethyltryptamine	H	CH_3	CH_3
Bufotenine	OH	CH_3	CH_3

Fig. 2. The chemical structures of different indolealkylamines.

Distribution

A variety of techniques are available for the measurement of biogenic amines like NE and serotonin. Originally, bioassay procedures were used to measure the concentration of these substances. In these procedures, a pharmacological response produced by the substance in either a tissue extract or a biological fluid is compared with that produced by a standard amount of the substance. For example, the rise in blood pressure produced by NE in the pithed rat is a frequently used bioassay procedure for this compound. These methods offer great sensitivity; as little as 5×10^{-10} g NE can be detected by bioassay procedures. However, they are somewhat tedious to perform and do suffer from a relative lack of specificity. For these reasons, chemical methods have tended to replace bioassay procedures.

There is no doubt that the development of sensitive and relatively specific fluorimetric analyses for the catecholamines and serotonin, pioneered primarily by Bowman and by Udenfriend, was one of the key advances in our understanding of the neurochemistry of these compounds. Most laboratories measuring catecholamines do so primarily by means of the fluorescent trihydroxyindole reaction, in which the catecholamine undergoes initial oxidation, followed by cyclization in an alkaline medium to produce a highly fluorescent compound. Such fluorescent procedures have yielded valuable information about the concentrations of biogenic amines in various tissues, and the influence of drugs and surgical procedures on these levels. However, questions now being asked by investigators require measurement of amine concentrations below the level of sensitivity of the fluorimetric assays. For example, it is generally not possible to measure basal plasma catecholamine concentrations very accurately using fluorimetric techniques. Also, the amount of biogenic amines in discrete brain nuclei are below the limits of sensitivity of most techniques employing fluorimetry.

To measure such small amine concentrations use has been made of radioactive tracers. In these radiochemical analyses, enzymes are used to produce labelled products, starting with either labelled substrates or cofactors. Such analyses, then, also offer the selectivity inherent in enzymatic reactions. Several different enzyme-isotopic assays are available. In one such analysis norepinephrine is converted to radioactive epinephrine by the action of the enzyme phenylethanolamine-N-methyltransferase and the addition of a radioactive cofactor, S-adenosylmethionine. This technique can measure as little as 2.5×10^{-11} g norepinephrine, whereas the limit of sensitivity for this catecholamine with the fluorescent trihydroxyindole reaction is about 1×10^{-9} g. Serotonin can also be measured by enzymatic-isotopic analysis, to a detection limit of about 5×10^{-11} g. Radiochemical analyses offer great potential in the accurate measurement of basal concentrations of these amines in plasma as well as in small, discrete brain areas.

Use has been made of bioassay and chemical techniques to measure the concentration of dopamine, norepinephrine and serotonin in different areas of the brain. Dopamine is found in highest concentration in the corpus striatum with much smaller levels in the hypothalamus and very small amounts in the other major areas. In most of the gross anatomical parts of the brain, the distribution pattern for NE and serotonin is similar. Their concentrations in subcortical regions is higher than in the cortex.

Another major advance in the investigation of catecholamine and serotonin mechanisms in the brain was the development of a histochemical method for their visualization, by a series of steps in which Eranko, in Finland, and Falck and Hillarp, in Sweden, played a large

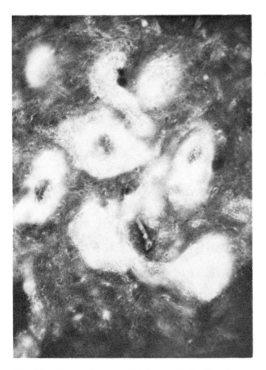

Fig. 3. Dopamine-containing cell bodies in the substantia nigra fluoresce brilliantly because of their content of dopamine in this histofluorimetric preparation. (Kindly supplied by Dr. Alan Laties, University of Pennsylvania.)

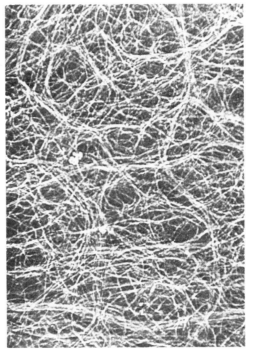

Fig. 4. Typical adrenergic innervation plexus as seen in the iris. Note multiple, fine varicose fibers. (Kindly supplied by Dr. Alan Laties, University of Pennsylvania.)

part.

In brief, the tissue in which catecholamines are to be visualized is first freeze-dried. This prevents the catecholamines from diffusing away from their localization *in vivo* while the tissue is dried. The dried tissue is then exposed to hot paraformaldehyde vapor under controlled humidity. The catecholamines convert into highly *fluorescent* isoquinoline derivatives which emit a greenish fluorescence under appropriate conditions. Serotonin can be converted by a similar process into a beta-carboline derivative which has a yellow fluorescence. Since fluorescent products often have their own characteristic fluorescent spectra, they may be distinguished from each other on this basis. An example of the final product of this technique is presented in Fig. 3. This method has been widely adopted by a number of in-

vestigators.

Application of this technique to the CNS revealed, firstly, that the amines were located within neurons. Secondly, the amines were shown to have a particular distribution within the neuron. Highest amine concentrations are found in the nerve terminal regions, which appear as small varicosities in a fluorescent micrograph (see Fig. 4). These varicosities are thought to represent the presynaptic structures involved in monoamine synthesis, storage, release, and re-uptake. In the soma and axon, however, amine concentrations are about one-hundredth fold lower than in the terminal region.

Finally, in conjunction both with nerve sectioning experiments and pharmacological manipulations, the histochemical fluorescent technique has permitted the amine pathways in the brain

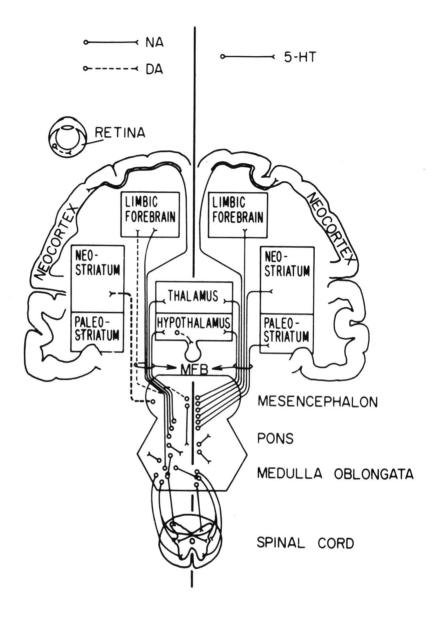

**Fig. 5.   Schematic representation of cate-
cholamine- and serotonin-containing neuron
systems in the central nervous system
(from Anden et al., 1966).**

to be established. A schematic representation of these pathways is shown in Fig. 5.

The cell bodies for DA, NE and serotonin neurons are localized almost exclusively in the tegmentum of the midbrain, the pons and medulla oblongata, with the exception of certain catecholamine cell groups found in the hypothalamus. The amine terminal systems present in other areas of the brain (e.g., limbic system, cerebellum, and spinal cord) arise from long axons whose cell bodies are found in the lower brain stem. Furthermore, collaterals arise from these axons so that a single soma may give rise to terminal innervation of anatomically distinct areas of the brain. For example, from norepinephrine-containing cell bodies in the locus coeruleus (area A_6 of Dahlström and Fuxe), axons arise that innervate the cerebral cortex, the cerebellar cortex, and the periventricular and paraventricular nuclei of the hypothalamus. The following types of norepinephrine and serotonin neurons have been shown to exist:

(1) Long, descending, partially crossed bulbo-spinal neurons originating from the most caudal cell groups in the medulla oblongata; these innervate the gray matter of the spinal cord. Serotonin nerve terminals are particularly concentrated in the lumbar and sacral part of the spinal cord, whereas NE nerve terminals are fairly evenly distributed throughout the cord. Dopamine nerve terminals have not been visualized in the spinal cord.

(2) Long, ascending neuron systems innervating the telencephalon and diencephalon. The NE pathway has been divided into two pathways:

(a) Ventral pathway—from cell groups in the medulla and pons that are caudal to the locus coeruleus. These neurons ascend in the medial forebrain bundle (MFB) to innervate the diencephalon. There are also shorter fibers in this ventral pathway, which innervate brain stem nuclei and the mesencephalon.

(b) Dorsal pathway—from cell bodies in the locus coeruleus. Ascending fibers enter the MFB, as is the case with the ventral pathway, and innervate thalamic nuclei, cerebral cortex, hippocampus, and hypothalamus.

A descending pathway that innervates lower brain stem nuclei as well as a lateral pathway that innervates the cerebellum also arise from the locus coeruleus. From this small cell group, then, NE fibers arise that terminate in practically all areas of the brain.

Ascending serotonin pathways arise from raphe nuclei lying in the midportion of the lower pons and upper brain stem. These fibers run along the most ventral part of the MFB and terminate in the thalamus, limbic forebrain, and hypothalamus. Raphe nuclei also give rise to neurons innervating areas of the lower brain stem.

The fiber tracks of the dopamine systems of the brain are distinct from those of norepinephrine (Fig. 6). There are three major dopamine systems:

(i) Nigro-striatal pathway—from cell bodies in the zona compacta of the substantia nigra in the midbrain. Fibers ascend in the lateral hypothalamus to terminate in the corpus striatum (caudate nucleus, globus pallidus, and putamen) and the central amygdaloid nucleus. It is within this pathway that degenerative lesions occur in Parkinson's Disease.

(ii) Meso-limbic pathway—from cell bodies in the ventral tegmental area, just dorsal to the interpeduncular nucleus. These fibers ascend together with axons of the nigro-striatal pathway and fibers of the MFB to innervate the accumbens nucleus and the olfactory tubercle, and possibly the cerebral cortex as well. The MFB, then, contains noradrenergic, dopaminergic, and serotonergic fibers.

(iii) Tubero-infundibular pathway—from the only monoaminergic cell bodies located above the midbrain. These cell bodies are in the arcuate nucleus of the hypothalamus and innervate the external layer of the median eminence. This fiber tract is presumed to be involved in neuroendocrine regulation (Chapter 4).

In addition to these dopamine systems, Glowinski and his associates in France have described recently a meso-cortical dopamine system. The terminals of this system are primarily in the deeper regions of the frontal, cingulate, and enterorhinal cortex.

Recently, another method has become available to localize NE-containing fibers. This is an immuno-fluorescent technique, developed by Hartman and Udenfriend. Purified antibodies to the enzyme dopamine β-hydroxylase, which is located in NE neurons, are prepared and conjugated to a fluorescent marker. Reaction of the enzyme with the tagged antibody results in a fluorescent precipitation product. Immunologic techniques like this are proving to be valuable "tools" in pharmacological investigations. In general, the pathways visualized by

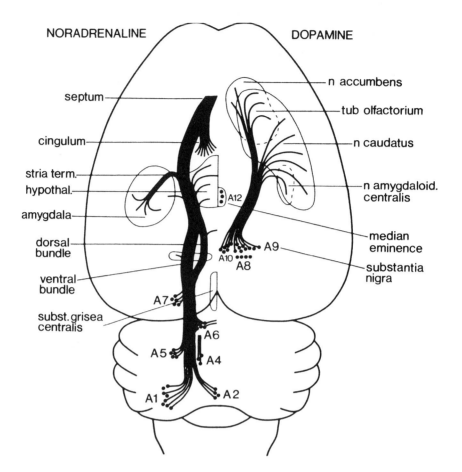

NORADRENALINE   DOPAMINE

septum

cingulum

stria term.
hypothal.

amygdala

dorsal
bundle

ventral
bundle

subst. grisea
centralis

n accumbens

tub olfactorium

n caudatus

n amygdaloid.
centralis

median
eminence

substantia
nigra

A12

A9
A10
A8

A7

A6

A5   A4

A1   A2

Fig. 6. Horizontal projection of the ascending norepinephrine and dopamine neuronal pathways in the brain. Note dopamine cell bodies in arcuate nucleus (area A12) of hypothalamus (from Ungerstedt, 1971).

this method agree with those found using fluorescent histochemistry.

While it has been estimated that there are no more than several thousand NE cell bodies in the brain, and a like number of serotonin soma, the terminal networks of these systems are rather diffuse. The terminal innervation of these systems is weighted heavily toward the reticular activating system and the limbic system. It is not surprising, then, that these compounds are thought to play key roles in the regulation of emotion and behavior (Chapter 14) and many generalized brain functions (e.g., sleep, Chapter 6; neuroendocrine regulation, Chapter 4).

The nigro-striatal DA system is involved with regulation of motor function (extra-pyramidal system). The function of the mesolimbic DA system is unclear at present; it has been hypothesized to be involved in schizophrenia (Chapter 12).

Biosynthesis

Catecholamines — Norepinephrine-containing neurons synthesize their endogenous amine from the amino acid L-tyrosine, by a pathway first suggested in 1939 by Blaschko (Fig. 7). Direct

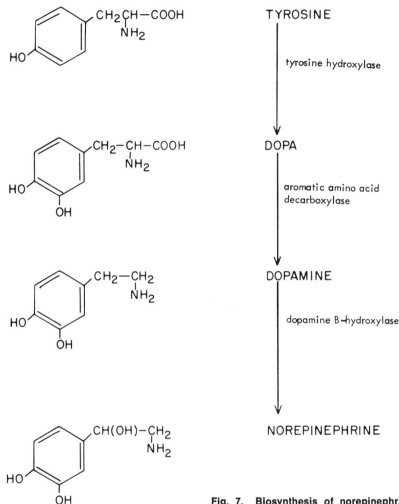

Fig. 7. Biosynthesis of norepinephrine from tyrosine.

evidence for this pathway came from studies showing that the adrenal medulla was capable of converting labelled L-tyrosine, or 3, 4, dihydroxyphenylalanine (DOPA) into DA, NE and epinephrine, both *in vitro* and *in vivo*. The same pathway has been demonstrated in brain tissue when exposed to radioactive L-tyrosine or DOPA. It should be noted that only a small percentage of available tryosine is utilized for catecholamine biosynthesis as compared with its other metabolic pathways.

The initial step in monoamine biosynthesis is the transport of amino acid precursors from the circulation to the intracellular sites where synthesis takes place. The transport of amino acids into brain is facilitated by temperature-sensitive catalytic mechanisms which are rapid, selective, and stereospecific. The enzymes involved in these uptake processes have been referred to as permeases, or somewhat more whimsically "here-to-there-ases." Since groups of amino acids are transported by the same mechanism, different amino acids within a group can compete with one another for transport (e.g., phenylalanine with tryptophan). This may be of importance in certain metabolic disorders which lead to high plasma concentrations of amino acids.

The initial enzymatic reaction in NE synthesis is the hydroxylation of tyrosine to DOPA. This reaction is catalyzed by tyrosine hydroxylase which is found in the adrenal medulla, brain, and all tissues receiving sympathetic innervation. Cutting the sympathetic nerves innervating the tissue and allowing time for degeneration of the nerve fibers to occur is termed "denervation." Since chronic denervation of adrenergically innervated tissue is associated with disappearance of tyrosine hydroxylase activity, the enzyme is considered to be localized within sympathetic nerves. Its precise subcellular localization in nerves remains obscure, as activity has been found in both the soluble fractions as well as in a particulate fraction following differential centrifugation. From data obtained upon assay of the particulate and soluble enzyme *in vitro*, it has been suggested that there may be two forms of the enzyme as the catalytic properties were not identical. In catecholamine areas of the brain containing primarily cell bodies, the enzyme exists primarily in a soluble form; in contrast, in areas rich in terminals of CA neurons, the enzyme is particle bound. An important question for future research is whether these two apparent forms of the enzyme really exist *in vivo*. It may be, for example, that the activity of tyrosine hydroxylase can be changed by a shift in its location from a free to a bound form.

The enzymatic reaction catalyzed by tyrosine hydroxylase is the rate-limiting step in catecholamine biosynthesis. This was first shown by Levitt and associates (1965) who found that addition of increasing concentrations of labelled DOPA or DA to the medium perfusing the isolated guinea pig heart produces proportionate increases in the rate of NE biosynthesis, such that the rate of NE synthesis greatly exceeds the normal *in vivo* rate. However, if labelled L-tyrosine is added to the system, the maximum rate of NE synthesis attained

is much lower than with DOPA or DA, that is, saturation of the system occurs when L-tyrosine is the substrate. Furthermore, the rate of catecholamine synthesis measured with L-tyrosine as the substrate was comparable to that measured *in vivo*.

Drug-induced blockade of the hydroxylation of tyrosine markedly reduces endogenous NE and DA in various tissues, as would be expected if this reaction is the rate-limiting step in catecholamine biosynthesis. Tyrosine analogues, such as α-methylparatyrosine (AMPT), inhibit tyrosine hydroxylase activity. Oral administration of AMPT to man is associated with as much as 70% inhibition of catecholamine production. Behavioral effects produced by this compound are discussed in Chapter 14.

The first catecholamine-synthesizing enzyme to be discovered was that which catalyzes the decarboxylation of DOPA to DA, and was consequently named DOPA decarboxylase. Since this enzyme was subsequently shown to act on all naturally occurring L-amino acids, it has been renamed L-aromatic amino acid decarboxylase. Pyridoxal phosphate (vitamin B_6) is required as a cofactor for enzyme activity as it is for other decarboxylases. Inhibition of this enzyme does not reduce endogenous catecholamine stores. Originally, α-methyl-DOPA, a compound that inhibits decarboxylase activity *in vitro* was thought to deplete catecholamine stores by this effect. This does not seem to be so. Its capacity to deplete catecholamine stores is due to its own decarboxylation to α-methylnorepinephrine which replaces endogenous intracellular NE stores, thus causing depletion of the naturally occurring transmitter.

The enzyme dopamine β-hydroxylase catalyzes the final reaction in NE biosynthesis. Denervation of sympathetic nerves causes a disappearance of dopamine β-hydroxylase activity; this indicates that the enzyme is localized within peripheral sympathetic nerves. In fact, the enzyme seems to be located in the granules or vesicles that store NE. Thus, the final step in the *de novo* synthesis of NE occurs in the storage granule in which it is concentrated.

A highly specific and sensitive isotopic assay has been developed for dopamine β-hydroxylase. By the use of this assay, it has been possible to demonstrate that dopamine β-hydroxylase activity in brain shows a good correlation to the regional distribution of NE. In addition, electrolytic or chemical lesioning experiments of brain areas indicate that the enzyme is located within NE-containing neurons.

5-Hydroxytryptamine (serotonin)—Serotonin is formed in the body by enzymatic conversion of the amino acid tryptophan. Very little tryptophan metabolism is directed toward serotonin synthesis, with most metabolism being toward nicotinamide formation.

The initial step in the synthesis of brain serotonin is the uptake of its precursor, tryptophan, into brain. Tryptophan uptake, similar to that of tyrosine, appears to occur by an active mechanism. As indicated in Fig. 8, after tryptophan is taken up into the neuron, it is hydroxylated to 5-hydroxytryptophan. This reaction is catalyzed by the enzyme tryptophan hydroxylase. Tryptophan hydroxylase may be present in the brain in both a soluble and particulate form. The soluble form occurs primarily in those areas of the brain rich in serotonin cell bodies, whereas the particulate form is located primarily in areas containing serotonin terminals. Recent evidence suggests that these two forms of the enzyme have different characteristics with regard to cofactor requirements and affinity for tryptophan. It may be, then, that changes in the physical state of tryptophan hydroxylase (soluble or particulate) can influence serotonin biosynthesis.

Inhibition of tryptophan hydroxylase reduces serotonin synthesis so that, over

time, there is a depletion of serotonin stores. This indicates that the hydroxylation of tryptophan is the rate-limiting step in serotonin synthesis. The compound most widely used to inhibit tryptophan hydroxylase is parachlorophenylalanine (PCPA). This agent initially produces competitive inhibition of enzyme activity but is then incorporated into the enzyme so as to produce irreversible inhibition *in vivo*. For this reason, recovery of serotonin synthesis, following administration of PCPA, requires the synthesis of new tryptophan hydroxylase. PCPA has been administered to animals and to man; it produces extensive depletion of serotonin stores. Its behavioral effects are noted in Chapters 7 and 14.

Conversion of 5-hydroxytryptophan to serotonin (Fig. 8) occurs rapidly by the action of L-aromatic amino acid decarboxylase. Originally it was thought that the decarboxylation of DOPA and of 5-hydroxytryptophan was catalyzed by the same enzyme. Recent data on the kinetics of these reactions, together with subcellular localization studies, suggest that this may not be so. Rather, it seems that there are two separate enzymes catalyzing these reactions, although these enzymes may have common immunogenic properties. As is the case in catecholamine synthesis, inhibition of decarboxylase activity is not an effective way to reduce serotonin biosynthesis.

Regulation of amine biosynthesis — It has been known for some time that prolonged stimulation of peripheral sympathetic nerves does not reduce the norepinephrine content of these nerves; yet norepinephrine has been released as a consequence of stimulation. What has happened to maintain norepinephrine stores is that the rate of norepinephrine synthesis rises to keep up with increased release of the transmitter substance.

This phenomenon has been studied extensively by Weiner and his associates who found that stimulation caused an

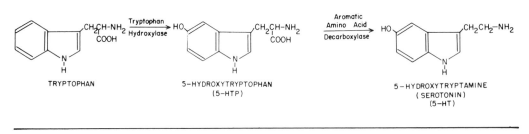

Fig. 8. Biosynthesis of serotonin from tryptophan.

increase in norepinephrine synthesis if tyrosine was the precursor but not if DOPA was precursor. Furthermore, the increased rate of synthesis was reduced by addition of norepinephrine to the medium bathing the test nerve. Also, the increased rate of synthesis was not associated with increased amounts of tyrosine hydroxylase protein. As catecholamines had been shown to inhibit tyrosine hydroxylase activity *in vitro,* it was hypothesized that stimulation causes the release of norepinephrine from a small, chemically undetectable compartment and that this removes endproduct inhibition of tyrosine hydroxylase by the catecholamine, so that norepinephrine synthesis is increased.

Quite recently, alternative explanations have been proposed to explain how stimulation increases catecholamine synthesis. It was found that calcium ions (which flow into nerves during stimulation) stimulate the activity of tyrosine hydroxylase isolated from either the adrenal gland or brain. Subsequent to this, Morgenroth and his associates (1974) found that either calcium ions or nerve stimulation changed the kinetic properties of tyrosine hydroxylase. Both treatments increased the affinity of the enzmye for its substrate, tyrosine, and for its cofactor; also, the affinity of the enzyme for its end-product inhibitor,

norepinephrine, was decreased by both treatments. These experiments, then, indicate that nerve stimulation produces an activation of tyrosine hydroxylase by changing the kinetic properties of the enzyme, possibly due to influx of calcium ions.

Whatever the actual mechanism is shown to be, the important point to remember is that NE-containing nerves possess a mechanism whereby shortterm increases in transmitter utilization are met by increased transmitter synthesis.

In other words, neurons should not be viewed as rigid filaments, but rather as dynamic structures that alter their total functional state in response to the requirements placed upon them. Demands for more transmitter to be released result in the transmitter being synthesized at an increased rate. Indeed, not only is there a mechanism whereby short-term increases in NE demand, but also long-term activity in adrenergic neurons produce an increase in NE synthesis. The mechanism is different, though. For example, increased adrenergic activity due to cold exposure, immobilization, or drugs, such as reserpine, produce an increase in NE synthesis. This increased rate of NE synthesis is due to enhanced activity of both tyrosine hydroxylase and dopamine β-hydroxylase; the increase in enzyme activity can be blocked by inhibitors of protein synthesis. This suggests that the increased enzyme activity is due to the accumulation of new enzyme molecules, and this has been confirmed by immunotitration techniques showing more enzyme protein in central noradrenergic neurons after reserpine administration. Whether the increase in enzyme protein in brain or in the periphery is due to enhanced synthesis or reduced degradation of enzyme molecules remains to be established. A normally functioning adrenergic neuron, then, has a variety of compensatory mechanisms which insure its capability to operate under a rather wide range of circumstances.

There are some differences between the regulation of NE synthesis and that of serotonin. Tyrosine hydroxylase is saturated with substrate at normal brain concentrations of tyrosine, so that increasing brain tyrosine concentration does not enhance catecholamine synthesis. Thus, L-DOPA is used in the treatment of Parkinson's Disease to increase dopamine concentration rather than tyrosine. In contrast, tryptophan hydroxylase does not seem to be saturated with its substrate at normal brain concentrations of tryptophan. Therefore, the overall rate of serotonin synthesis may be dependent, in part, on the availability of brain tryptophan. Administration of loading doses of tryptophan to rats increases brain serotonin concentrations, whereas elimination of tryptophan from the diet reduces the concentration of the indolealkylamine in brain. Therefore, factors influencing the transport of tryptophan into brain (e.g., extent of its binding to plasma protein; the concentration of other neutral amino acids in plasma, which compete with tryptophan for transport into brain) can regulate the rate of serotonin synthesis. Thus, while there are similarities in catecholamine and serotonin synthesis, some differences do exist.

Turnover

Since amine synthesis keeps up with amine release due to stimulation, it is evident that measurement of static amine concentrations need not reflect the activity of adrenergic neurons. To provide a better index of the activity in monoamine neurons, most investigators measure amine "turnover." The turnover time is defined as the time interval required to synthesize an amount of a given monoamine equal to that normally stored in the tissue under investigation. Increased activity in amine neurons has been shown to decrease turnover time measurements, even though static amine concentrations may not change. Both isotopic and non-isotopic methods are available to measure amine turnover. It has been found that the turnover of serotonin in brain is several fold faster than that of norepinephrine.

Storage

In the central nervous system, as in the chromaffin cells of the adrenal medulla and in sympathetic nerve endings, NE is stored in a bound form. Binding of NE occurs in specialized subcellular particles called either "granules" or vesicles. Various types of vesicles have been visualized with electron microscopic techniques. Vesicles can range in size from about 250–1200 Å in diameter; some contain granular material which can appear as a dense core in the vesicle, whereas other vesicles appear "empty." In peripheral sympathetic nerves, small granular vesicles (400–600 Å in diameter) are the main storage sites of NE. This may be the case in brain as well although larger granules (800–1200 Å in diameter) are present there also. The evidence is inconclusive as to which is the main storage site of NE.

Binding of NE within the granule occurs through the formation of a tetracatecholamine-adenosine triphosphate (ATP) complex. The NE-ATP complex may be stabilized further in the granule by binding to proteins present in the vesicle, termed chromogranins. Due to this stabilization of the complex in the granule, it has been postulated that NE exists in the vesicle in a bound and a free form. The bound form would consist of an NE-ATP aggregate held in a gel-like matrix formed by chromogranin, whereas the free pool might consist of NE which has been newly synthesized in the granule.

The storage granule performs several important functions. First, it is the site of NE synthesis from dopamine, as the enzyme catalyzing this reaction, dopamine β-hydroxylase, is located in the granule. Second, by binding monoamines, the granule prevents their diffusion onto the enzyme monoamine oxidase and subsequent intraneuronal degradation. Third, they serve as the site from which transmitter is released in response to depolarization of the nerve terminal.

Within the neuron, the highest concentration of granules is found in the terminal area. However, the vesicles are not synthesized in the terminals; rather, they seem to be formed in the cell body and transported to the terminal region. Most norepinephrine synthesis, though, occurs in the nerve terminals in preformed granules coming from the cell body.

The preceding discussion makes it apparent that norepinephrine does not exist in the neuron in a single, homogenous state but rather in functionally different states, called "pools." This idea is consistent with numerous pharmacological experiments. The cellular location of these pools remains to be determined. One site is clearly the granule, but exactly how many "pools" of norepinephrine exist within the granule is uncertain. Also, some norepinephrine in the neuron is presumably extra-granular, which could constitute another "pool."

As with the catecholamines, storage of serotonin within the nerve occurs in vesicles, and also there is kinetic evidence for the existence of different "pools" of brain serotonin.

Release

Much of the information on norepinephrine release comes from studies on peripheral sympathetic nerves and the adrenal medulla. This is because it is very difficult with present techniques to investigate endogenous monoamine release in the central nervous system. Nevertheless, available data would suggest that there are qualitative similarities in the release process from these different sites.

Under normal conditions, the neuronal release of norepinephrine occurs primarily at the terminal. Conduction of the action potential down the nerve with subsequent depolarization of the terminal is necessary for normal monoamine release. There appears to be spontaneous release of norepinephrine from sympathetic nerve terminals, similar to the spontaneous release of the transmitter acetylcholine at the neuromuscular junction.

The site in the nerve terminal from which norepinephrine is released by depolarization of the terminal membrane is the storage granule. There are several lines of evidence that support this view. For example, reserpine is a drug that causes depletion of amines from nerves by interfering with the uptake and storage of monoamines in the granule. A reserpine-treated animal shows a blockade of adrenergic transmission due to depletion of norepinephrine from the nerve terminal. The time course for restoration of synaptic transmission in a reserpine-treated animal coincides temporally with restoration of the ability of granules to take up and store the catecholamine. Direct evidence that norepinephrine is released from the granule by nerve stimulation is the finding that not only is NE released but also ATP and the enzyme dopamine β-hydroxylase. As mentioned previously, these latter two substances are found in the storage granule together with norepinephrine. In fact, the proportionality between released norepinephrine, ATP, and dopamine β-hydroxylase is quite similar to that found in granule extracts. Furthermore, in reserpine-treated animals, stimulation of sympathetic nerves fails to elicit release of norepinephrine although there is a normal release of dopamine β-hydroxylase.

Following release of the transmitter agent and its interaction with "receptors" on the postsynaptic membrane, the physiological actions of norepinephrine within the synaptic cleft are terminated primarily by a process of re-uptake back into the presynaptic terminal.

Uptake

The ability of sympathetic neurons to take up physiological concentrations of exogenous catecholamines was first observed by Axelrod and his associates who found that intravenously injected radioactive catecholamines were rapidly accumulated in various peripheral tissues. Numerous investigators, utilizing different techniques, have subsequently demonstrated that the site of catecholamine uptake in these tissues is the sympathetic neurons. The uptake process into sympathetic nerves is temperature dependent, requires energy, and the presence of sodium ion in the external medium. This active uptake process, located in the axonal membrane of adrenergic neurons, is specific in favor of the naturally occurring L-isomer of NE and takes up norepinephrine more efficiently than epinephrine.

Various drugs, such as cocaine and tricyclic antidepressants (Chapter 10), inhibit this uptake process. In addition, agents which reduce the sodium gradient across the nerve membrane, such as ouabain and metabolic poisons, also inhibit norepinephrine uptake.

In addition to the uptake process described, norepinephrine is also taken up by non-neuronal tissue. This process was first observed by Iversen who termed it $Uptake_2$ to differentiate it from the neuronal uptake process ($Uptake_1$). This non-neuronal uptake process, also a membrane transport system, has a much lower affinity for norepinephrine than the neuronal uptake system does. It is not stereochemically specific, is less markedly sodium dependent than $Uptake_1$, and takes up epinephrine with greater affinity than norepinephrine. Inhibitors of $Uptake_2$ include O-methylated catecholamine metabolities, such as normetanephrine, as well as certain steroids, like testosterone, estradiol, and corticosterone.

It is widely accepted that the effects of norepinephrine released from adrenergic terminals are terminated by the process termed $Uptake_1$. Evidence in support of this concept is that local inactivation of norepinephrine released by low frequencies of sympathetic nerve stimulation is not prevented by inhibition of the enzymes that metabolize norepinephrine. Furthermore, inhibition of these enzymes is usually not associated with either potentiation or prolongation of the effects of adrenergic transmission. In contrast, inhibition of $Uptake_1$ by drugs, such as cocaine, enhance the effects of adrenergic transmission.

Originally, it was not thought that the process termed $Uptake_2$ had any significant role in the inactivation of norepinephrine released into the synaptic cleft. This view may have to be re-evaluated in light of recent evidence showing that this process assumes considerable importance at high frequencies of sympathetic nerve stimulation. It should be remembered that the brain contains non-neuronal tissue, i.e., glial cells, so that nonneuronal uptake of norepinephrine may occur in brain.

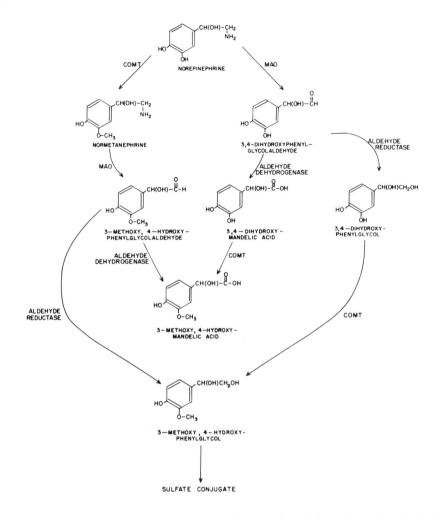

Fig. 9. Catabolism of norepinephrine. Note final product formation of either 3-methoxy, 4-hydroxymandelic acid (VMA) or 3-methoxy, 4-hydroxyphenylglycol (MHPG).

The uptake of monoamines by brain neurons has been studied extensively, in particular by the use of synaptosome ("pinched-off" nerve endings) preparations. Extensive studies on the specificity and kinetics of monoamine uptake by synaptosomes obtained from homogenates of different brain areas have been reported, especially by Snyder and his associates. It was found that the uptake process for norepinephrine by central NE-containing neurons is similar to that of peripheral sympathetic nerves, i.e., temperature sensitive, energy dependent and requiring sodium ions. Dopamine-containing neurons have a high affinity membrane transport system for this catecholamine that is also sodium dependent. A striking difference between norepinephrine and dopamine uptake is the relative insensitivity of the latter process to inhibition by tricyclic antidepressants. For example, the drug desipramine is about one thousand times less potent as an inhibitor of dopamine uptake than of norepinephrine uptake. Studies of serotonin uptake into brain neurons obtained from areas rich in serotonin terminals reveal, as with the catecholamines, a specific high affinity membrane transport system that is sodium dependent.

Metabolism

As just discussed, uptake of monoamines, as opposed to enzymatic degradation, appears to be the major route for terminating the activity of monoamines released into the synapse. Enzymatic degradation of monoamines does occur, however; this process is quite important in metabolizing monoamines released into the circulation.

Catecholamines are metabolized by a series of reactions involving 3-0-methylation and oxidative deamination (Fig. 9). The methylation reaction is catalyzed by catechol-3-0-methyltransferase (COMT) and oxidative deamination by monoamine oxidase (MAO). These enzymes are found in all catecholamine-containing tissues, with the highest activities observed in the liver, kidney, and gastrointestinal tract. About 65% of catecholamines entering the circulation, whether from endogenous or exogenous sources, are metabolized by both COMT and MAO, predominantly in the liver and kidney. This metabolism, coupled with tissue uptake, accounts for the fact that very little catecholamine (less than 5%) is excreted in the urine in a nonmetabolized form.

The enzyme COMT, first described by Axelrod and Tomchick, does not show any specificity toward the D- or L-isomers of norepinephrine. S-Adenosylmethionine is required for enzyme activity as is magnesium ion or some other divalent cation. Most COMT activity in peripheral tissues remains after sympathetic denervation. This suggests that most COMT activity is extraneuronal, although a small amount may be intraneuronal.

The enzyme monoamine oxidase is located in the outer lipoprotein membrane of mitochondria. As shown by denervation experiments, the enzyme is present both intraneuronally and extra-neuronally. Monoamine oxidase found in the neuron regulates the intraneuronal level of monamines, by promoting the degradation of monoamines in the axoplasm. In fact, because of the intraneuronal degradation of catecholamines, a considerable proportion of the norepinephrine leaving the neuron does so in a physiologically inert form as a deaminated metabolite. After inhibition of this enzyme with monoamine oxidase inhibitors, such as tranylcypromine or phenelzine (Chapter 10), the monoamine content of the brain increases markedly.

Perhaps the most important recent finding about monoamine oxidase is that it exists in multiple forms, usually referred to as isoenzymes. These multiple forms of the enzyme were first separated by Youdim and Sandler, using polyacrylamide gel electrophoresis. Four brain isoenzymes have been isolated. One of these isoenzymes appears to be highly specific in its ability to oxidize dopamine. These isoenzymes have marked differences in substrate and inhibitor specificity, and the activity of the different isoenzymes varies considerably from area to area in the brain.

In general agreement with electrophoretic data, the effect of selective inhibitors on MAO suggests two classes of enzymes, termed Type A and Type B enzyme. Norepinephrine and serotonin are metabolized by Type A enzyme but not Type B. In contrast, dopamine is oxidatively deaminated by both enzyme forms. Thus, administration of a drug, such as clorgyline, that inhibits the Type A enzyme, elevates brain concentrations of NE, DA, and serotonin. However, administration of an inhibitor of Type B monoamine oxidase, such as deprenyl, only elevates brain dopamine concentrations.

At the present time, those MAO inhibitors that are clinically useful in hypertension and in depression inhibit both types of MAO. It is anticipated that clinically useful selective inhibitors of the different forms of MAO will be developed. Such drugs might have somewhat different spectra of action than agents now available, and possibly produce less side effects.

As can be seen in Fig. 9, MAO converts catecholamines to their corresponding aldehyde derivatives. In peripheral tissues, the final product of norepinephrine (and epinephrine) metabolism is the acid, 3-methoxy-4-hydroxymandelic acid (VMA), formed by oxidation of the intermediate aldehyde. In brain, though, the intermediate aldehyde is reduced to an alcohol so that the major final product of norepinephrine in brain is 3 - methoxy - 4 - hydroxyphenylglycol (MHPG). Increasing attention is being focused on MHPG concentrations in urine and in cerebrospinal fluid of patients with psychiatric disorders (Chapter 14).

Dopamine is also metabolized by both MAO and COMT, to yield the primary dopamine metabolite homovanillic acid (HVA).

The metabolic degradation of serotonin is simpler than that of the catecholamines in that there is no methylation reaction involved. Serotonin is metabolized by monoamine oxidase to an aldehyde intermediate that is primarily oxidized to an acid derivative [5-hydroxyindoleacetic acid (5-HIAA)], but can also be reduced to the alcohol, 5-hydroxytryptophol. In addition, brain also contains an enzyme system, serotonin-sulfokinase, that catalyzes the sulfation of the indolealkylamine. However, under normal conditions, 5-HIAA is the principal metabolite of serotonin in brain, as the conversion of serotonin to 5-HIAA far outstrips the rate of sulfation of serotonin. Similar to the situation with the catecholamine metabolites MHPG and HVA, numerous investigators have studied the concentration of 5-HIAA in cerebrospinal fluid of psychiatric patients in an attempt to evaluate the status of serotonin nerve activity in such patients.

Receptors

The preceding discussions have been concerned primarily with what could be termed pre-synaptic aspects of monoamine or transmitter metabolism, namely synthesis, storage, release and uptake. However, the functional effects produced by transmitters are determined largely by their interaction with specific "receptors" on the post-synaptic cell. A receptor for the catecholamines, or any drug for that matter, is defined as a specific macromolecule (e.g., protein) with which they interact to produce their characteristic biological effect. Paul Erlich, in 1900, is usually credited with introducing the idea of receptors in his famous side-chain theory of immunity.

In peripheral tissues innervated by the sympathetic nervous system, two basic types of adrenergic receptors seem to exist. This idea was originally proposed by Ahlquist in 1948, based upon his observation on the relative potencies of six sympathomimetic amines (drugs that produce effects similar to those observed upon stimulation of peripheral noradrenergic neurons) in eliciting different adrenergic responses. He found two orders of potency among the amines in inducing the various responses and concluded that this was due to the drugs acting on two different types of receptors. Ahlquist termed these receptors either *alpha* (responsible for most excitatory actions) or *beta* (responsible for the majority of inhibitory actions). Ahlquist wisely cautioned that these two receptors cannot be classified simply as excitatory or inhibitory because each type of receptor may have either action depending on where it is located. Blocking agents specific for each type of adrenergic receptor in peripheral tissues (e.g., phentolamine for alpha receptors and propranolol for beta receptors) are now available and used clinically.

The importance of the receptor concept is that it emphasizes that a neurotransmitter can have either an excitatory or inhibitory action depending on the receptor activated, i.e., the receptor, not the transmitter, determines the nature of the response.

Whether adrenergic receptors in the brain are identical with peripheral adrenergic receptors is unclear. Certainly, some synaptic effects elicited by norepinephrine in the CNS can be antagonized selectively by either alpha or beta receptor blocking agents. Further research is needed, though, to better characterize the central adrenergic receptors.

Of course, the use of the Greek alphabet to classify drug responses does not increase our understanding of the molecular events between a transmitter substance or drug and a tissue. Ahlquist has stated that "when better knowledge of a receptor is obtained, for example, the exact identification of the enzyme or enzyme systems involved, the need for receptor vanishes." There are currently several hypotheses regarding those macromolecules which may serve as receptors for catecholamines. At different times, either the nucleotide ATP or the enzyme COMT has been proposed as a component of adrenergic receptors. At present, though, the evidence seems strongest in favor of the enzyme adenylate cyclase being a component of the receptor for catecholamines.

Adenylate cyclase, discovered by Sutherland and associates, is located in the cell membrane of most cells in the body. It catalyzes the formation of adenosine 3', 5'-monophosphate (cyclic AMP) from adenosine triphosphate. Cyclic AMP is known to mediate the cellular effects of many hormones in peripheral tissues. For example, hepatic glycogenolysis produced by epinephrine is known to be initiated by this substance first activating adenylate cyclase in the liver to increase the intracellular concentration of cyclic AMP. Cyclic AMP then acts as an intracellular "second messenger" to initiate processes that

ultimately result in the breakdown of glycogen in the liver. Quite recently, evidence has accumulated that cyclic AMP has a specific role in synaptic transmission due to transmitter activation of adenylate cyclase.

Firstly, it has been known for quite some time that brain contains very high activity both of adenylate cyclase and of phosphodiesterase, the enzyme that degrades cyclic AMP. More recently, Bloom and his associates have shown that the norepinephrine projection from the locus coeruleus to cerebellar Purkinje cells is inhibitory, i.e., it slows the rate of discharge of these cells by producing hyperpolarization of the membrane. When cyclic AMP was applied to these cells by iontophoresis (a technique whereby the passage of an electric current causes the displacement of charged molecules from glass capillaries or microelectrodes of very small diameter onto neurons), the effects observed were identical to those seen with either stimulation of the locus coeruleus or iontophoretic application of norepinephrine. As previous investigators had shown the cerebellum to posses an adenylate cyclase that was stimulated by norepinephrine, it was proposed that the synaptic effects of norepinephrine at the cerebellar Purkinje cell is due to activation of adenylate cyclase, producing an increase in the intracellular concentration of cyclic AMP. The results of subsequent pharmacological investigations, as well as those using an immunocytochemical method to visualize cyclic AMP, have provided additional support for this view.

Other evidence that adenylate cyclase may function as a catecholamine receptor in the brain comes from the study of a dopamine-sensitive adenylate cyclase in the caudate nucleus. As mentioned previously, this area of the brain contains a high concentration of dopamine nerve terminals. Dopamine functions primarily as an inhibitory transmitter at this site. In 1972, Greengard and his associates demonstrated the existence of an adenylate cyclase in homogenates of the caudate nucleus. Furthermore, the enzyme prepared from this site was much more sensitive to stimulation by dopamine than to stimulation by norepinephrine. The biochemical and pharmacological properties of this enzyme were similar to the reported properties of the dopamine receptor. In areas of the limbic system receiving a dopaminergic input, an adenylate cyclase has been isolated that appears similar to the dopamine receptor in these areas (See Chapter 10 for the effects of antipsychotic drugs on these adenylate cyclases, and Chapter 12 for the involvement of the mesolimbic dopamine system in the pathophysiology of schizophrenia). The mechanism whereby cyclic AMP produces the changes in membrane permeability that lead to the electrophysiological effects of the catecholamines is unknown, but may involve the phosphorylation of a protein in the cell membrane.

Much less is known about the molecular nature of the receptors for serotonin. In fact, available data indicate important differences between the receptors for serotonin in brain and those in smooth muscle. Thus, compounds like cinanserin and methysergide block the excitatory effect of serotonin on smooth muscle but do not block the inhibitory effect of iontophoretically-applied serotonin on neurons of the brain receiving a dense serotonergic input.

Conclusion

It seems safe to conclude that much more research is needed to clarify the cellular responses elicited by stimulation of the various monoamine systems. Nevertheless, there is a wealth of anatomical, biochemical and pharmacological data implicating these monoamines in various multicellular functions of the brain. Dopamine systems are clearly involved in extrapyramidal function and may also play some role in the regulation of certain behavioral states and of neuroendocrine processes. Norepinephrine- and serotonin-containing neurons may be involved in the regulation of mood as well as hunger and thirst, temperature, neuroendocrine processes, and sleep. Subsequent chapters will discuss the involvement of these amines in some of these functions in detail.

To summarize, there are many different transmitter substances in brain; three such substances, dopamine, norepinephrine, and serotonin have been selected for review. This is because methodology has been available that permits their detailed study. In general, it may be said that mechanisms are usually available for the synthesis, storage, release, and inactivation of transmitter substances. Certain similarities in these mechanisms are readily apparent for the different monoamines. Furthermore, these monoamine systems possess mechanisms whereby either acute or chronic demands on transmitter utilization can be met by compensatory changes in transmitter synthesis. These amine systems appear to be involved in many important and complex functions of the brain and, furthermore, appear to be involved in the pharmacological effects of several classes of psychotropic drugs.

Selected References

Ahlquist, R.P.: A study of the adrenotropic receptors. *Amer. J. Physiol.* 153:586-600, 1948.

Anden, N.E., Dahlström, A., Fuxe, K., Larrson, K., Olson, L., and Ungerstedt, U.: Ascending monoamine neurons to the telencephalon and diencephalon. *Acta Physiol. Scand.* 67:313-326, 1966.

Axelrod, J.: Noradrenaline: Fate and control of its biosynthesis. *Science* 173:598-606, 1971.

Cooper, J.R., Bloom, F.E., and Roth, R.H.: *The Biochemical Basis of Neuropharmacology.* Oxford University Press, New York, 1974.

Costa, E., Gessa, G.L., and Sandler, M.: *Serotonin-New Vistas, Histochemistry and Pharmacology.* Raven Press, New York, 1974.

Erlich, P.: On immunity with special reference to cell life. *Proc. Roy. Soc.* 66:424-448, 1900.

Falck, B., Hillarp, N.O., Thieme, G., and Torp, A.: Fluorescence of catecholamines and related compounds condensed with formaldehyde. *J. Histochem. Cytochem.* 10:348-354, 1962.

Frazer, A., and Stinnett, J.L.: Distribution and metabolism of norepinephrine and serotonin in the central nervous system. In *Biological Psychiatry.* J. Mendels, ed., John Wiley and Sons, Inc., New York, 1973, pp. 35-64.

Greengard, P.: Possible role for cyclic nucleotides and phosphorylated membrane proteins in postsynaptic actions of neurotransmitters. *Nature* 260:101-108, 1976.

Kebabian, J.W., Petzold, G.L., and Greengard, P.: Dopamine sensitive adenylate cyclase in caudate nucleus of rat brain and its similarity to the "dopamine receptor." *Proc. Nat. Acad. Sci. USA* 69:2145-2149, 1972.

Levitt, M., Spector, S., Sjoerdsma, A., and Udenfriend, S.: Elucidation of the rate-limiting step in norepinephrine biosynthesis in the perfused guinea-pig heart. *J. Pharmacol. Exp. Ther.* 148:1-8, 1965.

Morgenroth, V.H., Boadle-Biber, M., and Roth, R.H.: Tyrosine hydroxylase: Activation by nerve stimulation. *Proc. Nat. Acad. Sci. USA* 71:4283-4287, 1974.

Perkins, J.P.: Adenyl cyclase. *Adv. Cycl. Nucleot. Res.* 3:1-64, 1973.

Siggins, G.R., Hoffer, B.J., and Bloom, F.E.: Cyclic adenosine monophosphate: Possible mediator for norepinephrine effects on cerebellar Purkinje cells. *Science* 165:1018-1020, 1969.

Thierry, A.M., Blanc, G., Sobel, A., Stinus, L., and Glowinski, L.: Dopaminergic terminals in the rat cortex. *Science* 182:499-501, 1973.

Ungerstedt, U.: Stereotaxic mapping of the monoamine pathways in the rat brain. *Acta Physiol. Scand. Suppl.* 367, 1971.

Part II

Psychobiological Research Strategies

*I*NVESTIGATIONS *into the biological mechanisms associated with behavioral disorders has involved multiple research strategies and approaches. This is necessary both because of the complexity of the physiological aspects of brain function, and because of the intrinsic difficulties involved in conducting objective studies of human behavior.*

In this section, five approaches used in psychobiological research are presented: neuroendocrinology, genetics, sleep studies, animal models of behavior and clinical neurophysiological studies. A feature common to all of these strategies is the integration of basic biological principles and clinical issues. For example, the chapter on neuroendocrine techniques begins with a review of hypothalamic regulatory mechanisms of endocrine systems. Subsequently, the application of endocrine and neuroendocrine techniques to patients with a variety of psychiatric disorders is discussed.

An important advance has been the utilization of genetic principles in psychiatric research. Data obtained from genetic studies, described in the second chapter of this section, have provided strong support for the involvement of biological factors in these disorders. More recently, attention has been focused on pharmacogenetic aspects of psychotropic drugs, i.e., how clinical response and side-effects produced by these drugs is influenced by genetic factors.

In Chapter 6, the methodology involved in doing research on sleep is described. The sleep cycles of normal subjects and patients with various psychiatric disorders can be evaluated through objective measures such as the electroencephalograph (EEG). Abnormal sleep patterns have been reported in patients with psychiatric disorders. However, the biological significance of these abnormalities is not well understood, as the underlying neurochemistry of sleep is still being actively explored.

The field of animal models of behavior is a vast, complex Subject. Rather than review this entire area, Chapter 7 limits itself primarily to studies involving primates; the relationship of evoked behavioral abnormalities in these animals to psychopathology in humans is discussed. A particularly striking feature of this paradigm is the opportunity to study the interaction of such complex factors as environment, stress, and neurochemical deficits. By using animal models, such important interrelationships can be examined in a relatively direct manner not possible in studies involving humans.

Finally, the chapter on clinical neurophysiology represents an extension of the issue of brain organization and behavior described in Chapter 1. Methods available for obtaining information about functional aspects of brain organization in humans are outlined, and a discussion is presented of the application of this approach to schizophrenia, demonstrating the potential relevance of studies of brain organization to psychiatric disorders.

The psychobiological research strategies described in this section are representative of the kinds of investigative approaches that are currently being utilized. No one approach is likely to provide a complete understanding of any psychiatric disorder, but the effective utilization of multiple techniques offers considerable promise for extending our knowledge of biological-behavioral interrelationships.

Chapter 4

Neuroendocrinology: Applications to Psychiatric Disorders

Andrew Winokur

The endocrine system and the neural system work in concert to maintain the physiological stability of the body. Each of these systems is exposed to multiple sensory inputs from within and outside of the body, and each of these systems has extensive capabilities to respond to changes in the internal or external environment in such a manner as to defend the physiological equilibrium of the body. Communication and integration between endocrine and neural systems is necessary in order to assure that the overall goal of physiological stability is achieved. Thus, it has long been recognized that there are significant areas of overlap between endocrine and neural activity. It should be emphasized that these two systems have wider roles than simply maintaining homeostasis. For example, they are both involved in initiating important physiological and behavioral activities, frequently with highly integrated patterns of interaction in this capacity as well.

The endocrine system consists of a series of glands or organs which synthesize, store and secrete a variety of physiologically active hormones. Upon exposure of an endocrine organ to an appropriate stimulus, a hormone is secreted into the general circulation and is transported through the blood stream until it reaches its target organ. When a hormone interacts with its target organ(s), a physiological response ensues. The types of physiological responses that can be produced by the hormones are varied, and involve many of the important metabolic activities of the body. The organs comprising the endocrine system include the hypothalamus, the pituitary gland (which is actually made up of an anterior and posterior portion), the thyroid gland, the parathyroid glands, the adrenal glands (which are made up of two endocrine organs, the adrenal medulla and the adrenal cortex), the gonads (ovaries in women, testes in men), and the pancreas.

In light of the fact that the endocrine system represents one of the two major regulatory systems of the body, it is not surprising that there has been interest, for a number of years, in the involvement of the endocrine system in the physiological aspects of behavior. In the first half of the 20th century, Cannon and Selye demonstrated the importance of epinephrine and glucocorticoids (hormones secreted by the adrenal medulla and adrenal cortex, respectively) in the body's response mechanisms to stress. A great deal of subsequent research has provided further evidence for the involvement of epinephrine and glucocorticoids, as well as a number of other hormones, such as growth hormone and prolactin, in the body's response to a wide variety of physical, psychological and pharmacological stresses. A number of researchers have attempted to correlate the serum levels of various peripheral hormones (such as cortisol, thyroxine, testosterone or estrogen) with certain psychiatric disorders. This approach has generally not been fruitful in demonstrating specific relationships between variations in hormone secretion and psychiatric disorders because of the responsiveness of peripheral hormones to such a wide variety of stimuli. For example, there has been considerable interest in the relationship between cortisol levels and depression since Board et al. reported elevated cortisol levels in a group of depressed patients. However,

comparable elevations in plasma cortisol were subsequently also found in other groups, including schizophrenics, patients with various anxiety states, women awaiting reports of breast biopsies, and parents of terminally ill leukemic children. Thus, it was not possible to interpret the findings in the depressed patient group as reflecting a physiological variation that was specific for depression. In fact, it seemed that the finding of elevated cortisol levels was most closely associated with generalized anxiety, regardless of other characteristics of the subject groups. This is not to say that the hypothalamic-pituitary-adrenal cortex (HPA) axis does not have an important role in depression. In fact, recent studies employing more sophisticated techniques, such as measurement of 24-hour patterns of cortisol secretion and suppression of the HPA axis by the synthetic glucocorticoid, dexamethasone (Chapter 14), have provided data suggestive of significant abnormalities in depressed patients. The point to be emphasized here is that the straightforward technique of measuring serum levels at a single time point has not, on its own, been successful in teasing out specific correlations. Thus, investigators have had to turn to more sophisticated approaches in order to probe the relationships between endocrine systems and psychiatric disorders.

In this chapter, we shall review the current concepts of neuroendocrine regulatory systems, and then discuss the potential applicability of neuroendocrine techniques to the investigation of psychiatric disorders. Interest has focused on the central nervous system regulation of endocrine function because of the growing awareness of the role of the hypothalamus in regulating the endocrine system, as well as the development of new techniques, such as radioimmunoassay, to measure directly the activity of substances involved in neuroendocrine processes. Because of the importance of radioimmunoassay and other competitive

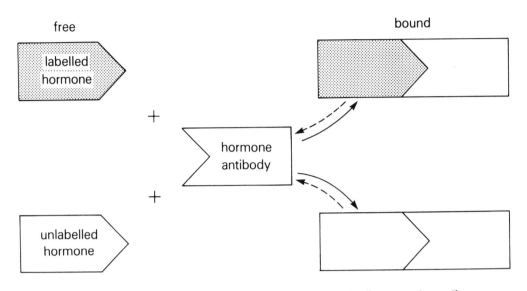

Fig. 1. This figure portrays the competitive nature of the radioimmunoassay technique. Labelled and unlabelled hormones compete to bind with the same antibody. Antigen-antibody complexes can be precipitated and the quantity of labelled complexes can be determined. With more unlabelled hormone in the assay system, the number of labelled hormone-antibody complexes decreases. From Vance (1971).

radioassay techniques to developments in endocrine research, these techniques will be discussed briefly.

The radioimmunoassay procedure, developed by Berson and Yalow, makes possible the detection and measurement of a large number of hormones and other compounds that are frequently present in very small quantities in biological fluids. The technique of radioimmunoassay is based upon two factors: (1) The ability of antibodies* to react with great sensitivity and specificity to hormones and

---

*Antibodies are produced as a result of stimulation of the body's immunological mechanisms in response to the injection of foreign substances, which may include hormones or hormones conjugated to larger, more antigenic molecules. After a period of several months, the serum of the injected animals (generally rabbits or guinea pigs) will contain antibodies to the injected substances. The antibodies can then be obtained by "bleeding" the animal.

other compounds, and (2) competition between radioactive and nonradioactive antigen for binding sites on the antibody (Fig. 1). Carrying out an assay involves incubating antibody, labelled hormone and non-labelled hormone (e.g., the sample containing the hormone to be measured). Hormone-antibody complexes are formed with both labelled and unlabelled hormone. With more unlabelled hormone in the sample, there is greater competition with labelled hormone for binding with the available antibody binding sites. Thus, as the amount of unlabelled hormone in the sample increases, the amount of labelled hormone-antibody complexes decreases. The hormone sample can be quantified by comparing the amount of binding in the sample assay to the binding obtained in a standard curve for known amounts of labelled hormone-antibody complexes.

Another variation of this technique, competitive radioassay, makes use of the selective binding of hormones to particular cellular constituents, their natural tissue reactors. As in the case of radioimmunoassay techniques, the quantity of labelled hormone-reactor complexes depends upon the amount of unlabelled hormones in the test sample. A number of hormones, such as thyroxine, cortisol and progesterone, are routinely measured by this technique. The contributions of the radioimmunoassay and other radioassay techniques both to research and clinical practice in endocrinology have been enormous. Moreover, they represent the kind of technological development that makes possible great advances in knowledge.

Until recently, the regulatory organization of several endocrine systems was thought of in terms of a direct relationship between the pituitary gland and the target organ. The pituitary gland is located just below the hypothalamus at the base of the brain. A number of hormones are stored in and secreted from the pituitary gland. Two of these, antidiuretic hormone and oxytocin, which are stored in the posterior pituitary, will not be discussed in this chapter. The anterior pituitary contains seven different hormones which will be considered later.

Structurally, the anterior pituitary hormones are characterized as being either polypeptides (long chains of amino acids) or glycoproteins (peptides linked to glycogen moieties). These hormones exert a regulatory influence upon many aspects of the metabolic processes of the body, either by acting on specific target organs, or by producing more generalized systemic effects (Fig. 2). There are considerable data suggesting that several of these anterior pituitary hormones exert their actions by affecting adenylate cyclase and, thus, activating the "second messenger" cyclic AMP system.

The adrenal cortex is acted upon by adrenocortical-stimulating hormone (ACTH) to induce secretion of glucocorticoids (cortisone-like hormones) and aldosterone (a hormone involved in the regulation of ion and fluid balance). Thyroid-stimulating hormone (TSH) causes release of thyroid hormone from the thyroid gland. Follicle-stimulating hormone (FSH) enhances ovarian follicle growth in females, and is, by this means, involved in the production of estrogens. In males, FSH stimulates the seminiferous tubules of the testicles. Luteinizing hormone (LH) has a number of complex functions in the female, but is generally involved with the process of ovulation. In the male, LH acts upon the interstitial cells of the testicles to stimulate production and secretion of testosterone. Prolactin acts upon the mammary glands in females to stimulate and sustain milk production. These effects of prolactin occur only in the presence of estrogen and progesterone.

The five anterior pituitary hormones just described all have specific target organs upon which their actions are exerted. In the case of the other two hormones of the anterior pituitary gland, growth hormone (GH) and melanocyte-stimulating hormone (MSH), their effects are exerted widely throughout the body. As its name implies, growth hormone is involved with general body growth, including both skeletal structures and internal organs. GH is also involved in a wide variety of physiological processes, including control of protein, carbohydrate and fat metabolism. The functions of MSH in humans are not well understood. One action of the hormone appears to be stimulation of melanin production from certain cells of the skin.

Regulation of secretion of the anterior pituitary hormones is thought to occur largely by means of *feedback inhibition* control mechanisms. This concept implies that a hormone secreted from a target organ, as a result of stimulation by a pituitary hormone, can decrease the synthesis and/or secretion of the latter. The exact site where this feedback inhibition effect occurs is not known

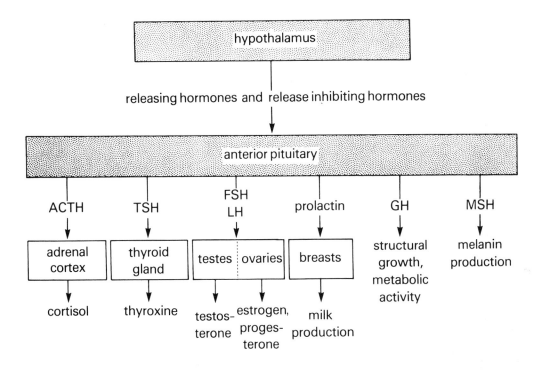

Fig. 2. A representation of the hypothalamic-pituitary-target organ endocrine systems.

for most of the hormone systems (see below). For example, in the case of the hypothalamic-pituitary-adrenal axis, data has been obtained indicating that feedback inhibition may come about as a result of effects of glucocorticoids at the pituitary, the hypothalamus or at other sites in the central nervous system (Fig. 3). The situation described in this example is often referred to as *long loop* feedback inhibition, indicating that a hormone secreted by a peripheral target organ is able to exert a regulatory influence upon the synthesis or secretion of the hypothalamic and/or pituitary hormones involved in the regulation of the target organ hormone. Later in this chapter, an example of *short loop* inhibition will be described, in which a pituitary hormone, itself, appears to regulate the release of its companion hypothalamic-releasing hormone.

In the 1920's and 1940's, Wislocki and King, Harris and a number of other investigators demonstrated an anatomical connection between the hypothalamus and the pituitary gland that led to an understanding of the physiological interactions between these two organs. While neural connections were not present, the hypothalamus was shown to be in contact with the anterior pituitary by means of an unusual form of circulation, a portal circulatory system (Fig. 4). A portal circulation exists when the venous outflow from one organ directly perfuses another.

In this case, the circulatory outflow from the hypothalamus was shown to perfuse the anterior pituitary. Chemicals secreted from the hypothalamus (especially from the median eminence region) into the portal vein would reach the pituitary gland, only a few millimeters away, in relatively high concentrations. Thus, the hypothalamus was situated anatomically in a position to exert a high degree of control over the pituitary gland, and the identification of this portal system provided a pathway by which such control could be humorally (i.e., chemically) mediated.

During the next few years, a variety of experiments demonstrated that the hypothalamus did, in fact, significantly modulate the secretory activity of the pituitary. With electrical stimulation of a number of areas within the hypothalamus, secretion of several of the anterior pituitary tropic hormones could be demonstrated. The hypothalamic control of pituitary hormone secretion was shown to occur through chemical rather than electrical stimulation. For example, a pituitary gland could be excised from a rat and transplanted into the hypothalamus or into the anterior chamber of the eye of a second rat. In each case, the secretory activity of the pituitary was maintained, indicating that chemical rather than neuronal influences of hypothalamic origin regulated the secretory activities of the pituitary. In summary, the presence of chemicals in the hypothalamus which control the secretion of pituitary tropic hormones was postulated on the basis of data obtained from a variety of experimental techniques.

In the past few years, a flurry of research activity has led to the demonstration of short-chain peptide substances that act as *hypothalamic hormones*. These neurohormones appear to be synthesized in the cell bodies of typical CNS neurons and are then transported down the axons of these neurons to be stored in vesicles within the nerve terminals which are located in the median eminence region of the hypothalamus. The neurons containing the hypothalamic-releasing hormones have the same neurophysiological characteristics as any other CNS neuron and are subject to the same multitude of influences as described in Chapters 1 and 2. Thus, the likelihood

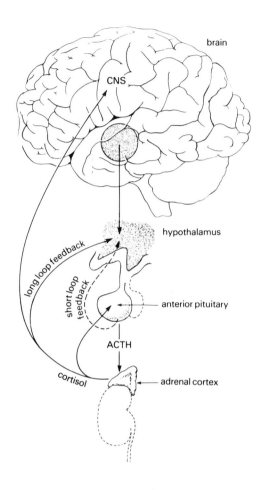

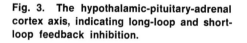

Fig. 3. The hypothalamic-pituitary-adrenal cortex axis, indicating long-loop and short-loop feedback inhibition.

that an action potential will be fired off, resulting in secretion of the neurohormone, is determined by the sum of the multiple neuronal inputs impinging upon the hypothalamic neuron at a given instant. When an action potential is fired off in these neurons, the excitation-secretion process results in the release of the neurohormones into the portal circulation (rather than into a synaptic space), from which point they pass directly to the pituitary gland where they activate appropriate target cells. Originally, it was believed that a very simple and specific relationship existed between the hypothalamic-releasing hormones and the anterior pituitary hormones. According to such concepts, a single hypothalamic-releasing hormone would stimulate secretion of a specific anterior pituitary hormone. However, subsequent investigation has proven that the situation is far more complex. Thus, some of the hypothalamic-releasing hormones stimulate secretion of more than one of the pituitary tropic hormones, while others inhibit release of the pituitary hormone. For example, thyrotropin-releasing hormone (TRH) has been demonstrated to stimulate secretion of TSH, prolactin and (in certain cases) growth hormone. Moreover, a single neurohormone, gonadotropin-releasing hormone (GNRH), appears to stimulate the secretion of both FSH and LH. Thus, there is not a direct one-to-one relationship between hypothalamic and pituitary tropic hormone secretion.

Three hypothalamic-releasing hormones have been identified which inhibit the secretion of their respective pituitary tropic hormones. These are prolactin, growth hormone and melanocyte-stimulating hormone release-inhibiting hormone. It may be that one or several of the pituitary hormones are under a dual control system, regulated by both a release-stimulating and release-inhibiting hormone.

Four of the hypothalamic releasing hormones, TRH, GNRH, MSH inhibiting hormone (MIH) and somatostatin (growth hormone release inhibiting hormone) (GHIH) have been identified, characterized as being short-chain substances, and synthesized in biologically active form. In addition, highly sensitive and specific radioimmunoassay techniques are now available for the measurement of TRH, GNRH and somatostatin. The availability of these neurohormones and of convenient assay techniques has made possible investigations into the distribution and function of these peptides in brain. TRH, somato-

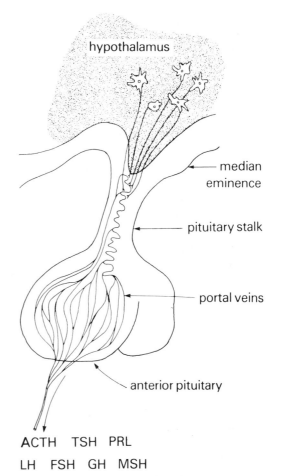

hypothalamus

median eminence

pituitary stalk

portal veins

anterior pituitary

ACTH   TSH   PRL
LH   FSH   GH   MSH

Fig. 4.   The portal circulation linking the median eminence region of the hypothalamus with the anterior pituitary gland. Hypothalamic releasing hormones are secreted from the median eminence region into the portal vessel where they are carried directly to the anterior pituitary. At this location they produce release (or inhibition of release in some cases) of pituitary hormones.

statin and perhaps prolactin-inhibiting hormone (PIH) have been shown to be widely distributed throughout the brain, although they are most highly concentrated in the hypothalamus. Further, TRH, GNRH and somatostatin have all been found to exert behavioral effects in animals, that appear to be unrelated to their actions on pituitary tropic hormone secretion.

In addition to acting as regulators of pituitary tropic hormone secretion, some of the hypothalamic hormones may also serve other functions in the central nervous system, for example, acting as CNS neurotransmitter agents. Thus, TRH is highly concentrated in the synaptic region, and appears to be stored in synaptic vesicles. When administered iontophoretically to hypothalamic neurons, TRH can alter neuronal firing rates. These observations, together with the reports of its behavioral effects, support the idea that TRH may function as a neurotransmitter. In addition, TRH has been found to be present in high concentration in the brain of the *Axolotl* (a Mexican salamander), a species in which it does not produce release of TSH. Thus, it is possible that TRH has long had a role as a CNS neurotransmitter, while its function as a regulator of pituitary hormone secretion may have evolved relatively recently. While considerable additional data is needed to support this hypothesis, the development of such powerful research techniques as the radioimmunoassay has provided vast new opportunities to undertake the necessary studies. Investigation into the possible roles of peptide hormones as neurotransmitter agents is an exciting and promising area for future research.

With the demonstration that hypothalamic hormones, which act as regulators of various endocrine systems, may also be directly involved in central neural activity, it is apparent that the degree of overlap between endocrine and neural systems is even greater than previously believed. This degree of integration be-

comes heightened with the recognition that the activity of neurons containing the neurohormones are modulated by the major CNS neurotransmitter agents, acetylcholine, dopamine, norepinephrine and serotonin. There has been a great deal of research in the past few years, directed toward establishing the neurotransmitter controls over secretion of the hypothalamic-releasing hormones. While this is an issue of great interest, it has also proven to be a difficult one to sort out. In the case of thyrotropin-releasing hormone, for example, little is known about the neurochemical control mechanisms. On the other hand, acetylcholine, serotonin and norepinephrine have all been implicated as having a potential role in the regulation of corticotropin-releasing hormone.

Several different strategies have been employed to explore the manner in which the CNS neurotransmitters may regulate the secretion of the hypothalamic-releasing hormones. One such strategy involves the administration of a number of drugs that effect CNS neurotransmitter activity. After the administration of these drugs to humans, the effects on hypothalamic-pituitary responsiveness can be studied. Results of such studies indicate that alteration in hypothalamic-pituitary function can be produced by these drugs. Numerous instances have been observed in which hypothalamic-pituitary function was significantly altered by the administration of drugs that effect neurotransmitter activity. A specific example of this involves the effects of various drugs on the release of prolactin. The release of prolactin from the pituitary appears to be regulated primarily by a hypothalamic-inhibitory neurohormone known as prolactin-inhibiting hormone (PIH). Evidence indicates that PIH secretion is controlled by catecholamine activity, especially by dopamine. Thus administration of L-DOPA, the precursor of dopamine and norepinephrine, results in reduced secretion of prolactin, presumably due to increased

Table 1. Drugs that alter prolactin secretion

Drugs Increasing Prolactin Secretion	Drugs Decreasing Prolactin Secretion
Alpha-methylDOPA (inhibits synthesis of DA and NE)	L-DOPA (increases DA and NE synthesis)
Reserpine (depletes nerve terminals of DA and NE)	Apomorphine (direct DA receptor agonist)
Chlorpramazine (DA receptor blocker)	

PIH secretion (Table I). In this system, activation of a dopamine neuron leads to release of dopamine, which stimulates the PIH-containing neuron. PIH would then be released from the nerve terminal of the hypothalamic hormone neuron, be secreted into the portal circulation, and pass directly to the anterior pituitary, where it would produce its effects of inhibiting release of prolactin.

The direct dopamine receptor agonist (stimulant) apomorphine causes release of PIH from the hypothalamic neuron, which results in decreased prolactin secretion. In contrast, drugs that interfere with catecholamine activity, such as alpha-methyl-DOPA or reserpine (Chapter 3) cause an increase in prolactin secretion, presumably by inhibiting release of PIH from the hypothalamus. Chlorpromazine, which has significant dopamine receptor blocking activity, also produces a marked increase in prolactin activity.

In summary, drugs that enhance dopamine activity produce a decrease in prolactin secretion, while drugs that diminish dopamine activity increase prolactin secretion (Table I). Studies employing similar strategies have been conducted to investigate the neurotransmitter control of other hypothalamic hormones. Much additional work is needed to clarify the influences of neurotransmitters on the secretion of these neurohormones. Nevertheless, it appears that the functional activity of the various hypothalamic-pituitary-target organ axes may be modified by the actions of the CNS neurotransmitters.

Information obtained from this type of neuroendocrine research has numerous clinical implications. For example, knowledge about the neurotransmitter regulation of prolactin secretion has led to new treatments for galactorrhea, a condition characterized by inappropriate lactation caused by hypersecretion of prolactin. Treatment with L-DOPA has been found to be effective in restoring prolactin levels to normal in these patients, resulting in improvement of the galactorrhea. Advances in research technology and information obtained from neuroendocrine studies are expected to contribute in a significant manner to the diagnosis and treatment of a number of endocrine, neurological, psychiatric and other medical disorders.

Another facet of endocrine-CNS interactions involves the effects of peripheral hormones on central nervous system activity. It has become increasingly well demonstrated that neural activity and the secretion of the hypothalamic hormones can be influenced by feedback effects of the peripheral hormones. For example, ACTH appears capable of inhibiting the secretion of its hypothalamic hormone (CRH) through a direct, short-loop feedback effect on the hypothalamus (Fig. 3). Additionally, after administration of radioactively-labelled estradiol peripherally, much of the labelled estrogen is found concentrated in the anterior portion of the hypothalamus, suggesting that this may be the site of feedback inhibition for this system. It is also of interest that peripherally-administered glucocorticoids have been found to be concentrated to a large extent in other limbic structures, such as the hippocampus and amygdala. Thus, the effects of peripheral hormones on brain function need not be limited to the hypothalamus.

The effects of hormones on central nervous system activity may be expressed in a number of ways. For example, glucocorticoids may alter neuronal activity through a variety of mechanisms: alteration of ion distribution across the neuronal membrane, effects on enzymes (such as tyrosine hydroxylase) which are involved in neurotransmitter synthesis, or alteration in catecholamine uptake. Thyroid hormone has been postulated to produce a sensitizing effect on postsynaptic adrenergic receptors, both in the periphery and in brain tissue. However, the data on this point is controversial. Both glucocorticoids and estrogens have been shown to enter target cells in the hypothalamus and bind to specific cytoplasmic receptors. In some cases, the receptor-bound hormone is then transported into the nuclei of these cells, where the hormones appear to affect important metabolic functions of the cell, such as protein synthesis.

With the advances in understanding of neuroendocrine mechanisms, the development of radioimmunoassay techniques to measure pituitary tropic hormones in humans, and the availability of synthetic hypothalamic-releasing hormones for administration to subjects, it has been possible to undertake a series of investigations into the hypothalamic-pituitary responsiveness in patients with various psychiatric disorders. Most of the studies conducted to date have been carried out in depressed patients (Chapter 14). In fact, many of the physiological symptoms of depression (sleep disturbance, decreased appetite, decreased libido, anxiety and disturbed diurnal rhythms) could be explained on the basis of hypothalamic dysfunction. The functional state of the hypothalamic-pituitary axis in depressed patients can be evaluated by giving a number of drugs that are known to alter the activity of this axis. From such data, it may be possible to make inferences about the activity of various neurotransmitter agents in the hypothalamus. Such information is especially relevant in light of the interest in neurotransmitter activity in depression. A research strategy that is frequently employed involves the administration of drugs peripherally that are believed to alter the hypothalamic-pituitary axis through central actions, usually exerted on neurotransmitters. The effects of these drugs are monitored through the response of the pituitary hormone. Sachar has described this strategy as using the hypothalamus as a "window into the brain." An example of this approach is the use of drugs to study alterations in prolactin secretion.

To date, several instances of hypothalamic-pituitary dysfunction in depressed patients have been reported. For example, the rise in growth hormone levels normally seen after insulin-induced hypoglycemia (lowered blood glucose levels) has been reported to be blunted in some depressed patients. Dexamethasone, a synthetic glucocorticoid, normally produces a suppression of glucocorticoid secretion. However, in some depressed patients, this dexamethasone-suppression effect is lost. Additionally, the TSH response to the administration of TRH has been noted to be diminished in some depressed patients. At this point, it is not clear whether these types of observations in depressed patients represent epiphenomena, or whether they may provide important clues to the physiological states associated with depression. As more information is obtained about the neurotransmitter regulation of all of the hypothalamic hormones, it may be possible to interpret such studies in a much more meaningful way in terms of the state of neuro-transmitter activity. It may be that conducting a battery of tests on the various hypothalamic-pituitary systems would provide the most informative picture of the status of central nervous system neurotransmitter activity in depressed patients.

While much of the interest in neuro-endocrine approaches to psychiatric disorders has been focused on depression, relevant studies have been conducted on such disorders such as *anorexia nervosa*. Anorexia nervosa is generally seen in females in late adolescence. It is characterized by excessive concern about weight, weight loss of at least 25 percent of the ideal body weight, and loss of menstrual periods (amenorrhea). The weight loss is often so severe as to become life-threatening. There has been and continues to be considerable interest in the psychological and family dynamic aspects of anorexia nervosa. However, several investigators have speculated that this disease may reflect some aspects of hypothalamic dysfunction. Thus, the cardinal symptoms of the disease, eating problems and disorders of reproductive cycles, could both be explained on this basis. Moreover, in a small pilot study, patients with anorexia nervosa were reported to manifest problems with temperature regulation, again a possible reflection of some hypothalamic dysfunction.

The status of various endocrine systems in patients with anorexia nervosa has been evaluated in several studies. Some of the abnormalities that have been observed appear to be due to the effects of starvation and malnutrition. For example, growth hormone has been reported to be markedly low in anorexia nervosa patients who were malnourished, but normal in well-nourished anorectic patients. Moreover, when the malnourished patients were treated and normal body weight was restored, growth hormone levels returned to a normal range. On the other hand, serum LH and FSH

levels have been reported to be low in patients with this disease, independent of the nutritional state. Administration of GNRH to such patients produced normal elevations of both gonadotropic hormones (LH and FSH). The observation that the pituitary response to GNRH administration was normal suggests that the low serum levels of LH and FSH in these patients reflect a hypothalamic deficit. Additionally, Halmi examined, at autopsy, the pituitary glands of patients with anorexia nervosa. No abnormalities were seen in the secretory cells for TSH, GH, ACTH or prolactin. However, gonadotrophin secretory cells stained more faintly than normal, a finding that was consistent with the reduced levels of gonadotrophin hormones that have been observed in other studies.

Another strategy of neuroendocrine research has been applied to investigations of anorexia nervosa, in this case, measurement of 24-hour patterns of hormone secretion. Sachar and Weissman have shown that many hormones are secreted in episodic bursts throughout the day (Chapter 14). Katz and co-workers have studied the 24-hour pattern of secretion of luteinizing hormone in patients with *anorexia nervosa*. LH secretion patterns in these patients most closely resembled that of a pre-adolescent girl. This pattern may not reflect simply a starvation effect since a small number of female subjects with marked weight loss from other causes did not show a comparable change in LH secretion patterns. The data obtained from patients with anorexia nervosa is suggestive of a hypothalamic basis for the alteration in pattern of LH secretion. However, further studies are necessary to substantiate this hypothesis.

Some work has been conducted on the endocrine aspects of alcohol and drug abuse; however, the application of neuroendocrine techniques of investigation to these conditions has begun only recently. A feature common to both alcohol and drug abuse is a decreased interest in sex and an impaired ability to perform sexually. While these symptoms may be related to a number of nonspecific psychological and physiological factors, the possibility that they may reflect a specific endocrine response to chronic drug or alcohol use has attracted some interest.

An example of work in this area involves studies of the effects of narcotic agents on the physiology of sexual behavior. Chronic morphine administration has been reported to disrupt estrus in rabbits and to interfere with the menstrual cycle in humans; while acute morphine treatment blocks ovulation in the rat and the rabbit. Cicero has demonstrated that morphine implants produce atrophy of the secondary sexual organs including the prostate and seminal vesicles, and also causes a decrease of serum testosterone levels as a result of inhibitory effects on the hypothalamic-pituitary axis, causing a reduction in secretion.

Cicero and coworkers have also conducted clinical studies on the effects of chronic morphine and methadone usage on sexual activity. Addicts were found to have frequent problems, including impotence, loss of libido, and delayed ejaculation. Significant decreases in serum testosterone levels were found in chronic methadone users but not in heroin addicts. Considerably more work is needed to clarify the mechanisms underlying these observations. Nevertheless, the application of neuroendocrine techniques to the study of this issue and to other aspects of drug abuse may provide considerable information about the interaction of physiological and behavioral factors in these conditions.

Recently an interesting application of neuroendocrine techniques to schizophrenia has been described. There has been considerable interest in the idea that schizophrenia is related to hyperactivity of certain dopamine systems in the brain, and that the therapeutic effects of antipsychotic agents may be related to their dopamine-receptor block-

ing actions (Chapters 10 and 12). Earlier in this chapter, it was pointed out that dopamine has been noted to stimulate PIH secretion, resulting in an inhibition of prolactin release. Sachar and Meltzer studied the levels of prolactin in schizophrenic patients and found no differences from control groups. After the administration of antipsychotic agents, a profound increase in prolactin levels was observed. They found that this rise in prolactin occurred after the administration of a variety of antipsychotic agents with widely differing chemical structures. Structurally related drugs that were not efficacious in the treatment of psychosis did not produce a rise in prolactin levels. These results suggest that effective antipsychotic agents all have dopamine-receptor blocking properties, as revealed by the increase in prolactin after administration of these agents. A number of investigators are currently exploring the possibility of using prolactin levels as an indication of the effectiveness of antipsychotic drug therapy. They suggest that it may be possible to utilize the rise in prolactin levels as an indication of appropriate response to antipsychotic treatment.

In summary, the multiple points of integration between endocrine and neural systems have been discussed. In recent years, the involvement of the hypothalamus and other central nervous system structures in the control of endocrine function has been elucidated. The demonstration, characterization and isolation of hypothalamic hormones has represented a significant advance in understanding neuroendocrine physiology. It is now necessary to consider both the effects of CNS neurotransmitters in regulating hormone systems through effects on hypothalamic hormones, and the effects of peripheral hormones on central neural activity. The advances in understanding of neuroendocrine physiology, the development of new techniques, such as radioimmunoassay procedures for pituitary and hypothalamic hormones, and the availability of synthetic hypothalamic hormones have made possible new approaches and strategies for conducting clinical neuroendocrinological investigations. The utilization of techniques of modern neuroendocrinology may have particular relevance to the investigation of biological mechanisms associated with various psychiatric disorders.

Selected References

Brown, G.M.: Psychiatric and neurologic aspects of endocrine disease. *Hosp. Pract.* 10(8): 71-79, 1975.

Frohman, L.A.: Clinical neuropharmacology of hypothalamic releasing factors. *New Eng. J. Med.* 286:1391-1397, 1972.

Guillemin, R., and Burgus, R.: The hormones of the hypothalamus. *Scient. Amer.* 227:24-33, 1972.

Mason, J.W.: A review of psychoendocrine research on the sympathetic adrenal medullary system. *Psychosom. Med.* 30:631-653, 1968.

Mason, J.W.: A review of psychoendocrine research on the pituitary-adrenal cortical system. *Psychosom. Med.* 30:576-607, 1968.

McEwen, B.S.: The brain as a target organ of endocrine hormones. *Hosp. Pract.* 10(5): 95-104, 1975.

Prange, A.J., Jr. (Ed.): *The Thyroid Axis, Drugs and Behavior.* Raven Press, New York, 1974.

Sachar, E.J.: Endocrine Factors in Psychopathological States. In *Biological Psychiatry,* J. Mendels, ed., John Wiley and Sons, New York, 1973.

Sachar, E.J.: Hormonal changes in stress and mental illness. *Hosp. Pract.* 10(7):49-55, 1975a.

Sachar, E.J. (Ed.): *Topics in Psychoendocrinology.* Grune and Stratton, New York, 1975b.

Vance, J.E.: Principles of radioimmunoassay of hormones. In *Laboratory Diagnosis of Endocrine Disorders.* F.W. Sunderman and F. Sunderman, eds. Warren H. Green, Inc., St. Louis, 1971, pp. 123-129.

Chapter 5

Applications of Genetic Techniques to Psychiatric Research

J. Mendlewicz

Interest in the question of whether genes play a role in the development of psychiatric disorders has existed since the time that investigators began systematically to categorize the latter. The demonstration that drugs were effective in the treatment of major psychiatric disturbances such as schizophrenias and the affective disorders, stimulated interest in the biological aspects of these illnesses, and, as a consequence, in more extensive genetic studies. Data obtained from these investigations have provided important support for the existence of a biological component in the major psychiatric disorders. Currently, the interplay between biological and environmental factors represents a major area of research in this field.

Basic Genetic Principles

Prior to discussing particular aspects of genetic research in psychiatry, *a brief review of basic genetic principles* might be useful. A gene is made up of a series of molecules of deoxyribonucleic acid (DNA) in a sequence that designates the synthesis of a specific polypeptide (i.e., a string of amino acids). Genes, therefore, control the synthesis of proteins (including enzymes, protein hormones and structural proteins for cell membranes) which are involved in a wide range of physiological activities. Some genes may determine the structure of proteins, while others control the rate of protein production. In view of the fact that genetic influences are expressed in terms of physiological processes, the demonstration of a genetic component in a psychiatric disorder is of considerable importance in establishing a physiological contribution to that disorder.

Genetic influences are transmitted to the child by elements in the parents' germ cells. A male and a female germ cell (gamete) from each parent must fuse to produce the single cell (zygote) from which the new individual develops. The basic elements of hereditary transmission are the chromosomes, which are linear structures in the cell tissues. In humans, each cell in the body contains 46 chromosomes which are present in pairs. There are 22 pairs of non-sex chromosomes (autosomes) and one pair of sex chromosomes. In the male, the sex chromosomes pair is an X chromosome and a smaller Y chromosome. Females have one pair of X chromosomes.

The process of cell division ending in egg or sperm formation is termed *meiosis*. Several pertinent processes occur during meiosis: (1) each chromosome duplicates itself by longitudinal division into daughter chromatids, thus doubling the total number; (2) exchanges of genetic material may take place when the chromosomes split into chromatids. This process is termed *crossing over* and *recombination*. As a consequence of "crossing over," the chromosomes resulting from this first division are not exact replicas of parent chromosomes. Crossing over involves only a few exchanges of relatively large, unpredictable chromosome segments. Crossing over and recombination are important mechanisms for producing hereditary variation. Fur-

thermore, this process contributes to the pairing of certain genetically-determined characteristics within members of a family. Use has been made of the pairing of genetically-determined traits in what are termed *linkage* studies. Linkage studies have been used by geneticists investigating psychiatric illnesses and examples will be described later; (3) finally, the cell divides and each of the two new cells also divide, forming four gametes (egg or sperm), each with 23 unpaired chromosomes. With fertilization, a zygote with a full complement of 46 chromosomes is formed.

In classical genetics, single genetic factors are determined by genes and the genetic constitution of an individual is called genotype, while its appearance is the phenotype. Single-gene inheritance may be of *dominant or recessive* type, when the gene is carried in a non-sex chromosome. Dominant conditions are manifested in the presence of one specific gene, the other gene of the pair being normal. Simple dominant traits are usually incompletely expressed and should be present theoretically in about 50% of the offspring of one affected parent. The transmission of dominant genes can be traced in families without "skipping" a generation. In contrast, the appearance of recessive conditions depends on the presence of two matching genes, one coming from each parent. Individuals who possess these genes in a double dose are called *homozygotes,* whereas individuals having only one of the genes in question are termed *heterozygotes*. In simple recessive traits, then, transmission from both parents is necessary since the latter are usually heterozygotes and unaffected. Roughly 25% of sibs of patients with recessive forms of genetic defects may be expected to be affected. Furthermore, half of the sibs in a sibship containing an individual with a recessive defect will be apparently symptomless carriers. With recessive transmission, marriage between blood relatives increases the risk of mating between carriers of the recessive gene, as such individuals may have a number of genes in common. The likelihood of offspring having the recessive condition is, therefore, increased by consanguinity.

In addition to single-factor inheritance, some traits are determined by the complex interaction of several genes, a type of inheritance called *polygenic*. This is the case when we are dealing with characteristics in which there is quantitative variation, like weight, intelligence, and longevity.

The above discussion of inheritance was concerned with transmission by non-sex linked or autosomal genes. Transmission of inherited disorders by the sex chromosomes also occurs, and is referred to as *sex-linkage*. For example, the aberrant gene can be carried by one of the X chromosomes. Most genes of this type are recessive and have, consequently, little or no effect in the heterozygous female, but demonstrate their full effect in the male. A family afflicted by a sex-linked disorder, such as hemophilia A, will show a characteristic pedigree, with the disease appearing in alternate generation males. Thus, an affected male passes the gene to all of his daughters, who are carriers but are not affected by the illness. However, the disorder will appear in half of the daughters' sons.

There are several methods available to study genetic phenomenon. The *pedigree method* provides data on the familial distribution of pathological traits in successive generations, but these data are usually limited and difficult to interpret. Family studies are more useful, if performed on a large scale and if one selects a sample of families in a non-biased manner. The aim of the method is to compare *morbidity risks* (i.e., lifetime risks) for a given condition among relatives of affected patients with the risks in the general population, or in relatives of controls. The *twin method* was initiated by Galton, and is based on a comparison between concordance rates for a certain condition in monozygotic (identical) versus dizygotic (fraternal) twins. Concordance occurs when both members of a pair show the same trait. This method provides a unique opportunity to investigate intra-family variations and to reduce uncontrolled variables. Since both types of twins share the same environment, but only the monozygotic twins have essentially the same genetic material, data showing that the concordance rate for a disease is significantly higher in monozygotic as compared to dizygotic twins can be taken as evidence for a genetic factor. This postulate, however, does not give full consideration to the facts that, on the one hand, identical twins may share a more similar postnatal environment than non-identical twins and, on the other hand, that prenatal conditions (twin position, circulatory, and others) are often more disparate in monozygotic than in dizygotic twins. It is also conceivable that being an identical twin may increase the liability to some conditions, so one has to ascertain that the condition being studied is no more frequent in twins than in the general population. Nevertheless, the twin method is of great value for estimating the heritability of a phenomenon.

Genetic Studies of Psychiatric Disorders

One of the problems inherent in the above genetic methods is the difficulty to separate environmental from hereditary influences. Two other methods are able to separate biological from rearing influences. The *adoption study* method is based on investigating children raised since early childhood by non-biologically related parents. This technique has been used to discriminate between genetic

**Table 1. Concordance rates for
manic-depressive illness in twins**

Author	MZ Concordance rate	DZ Concordance rate
Rosanoff et al.	59.6%	16.4%
Kallmann	92.6%	23.6%
Da Fonseca	71.4%	38.5%
Harvold and Hauge	50.0%	2.6%
Kringlen	33.3%	0.0%

and environmental factors. The *linkage method* analyzes individual families to determine whether the conditions studied tend to assort in a dependent fashion with a known genetic marker. Some of these methods have been applied to genetic research in the major psychoses. Table 1 provides concordance rates for *affective disorders* in monozygotic (MZ) and dizygotic (DZ) twins according to some recent studies. The concordance rates in MZ twins vary between 33% and 92.6%, as compared to 0–38.5% in DZ twins. These results indicate that genetic factors play a role in the etiology of manic-depressive illness. There are also a few pairs of identical twins who had been reared apart since early childhood and of whom at least one twin had been diagnosed as suffering from an affective disorder. Among twelve such pairs, eight were concordant for the disease, an observation suggesting that the early environment may not be that important in the clinical expression of the disturbance.

A re-analysis of twin data, based on the bipolar-unipolar classification (see chapter 13 for discussion of this classification), made it possible to ascertain 50 MZ pairs concordant for one type of affective illness. Among all pairs, 43 were concordant for one of the other forms of the illness (i.e., bipolar or unipolar) and 7 (14%) were discordant for

the type of disorder. This observation would indicate that separate genetic influences might contribute to the unipolar and bipolar forms of the illness but that there is some genetic overlap between these two conditions. The twin data, then, are indicative of a genetic etiology in affective disorders, but they do not allow any further interpretation.

Family studies of affective disorders are also contributing to the genetic hypothesis. The morbidity risk for a disease is the probability to have this disease during a life-time, i.e., if one lives long enough to survive the risk period for this disease. Most of the family studies on manic-depressive illness have shown that this disorder tends to run in families, and that the risk in relatives is significantly higher than in the general population. The risks published by Kallmann (1953) for parents of manic-depressive patients is 23.4% and for sibs 22.7%. For the general population, the morbidity risk for manic-depressive illness is much lower, with values ranging from 0.6 to 2.7%. Two recent independent studies have investigated separately morbidity risks among bipolar and unipolar patients. Both studies found that the morbidity risks for affective disorders were significantly larger in the relatives of bipolar as compared to unipolar patients. Bipolar and unipolar illness was present in the relatives of bipolar patients while only unipolar illness was found in the relatives of unipolar patients. These results have now been confirmed by other investigators, including ourselves. In studying the *first degree* relatives of 134 bipolar manic-depressive patients, we have found that the relatives of bipolar patients manifest both the unipolar and bipolar forms of the illness (Table 2). The risks of unipolar illness are indeed quite significant in these relatives. The overall rates for affective illness are similar in sibs and parents; however, sibs are more likely to manifest bipolar illness than parents. It can also be seen from Table 2 that

Table 2. Morbidity risks for affective illness in relatives of bipolar manic-depressive patients (N = 134)

	All Affective	Bipolar	Unipolar
Parents	33.7 ± 2.9%	12.1 ± 2.0%	22.0 ± 2.6%
Sibs	39.2 ± 3.0%	21.2 ± 2.5%	18.6 ± 2.5%
Children	59.9 ± 6.0%	24.6 ± 5.0%	41.3 ± 6.7%

children of bipolar probands constitute a high-risk group. After reviewing family studies, one can estimate the risk for *bipolar illness* in the various types of first-degree relatives of affected patients to be between 15 and 35%. This observation is consistent with a single dominant mode of transmission, although the penetrance is obviously less than 100%.

It seems, then, that genetic factors are involved in the etiology of the affective disorders. Different models have been proposed to explain the precise mode of inheritance. Although there is no final consensus on the exact type of inheritance operating in affective illness, there are, however, certain genetic models which can be ruled out from the data available today. Autosomal recessive inheritance is very unlikely in manic-depressive illness since it can not account for the appreciable number of families showing the presence of the illness in *successive* generations. Furthermore, there have been no reports of an increased risk in the sibs of affected patients nor in the children of consanguineous marriages of affected patients, which would be expected under such a type of heredity. Sex-linked recessive inheritance is also very unlikely because no studies have reported an excess of affective males over females. In fact, the opposite has generally been observed.

In favor of a single dominant type of inheritance are the following arguments: (1) the presence of the illness in successive generations, and (2) comparable morbidity risks in parents, sibs and chil-

dren, the observed risks being consistent with those expected under a single dominant type of inheritance. Polygenic inheritance however cannot be ruled out for affective illness, and this has been suggested by some investigators; but it cannot account for the sex ratio differences (an excess of females) generally found in patients and affected relatives. This sex ratio is unexplainable according to an autosomal dominant model, unless one takes into consideration sex-linked hormonal factors.

Finally, based primarily on data obtained by Winokur and his associates (1969), an X-linked dominant mode of transmission of affective illnesses has been proposed. The main support for this hypothesis was the absence of father-to-son transmission in the group of patients studied by Winokur. Furthermore, linkage studies provide some support for X-linked dominant transmission. As was mentioned, *linkage* results from the proximity of two traits on the same chomosome leading to their dependent assortment during the process of meiosis. This method has been used to test the hypothesis of X-linkage in manic-depressive illness. Fig. 1 illustrates the pedigree of a family used for linkage analysis between color blindness and affective illness. In this pedigree, the genetic marker is protanopia (an X-linked recessive form of color blindness); this family provides an illustration of *X-linked transmission*. Both the marker and the illness are assorting in a dependent fashion across successive generations. The relatives are either affected and color blind or nonaffected with normal color vision. In other words, all subjects carry both traits together or none of them. Similar observations, subsequently reported by other centers suggest that an X-linked dominant factor is involved in the transmission of the manic-depressive phenotype in at least some families. However, the X-linked theory cannot be generalized to all families. For example, there are several observations of male-

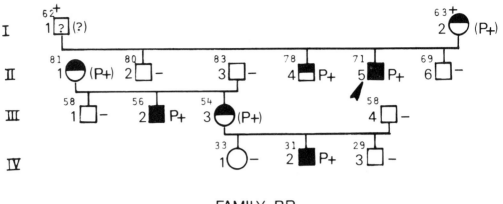

FAMILY BR

Fig. 1. A family pedigree showing a linkage analysis between color blindness (P+) and affective illness (shaded area). This is an example of X-linked transmission.

to-male transmission of the disease in some families, a pattern clearly inconsistent with X-linkage. Also, the sex distribution, i.e., the excess of females among afflicted relatives of affectively ill patients is not a universal finding. Nevertheless, the X-linked dominant transmission is present in a respectable number of families with manic-depressive illness, but it also seems quite clear that there are other genetic entities in this disease.

The genetic studies on *schizophrenia* have not yet contributed to the recognition of specific genetic models for this syndrome. In a large family study conducted in Berlin, Kallmann (1953) found the expectancy rates for sibs of schizophrenics to be 11 percent. Zerbin-Rüdin (1969) reviewed 25 genetic investigations on schizophrenia and concluded that the overall risk in sibs was 8.7%. The risk in children with one affected parent was 12%, while the minimal risk for children when both parents were schizophrenic was about 35%. All these figures are consistently greater than the one expected for the general population (about 1–2%, see Table 3). Twin studies

cannot establish the mode of inheritance of a disease, but they give some indication on the relative contribution of nature and nurture to the etiology of the disease. Kallmann (1953) has shown in a large series of index cases the concordance rates (with age correction) to be 86% for monozygotic twins as compared to 14% for dizygotic twins. These findings anticipate some of the more sophisticated twin studies in Scandinavia, England and the United States. These recent investigations are more representative since their samples are based on general population registers or on clinic and day hospital patients. In other words, less severe and nonchronic cases of schizophrenia are included in these surveys. These studies also benefit from more reliable methods of zygosity analysis, in particular, blood group typing, thus reducing possible sources of error in data analysis. The largest of the more recent studies was carried out by Kringlen in 1967 and was based on 25,000 twin pairs born in Norway. Concordance rates for schizophrenia in monozygotic twins was about 38% as compared to 10% for dizygotic twins (Table 4).

Table 3. Morbidity risks for schizophrenia in relatives of schizophrenic patients

Author	Parents	Sibs	General Population
Strömgren	0.7%	6.7%	0.5%
Kallmann	9.2%	14.3%	0.35%
Slater	4.1%	5.4%	
Garrone	7.0%	8.6%	2.4%

Table 4. Concordance rates for schizophrenia in twins

Author	MZ Concordance rate	DZ Concordance rate
Rosanoff et al.	61.0%	10.0%
Kallmann	86.2%	14.5%
Slater	74.7%	14.4%
Gottesman and Shields	41.7%	9.1%
Kringlen	38.0%	10.0%

Perhaps the most convincing evidence in favor of genetic factors in schizophrenia is provided by the adoption studies. As mentioned previously, this technique is utilized in an attempt to distinguish between genetic and environmental factors in the development of a given disorder. Heston and others have demonstrated that children of schizophrenics who were adopted in early infancy and raised in adoptive or foster homes develop schizophrenia as frequently as do children raised by their biological, schizophrenic parents. Kety and his group have utilized an even more complex research design, taking advantage of the extensive public health records maintained by the government of Denmark. They identified schizophrenics who had been given up for adoption by their biological parents soon after birth. The prevalence of schizophrenia and related disorders in the biological relatives of these adopted schizophrenics was found to be significantly higher than in the adoptive relatives; and this prevalence of schizophrenia was also significantly greater than in biological relatives of a matched control group of non-schizophrenic adoptees. Furthermore, Heston and Rosenthal have reported complementary findings by showing

higher rates for schizophrenia in the children of schizophrenic parents than in the children of non-schizophrenic parents, regardless of the rearing environment, i.e., even when the children were not raised by their biological parents, but in adoptive homes.

Regarding the mode of inheritance of schizophrenia, Kallman (1953) hypothesized that a single genetic factor was responsible for this disorder and that this factor was autosomal recessive, but subject to modifying genes causing variations in the expressivity of the disorder. Other hypotheses include a dominant type of inheritance with incomplete penetrance or a polygenic form with a threshold. An heterogenic model with a variety of separate genes, dominant or recessive, any one of which might be involved, should also be considered in the etiology of schizophrenia. The variety of hypotheses seems to indicate that no conclusive mode of inheritance can be retained for schizophrenia until more specific and sophisticated methods can be applied to genetic research in schizophrenia.

Pharmacogenetics

Not only do genes contribute to the etiology of psychiatric illnesses, but there is also evidence that genetic and environmental factors interact, affecting both drug metabolism and drug response. Recent kinetic studies show that the *rates of metabolism of drugs vary widely between unrelated individuals,* while they are rather constant within the same individual. Twin and family studies indicate that interindividual variations of drug biotransformation rates are *determined by hereditary factors to a significant extent.* Environmental factors such as diet and drug interaction also play a role, although the relationship between environmental and genetic factors is still poorly understood.

Most drugs are metabolized by enzymatic systems constituting complex proteins whose rate of synthesis and degradation are controlled by genes. Gene mutations or modifications may produce a qualitative change in these metabolizing enzymes or a quantitative one by reducing or suppressing their activity. This would account for the genetic basis of drug metabolism.

The therapeutic actions of drugs are dependent on physical, biochemical and physiological processes, such as drug absorption, binding to proteins, membrane transfer, and interaction with receptor cells before being metabolized and excreted. Enzymatic systems play an important role in these operations which are thus subject to genetic mechanisms. Most investigators in this field believe that a large number of enzymes in man are present in more than one form (i.e., polymorphic forms). More than one gene is responsible for the synthesis of polymorphic forms of an enzyme. As a result, enzyme variants, termed isoenzymes, are formed which can be separated by techniques such as electrophoresis. These variants may have differing susceptibilities to drugs, a phenomenon which would explain the various responses to specific drugs.

It is of great interest to describe some recent genetic advances in our understanding of the *metabolism of tricyclic antidepressants,* since these drugs are so widely used today (see Chapter 10). Hammer and Sjöqvist (1967) measured the plasma levels of tricyclic antide-pressant drugs and were able to show that large interindividual differences (sometimes 40-fold) exist in the steady-state plasma levels of the drugs desmethylimipramine and nortriptyline hydrochloride. Steady-state plasma concentrations occur after a certain delay and result from a balance between drug intake and excretion. Therefore, it is now clear that a certain oral dose does not assure that a patient has received adequate tricyclic treatment, but that individual plasma levels should be monitored.

Alexanderson et al. (1969) investigated the effect of genetic factors on plasma levels of tricyclic antidepressant drugs. They used the twin method and were able to study 19 monozygotic and 20 dizygotic twins who were given the drug, nortriptyline, orally. The intra-pair difference in steady-state plasma concentrations was found to be insignificant in identical twins, while this was not the case in fraternal twins. These investigators concluded that most of the variability in nortriptyline steady-state plasma concentrations between unrelated persons was genetically determined.

A better knowledge of how the genetic-environmental interactions affect the metabolism of antidepressant drugs will no doubt result in a more rational approach to the pharmacological treatment of depression.

Let us now turn to the *relationship between genetic factors and drug response in some psychiatric disorders.* Genetic factors have been studied quite extensively in the schizophrenias and the affective disorders, but the possible relationship between hereditary factors and the outcome of pharmacological treatments is still an area requiring a great deal of research. Our present knowledge of the genetics of the major psychoses would indicate that familial data could predict response to treatment. For example, a positive family history of schizophrenia in the relatives of a patient presenting an unclear clinical picture, including depressive symptoms, is an indication that this patient's illness may be genetically related to schizophrenia and would probably not benefit from antidepressive therapy alone.

A recent collaborative study sponsored by the National Institute of Mental Health has shown that a positive family history of mania can predict both the clinical picture of bipolar manic-depressive illness and the efficacy of the drug lithium carbonate in altering the natural course of affective disorders.

The relationship between familial factors, the course of the illness and the effectiveness of lithium therapy in manic-depressive illness has been investigated in a series of studies. The author and his associates have studied 89 manic-depressive patients who were followed in a double-blind study of lithium maintenance treatment for periods up to 48 months. Sixty-six percent of successfully treated lithium cases had at least one first-degree relative with bipolar manic-depression as compared to 21% of lithium failures. No relationship was found between long-term lithium response and the presence of unipolar illness in the patients' families. Such findings underscore the need for correlating a patient's response to lithium with his family background in order to predict the long-term response of patients on lithium maintenance therapy.

The correlation of familial factors with the response to psychotropic medication seems to represent a promising new approach to the problem of therapy and needs to be expanded to other drugs and disease states.

Another area of great interest in psychopharmacogenetics is the role played by a hereditary predisposition to drug-induced syndromes. This question has been examined, for example, in a study of parkinsonian patients experiencing affective syndromes (depression or mania) while treated with the drug L-Dopa. Thirty such cases were matched with 30 controls (i.e., parkinsonian pa-

tients with no psychiatric reaction while on L-Dopa), and family studies were conducted blind on both groups. The risks for affective illnesses in the first-degree relatives of the cases exhibiting an affective episode were significantly greater than in the relatives of the controls. The patients with the L-Dopa-induced affective syndrome also had more affective episodes in their past than did the controls. These results suggest that patients with Parkinson's disease presenting affective syndromes on L-Dopa may be genetically predisposed to affective illness.

Phenothiazine induced parkinsonism (see Chapter 10) in psychiatric patients has also been extensively studied. The incidence of Parkinson's disease was significantly higher in the relatives of these patients as compared to controls, a finding suggesting that there may be a hereditary susceptibility to parkinsonism induced by phenothiazine drugs.

In conclusion, application of techniques of genetic research to psychiatric disorders has provided strong evidence for a biological component in the case of both the schizophrenias and the affective disorders. It is anticipated that further genetic studies of these disorders will provide additional information about such issues as diagnostic subgroups, predictive factors for prevalence in relatives, and modes of transmission of the illness. Furthermore, investigation of the contributory effects of genetic and environmental influences on drug metabolism and drug response (both clinical efficacy and side effects) represents an essential area of research that will hopefully lead to the establishment of predictive factors in drug treatment responses.

Selected References

Alexanderson, B., Evans, D.A.P., and Sjoqvist, F.: Steady-state plasma levels of nortriptyline in twins: Influence of genetic factors and drug therapy. *Brit. Med. J.* IV: 764-768, 1969.

Fieve, R.R., Rosenthal, D., and Brill, H. (Eds.): *Genetic Research in Psychiatry.* The Johns Hopkins University Press, Baltimore, 1975.

Hammer, W. and Sjoqvist, F.: Plasma levels of monomethylated tricyclic antidepressants during treatment with imipramine-like compounds. *Life Sci.* 6: 1895-1903, 1967.

Kallmann, F.J. (Ed.): *Heredity in Health and Mental Disorder.* W.W. Norton & Company, Inc., New York, 1953.

Mendlewicz, J.: Genetics and psychopharmacology. In *Modern Problems in Pharmacopsychiatry*, T.A. Ban, F.A. Freyan, P. Pichot, and W. Pöldinger, eds., S. Karger, Basel, 1975.

Mendlewicz, J., Fieve, R.R., and Stallone, F.: Relationship between the effectiveness of lithium therapy and family history. *Am. J. Psychiat.* 130:1011-1013, 1973.

Mendlewicz, J., and Rainer, J.D.: Morbidity risks and genetic transmission in manic-depressive illness. *Am. J. Hum. Genet.* 26: 692-701, 1974.

Neel, J.V., and Schull, W.J. (Eds.): *Human Heredity.* University of Chicago Press, Chicago, 1954.

Rosenthal, D. (Ed.): *Genetic Theory and Abnormal Behavior.* McGraw-Hill Book Company, New York, 1970.

Rosenthal D., and Kety, S.S. (Eds.): *The Transmission of Schizophrenia.* Pergamon Press, Oxford, 1968.

Slater, E., and Cowie, V. (Eds.): *The Genetics of Mental Disorders.* Oxford University Press, London, 1971.

Winokur, G., Clayton, P.J., and Reich, T. (Eds.): *Manic-Depressive Illness.* C.V. Mosby, St. Louis, 1969.

Zerbin-Rüdin, E.: Zur Genetik der depressiven Erkrankungen. In *Das Depressive Syndrom*, H. Higgins and H. Selbach eds. Urban und Schwarzenberg, Munich, 1969.

Chapter 6

Human Sleep: Basic Mechanisms and Pathologic Patterns

Robert T. Rubin
  and
Russell E. Poland

Over the last twenty years, investigators of varied backgrounds, including anatomists, physiologists, pharmacologists, psychologists and psychiatrists, have devoted their talents to the scientific study of sleep. Thousands of reports about sleep have been published. They include studies of both laboratory animals and man, and they cover a broad range, from the neurochemistry of specific brain areas controlling sleep to the psychological interpretation of dream content. The development of the sleep laboratory, with its sophisticated equipment for the objective identification of the stages of sleep, has encouraged the study of normal subjects, psychiatric patients, and persons with primary complaints of sleep disturbance.

From the results of these investigations, we can conclude that sleep is an active, complex process involving the participation of specific areas of the brain stem for its control, and encompassing at least two very different states of brain activity. Unfortunately, sleep deprivation studies and other manipulations of sleep have not provided us with any specific insights into the function of sleep, other than that all higher organisms must have it to survive.

This chapter will trace the development of sleep research techniques and will touch upon normal sleep neuro-physiology, neurochemistry, and neuro-endocrinology, as well as the alterations in sleep patterns that occur in psychiatric illness and in the primary disorders of sleep. Of necessity, many areas of sleep research that have been studied in depth will be mentioned only briefly in this chapter; for further information the reader is referred to the general references listed, which contain more specialized and definitive bibliographies.

The Sleep Laboratory

The investigation of sleep physiology and pathology is conducted in a laboratory which permits the subject to sleep comfortably in a quiet, climate-controlled room. Electroencephalographic (EEG), electrooculographic (EOG), and electromyographic (EMG) recordings are made to quantitate sleep stages; the subject has disc electrodes attached to the scalp, the corners of the eyes, and under the chin for this purpose. The subject's head is wrapped with soft gauze to hold the electrodes firmly in place. The electrode wires are attached to a junction box at the head of the bed, which in turn is connected to a standard EEG recording machine in an adjoining room. The laboratory area must be free of stray electrical fields that might interfere with the small potentials generated by the EEG. If blood studies are performed while the subject is sleeping, a long flexible plastic catheter is placed in an arm vein, taped to the subject's arm and neck, and carried along with the EEG cable through a wall port into the adjoining equipment room. Thus, blood samples may be taken periodically during the night, without disturbing the sleeping subject.

The electrophysiologic recordings (EEG, EOG, EMG) are made continuously throughout the night. Usually, three channels of EEG, two of EOG, and one of EMG are recorded. Extra electrodes are placed on the subject in the event that one loses contact during the night. The recording machine can then be switched to the spare electrodes as needed. During a typical eight-hour sleep session, approximately one-quarter mile of six-channel tracing is produced, which must be scored for several sleep stages by a specially trained technician. With practice, careful scoring of an eight-hour record can be done in two hours.

The Electrophysiologic Stages of Sleep

Fig. 1 illustrates the electrophysiologic characteristics of the various stages of sleep, and Fig. 2 shows the normal patterns of sleep staging for children, young adults, and elderly subjects. From these figures it can be seen that, initially, the subject progresses from the awake stage through stage 1 and stage 2 of sleep, and then into stages 3 and 4, which are called *slow-wave* or *deep sleep*. Periodically, throughout the night, the subject enters a *rapid eye movement* (REM) or *dreaming sleep* episode, which is characterized by a specific EEG, EOG, and EMG pattern (Fig. 1). Persons awakened from this stage of sleep frequently recall many vivid dreams. Following the REM sleep episode, there again is a progression through the non-REM stages of sleep (1 through 4) until the next REM episode occurs.

Throughout the night, there is an orderly cycling of non-REM and REM sleep stages, with a frequency of 80–110

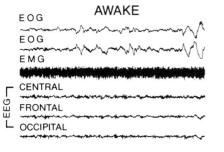

AWAKE

EOG
EOG
EMG
CENTRAL
FRONTAL
OCCIPITAL

EEG

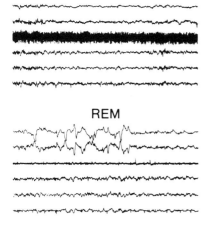

STAGE 1

REM

STAGE 2

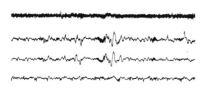

STAGE 3

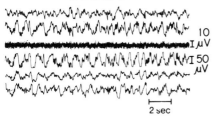

STAGE 4

10 I μV
I 50 μV

2 sec

Fig. 1. Electrophysiology of sleep stages. The same six channels are used throughout, as labeled in the AWAKE record. Electrooculogram (EOG) records eye movements; electromyogram (EMG) records muscle tonus from beneath the chin; electroencephalogram (EEG) records from areas noted. AWAKE is characterized by high EOG and EMG activity and low amplitude, fast frequency EEG activity. STAGE 1 sleep is characterized by a quiescent EOG and a low-amplitude, fast EEG; the subject is somewhat relaxed in muscle tonus but easily aroused. STAGE 2 sleep is characterized also by a primarily low amplitude, fast EEG, but with the occurrence of 12-16 Hz sleep spindles and high amplitude, slow K complexes; most of this stage occurs in the latter part of the night. STAGE 3 and 4 sleep are characterized by high amplitude slow waves covering more than 20% of the record; stage 4 is reached when the slow waves exceed 50% of the record. Stages 3 and 4 are the deepest stages of sleep and occur in the early hours of the night. REM sleep is characterized by bursts of eye movements (EOG), sharply reduced muscle tonus (EMG) and a low amplitude, fast frequency EEG. Four to five progressively longer REM periods occur cyclically throughout the night (see text). [From Kales, A. (1968) Ann. Intern. Med. 68:1078-1104, with permission.]

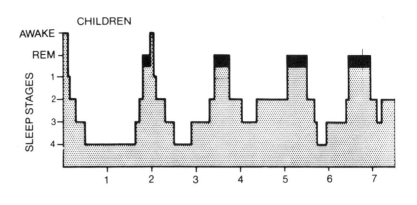

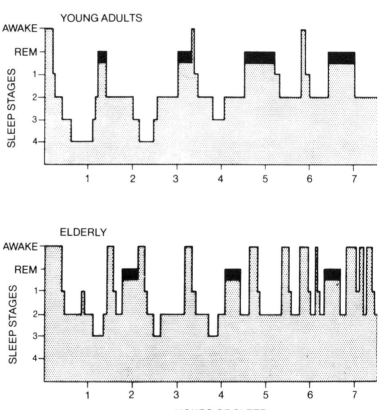

HOURS OF SLEEP

Fig. 2. Sleep cycles of normal subjects.
Children and young adults show early appearance of slow wave (stages 3 and 4) sleep,
progressive lengthening of the first three
REM episodes, and infrequent awakenings.
Elderly adults show reduced slow-wave sleep,
fairly uniform REM episodes, and frequent
awakenings. [From Kales, A. (1968) Ann.
Intern. Med. 68: 1078-1104, with permission.]

minutes, depending on the subject (Fig. 2). This appears to be the nocturnal part of a basic, approximately 90-minute rest-activity cycle that occurs during the entire 24 hours. Infants have relatively high amounts of REM sleep; by the age of one year, the amount of REM has decreased to 25–30% of total sleep, which remains approximately the same throughout life. Slow-wave sleep (stages 3 and 4), on the other hand, declines throughout life, comprising 20–30% of the sleep of children, 10–15% of the sleep of young adults, and occasionally being completely absent in the elderly. There also is a gradient of sleep staging during the night, with slow-wave sleep occurring early in the sleep period and REM sleep being more frequent in the hours prior to awakening.

The Neurochemistry and Neuroendocrinology of Sleep

Several chemical substances present in the central nervous system (CNS) are thought to be synaptic neurotransmitters in areas of the brainstem involved in the triggering and maintenance of sleep stages. In the cat, the animal in which most neurochemical sleep research has been done, many experiments suggest that slow-wave sleep is triggered by serotonin-containing neurons in the median raphe nuclei and that REM sleep is primed by a serotoninergic mechanism. The maintenance of REM sleep appears to depend on pontine noradrenergic and cholinergic mechanisms located in the locus coeruleus. These neurochemical data from cats, however, are at some odds with human neuropharmacologic studies of sleep. In humans, decreasing brain serotonin or increasing brain catecholamines (dopamine, noradrenaline) decreases REM sleep, while decreasing brain catecholamines increases REM sleep. Clearly, then, only limited inferences about the role of specific postulated neurotransmitters in human sleep staging may be drawn from the animal work.

The same neurotransmitters that appear to be involved in the triggering and maintenance of sleep stages also play a prominent role in the CNS regulation of pituitary hormone secretion, via the hypothalamic releasing and inhibiting factors. Fig. 3 illustrates the typical secretion patterns (plasma levels) of five of the anterior pituitary hormones (ACTH, GH, LH, FSH, and PRL) as well as ADH (a posterior pituitary hormone), testosterone (an androgenic gonadal steroid) and aldosterone (an adrenal mineralocorticoid) in young adult men. The various hormones have unique secretion patterns, some of which are closely linked to the sleep-wake cycle and the stages of sleep. ACTH has a prominent 24-hour rhythm, with lowest blood levels in the early hours of the sleep period and rapidly increasing levels in the latter few hours of sleep, which reach a maximum about the time of awakening. The similarity between the ACTH and aldosterone rhythms suggests that ACTH is an important regulator of adrenal mineralocorticoids as well as adrenal glucocorticoids (cortisol).

GH, in contrast to ACTH, is released soon after sleep onset and is closely linked to the first slow-wave sleep episode of the night. This slow-wave sleep-related release of GH is normally its major secretion during the entire 24-hour period. While the ACTH rhythm does not change rapidly in response to alterations of sleep, GH immediately responds to a shifted sleep schedule, being released at the new time of onset of slow-wave sleep.

The gonadotropins, LH and FSH, have no 24-hour rhythm in normal adult men, whereas both PRL and testosterone show increasing plasma levels during sleep. The similarity between the PRL and testosterone rhythms suggests that

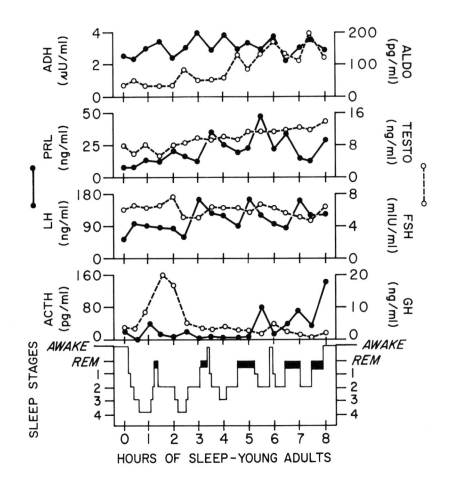

Fig. 3. Composite representation of the typical secretion patterns (plasma levels) of eight hormones during a normal eight-hour sleep period in a young adult man. REM = rapid eye movement sleep; ACTH = adrenocorticotropic hormone; GH = growth hormone; LH = luteinizing hormone; FSH = follicle stimulating hormone; PRL = pro-lactin; TESTO = testosterone; ADH = anti-diuretic hormone; ALDO = aldosterone. Hormones named on left side of figure depicted by dots and solid line; those named on right side depicted by open circles and dashed line.

PRL may be another pituitary hormone (in addition to LH) that is influential in the secretion of testosterone in men. Finally, Fig. 3 also illustrates that the posterior pituitary hormone, ADH, is secreted episodically, like the anterior pituitary hormones, and that its plasma levels bear no relationship to sleep stages.

Effects of Sleep Deprivation

Early sleep deprivation studies were undertaken with the hope that the resulting effects would be important indicators of why we sleep. When the first sleep-deprived subjects showed mental aberrations suggestive of psychosis (visual illusions, etc.), it was thought that a basic function of sleep was to discharge normal "psychotic-like" brain activity, so that the waking hours would remain clear for logical thinking and reality testing. Further studies, however, disallowed such a simplistic view of the functions of sleep. It was shown that even after eight days of total sleep deprivation, subjects did not become regularly psychotic. They did become irritable, had misperceptions of their environment, lost the ability to concentrate, had lapses of attentiveness, on occasion had frank visual hallucinations, and were consistently very sleepy. If anything, their symptoms resembled more a toxic type of psychosis than a schizophrenic-like episode. They showed decrements in performance and memory but were responsive to interpersonal support from the experimenters. Thus, total sleep deprivation studies have permitted only the general conclusion that sleep is necessary for optimal individual health, and, conversely, that sleep loss can result in irritability, reduced attention span, poor work performance, and generalized ill feeling. Attempts to selectively deprive subjects of the individual stages of sleep similarly have not shed light on the specific importance of the individual sleep stages. Effects resembling those of total sleep deprivation occurred when slow-wave sleep or REM sleep were selectively deprived. Suppression of REM sleep by antidepressant medication in depressed patients for periods of several months has produced no detectable ill effects. Therefore, all the sleep-deprivation studies performed to date permit inferences only about the general ill effects of sleep loss, in spite of the large amount of theoretical speculation surrounding these studies.

Sleep Patterns in Psychiatric Illness

Many psychiatric disorders have disturbances of sleep as part of their symptomatology. The patterns of sleep pathology associated with mental illnesses are varied, and there is no unique pattern of sleep disturbance for any given psychiatric disorder. Indeed, generalized anxiety reactions in normal persons during periods of increased life stress may have concomitant sleep disruptions that are quite similar to those occurring in major mental illnesses. As a corollary, it is possible that some of the sleep disturbance associated with psychiatric illness may be related to the non-specific anxiety which accompanies it. On the other hand, it is also possible that functional CNS neurotransmitter disturbances in certain psychiatric conditions, e.g., severe depressions, may alter sleep staging at a neurochemical level. This remains a speculative area.

The general changes in sleep patterns accompanying psychiatric illness include: (1) increased sleep latency (time to fall asleep), (2) more frequent awakenings during the night, (3) foreshortened sleep (early morning awakening), (4) decreased amount and percentage of slow-wave (stages 3 and 4) sleep, and (5) reduced REM sleep, although this latter finding is inconstant.

Schizophrenic patients may show, in addition to the above-mentioned general changes, intermediate stages of sleep having characteristics of stage 1, stage 2 and REM (admixtures of low voltage, fast EEG activity, sleep spindles, and variable amounts of eye movements and muscle tonus). These intermediate sleep stages have not been consistently confirmed by independent laboratories, however. Schizophrenic patients also may show a lack of REM rebound following REM sleep deprivation. In contrast, a compensatory rebound of REM sleep does occur in psychotically depressed patients and in alcoholic withdrawal syndromes.

The hallucinations reported by some schizophrenics may have an approximate 90-minute periodicity, reminiscent of the general basic rest-activity cycle. It has been suggested that schizophrenic hallucinations may represent the intrusion of dream mechanisms into the waking state, but there is little evidence to support this hypothesis at present. An analogous phenomenon is the marked REM rebound that some subjects manifest when withdrawing from REM-suppressing drugs such as barbiturates and alcohol. The severe nightmares, extensions of dream-like mental activity into wakefulness, and vivid visual hallucinations that can accompany REM rebound might be based on neurophysiologic dream mechanisms similar to those in schizophrenic reactions.

With reference to the major affective psychoses, manic patients tend to have sleep patterns similar to those of schizophrenic patients, with decreased total sleep time, frequent awakenings and decreased slow-wave sleep, the greatest disturbances occurring during the last third of the night. Early morning awakening may be a clinical hallmark of psychotic depression, but sleep laboratory studies indicate that some depressed patients do not have a clear early morning transition between sleep and waking, and that many will have at least fleeting episodes of sleep as long as they lie in bed. Conversely, some depressed patients may have hypersomnia during the active phase of their illness. Recently, it was reported that REM sleep deprivation in depressed patients resulted in clinical improvement compared to depressed control patients who were deprived of non-REM sleep. However, this improvement was short-lived, so that sleep deprivation appears to have little real therapeutic potential. Its effects, however, certainly are of research interest.

Primary Disorders of Sleep

Several primary disturbances of sleep patterns and behavior now have been identified, based on painstaking sleep laboratory studies of many patients. Table I lists the sleep laboratory findings, psychological evaluation, and principles of management and treatment for several of these disorders (somnambulism, enuresis, night terrors, nightmares, narcolepsy, and hypersomnia). Insomnia, in particular, is less a primary sleep disorder than it is a secondary symptom of psychological distress or psychiatric illness, such as depression. Treatment of the underlying pathology, such as the use of antidepressants, frequently results in improvement of the insomnia as well. The excessive and unwarranted use of hypnotic agents for complaints of insomnia is one of the major drug problems in the United States today.

Table 1. Sleep Disorders. [Modified from Kales, A., and Kales, J. (1974) N. Engl. J. Med. 290:487-499, with permission.]

	Sleep Laboratory Findings	Psychological Evaluation	Management and Treatment
Somnambulism	Incidents occur in stage 4 sleep. Critical faculties and reactivity are impaired during the incident.	In children psychiatric disturbances are infrequent, while in adults they are frequent.	Prophylactic measures, Parental reassurance that children frequently outgrow disorders. Psychiatric evaluation for adults.
Enuresis (Bedwetting)	Occurs in all sleep stages. Misconception that dreaming is a frequent causal factor.	Psychiatric disturbances are infrequent with primary enuresis. Psychological evaluation often indicated for enuresis. Associated with other psychological symptoms.	Parental counseling and reassurance is critical, so that parental mishandling does not create psychiatric problems. Pharmacological treatment (imipramine) may be indicated in older children.
Night Terrors	Occur in stage 4 sleep. Characterized by extreme vocalizations, motility and autonomic response. Recall is minimal or absent.	Psychiatric disturbances are infrequent in children but frequent in adults.	Reassurance of parents that children frequently outgrow the disorder. For adults, psychological evaluation is often indicated. Use of stage 4 suppressants (benzodiazepines) may be helpful.
Nightmares	Occur in REM sleep. Characterized by less motility and autonomic response. Recall is frequent and vivid.	Frequent nightmares in children or adults may indicate psychopathology.	Parental reassurance that nightmares in children are often transient. If they are frequent, psychological evaluation may be indicated
Narcolepsy (Sleep attacks)	Attacks of narcolepsy may be accompanied by 3 auxiliary symptoms: cataplexy, sleep paralysis and hypnogogic reverie. Cataplexy is accompanied by sleep onset REM periods.	Sleep attacks may be misinterpreted as laziness, irresponsibility, or emotional instability.	Establishing the diagnosis is critical. Stimulants are effective for sleep attacks. Imipramine is effective for auxiliary symptoms. There may be a danger in using both drugs simultaneously.
Hypersomnia	Sleep-stage patterns are normal but sleep is extended. Associated with post-dormital confusion and difficulty in awakening.	Often is a symptom of psychological disorder, e.g., depression.	Stimulant drugs are effective. Neurological and psychological evaluation is important in establishing a diagnosis.
Insomnia	Complaints of insomnic patients have been verified in the sleep lab. Sleep of insomniacs is more aroused, i.e., heart rate and respiration are increased. Most hypnotic drugs lose their effectiveness within two weeks.	Insomnia is most often a secondary symptom of psychological disturbance, and not a primary sleep disorder. Depression is a common feature.	When insomnia is secondary to medical conditions, pharmacological treatment may be useful. If psychological factors are primary, pharmacological therapy should be combined with psychotherapeutic techniques.

Summary

Sleep is a very active, complex bodily process that is controlled by specific areas of the brain. There are several stages of sleep in humans, identifiable by electrophysiologic recordings in the sleep laboratory. Sleep is divided primarily into non-REM and REM or dreaming sleep. Slow-wave or deep sleep is a part of non-REM sleep. Throughout the night, there are regular, cyclic repetitions of non-REM and REM sleep. Specific neurotransmitters in the CNS appear to be responsible for the transitions between sleep and wakefulness and the staging of sleep. The secretion patterns of several pituitary hormones are closely linked to sleep, highlighting the importance of the CNS in endocrine regulation. Many psychiatric disorders have concomitant non-specific alterations in sleep patterns, including frequent awakenings, reduced slow-wave sleep, and variably reduced REM sleep. Conversely, sleep deprivation produces symptoms of irritability, lapses in attention, distractability, and sometimes visual illusions and hallucinations, but these resemble more a toxic psychosis than a schizophrenic episode. A number of primary disorders of sleep have been identified, including somnambulism, enuresis, night terrors, nightmares and narcolepsy. Specific pharmacologic treatments for many of these sleep disorders are now available.

Selected References

Anders, T., Emde, R., and Parmelee, A. (Eds.): *A Manual of Standardized Terminology, Techniques and Criteria for Scoring of States of Sleep and Wakefulness in Newborn Infants.* UCLA Brain Information Service, NINDS Neurological Information Network, Los Angeles, 1971.

Broughton, R.: Neurochemical, neuroendocrine, and biorhythmic aspects of sleep in man: Relationship to clinical pathological disorders. In *Neurohumoral Aspects of Brain Function*, R.R. Drucker-Colin, and R.D. Myers, eds. Plenum Press, New York, 1974, pp. 1-37.

Chase, M.H. (Ed.): *The Sleeping Brain.* Perspectives in the Brain Sciences, Volume 1. Brain Information Service/Brain Research Institute, UCLA, Los Angeles. Proceedings of the Symposia for the Psychophysiological Study of Sleep, June 1971, 1972.

de Wied, D., and de Jong, W.: Drug effects and hypothalamic-anterior pituitary function. *Ann. Rev. Pharmacol.* 14:389-412, 1974.

Jouvet, M.: The role of monoamines and acetylcholine-containing neurons in the regulation of the sleep-waking cycle. *Ergebn. Physiol.* 64:166-307, 1972.

Kales, A., and Kales, J.: Sleep disorders: Recent findings in the diagnosis and treatment of disturbed sleep. *N. Engl. J. Med.* 290:487-499, 1974.

Kleitman, N.: *Sleep and Wakefulness.* University Chicago Press, Chicago, 1939.

Moruzzi, G.: The sleep-waking cycle. *Ergebn. Physiol.* 64:1-165, 1972.

Rechtschaffen, A., and Kales, A. (Eds.): *A Manual of Standardized Terminology, Techniques and Scoring System for Sleep Stages of Human Subjects.* Public Health Service, U.S. Government Printing Office, Washington, D.C., 1968.

Rubin, R.T.: Sleep-endocrine studies in man. In *Hormones, Homeostasis, and the Brain.* Progress in Brain Research, Volume 42, W.H. Gispen, Tj.B. van Wimersma Greidanus, B. Bohus, and D. de Wied, eds. Elsevier, Amsterdam, 1975, pp. 73-80.

Sleep Reviews: Brain Information Service/Brain Research Institute, UCLA, Los Angeles, 1967-1975.

Vogel, G.W.: A review of REM sleep deprivation. *Arch. Gen. Psychiat.* 32:749-761, 1975.

Holman, R.B., Elliott, G.R., and Barchas, J.D.: Neuroregulators and sleep mechanisms. *Ann. Rev. Med.* 26:499-520, 1975.

Chapter 7

Models of Human Psychopathology: Experimental Approaches in Primates

Helen L. Morrison and
William T. McKinney, Jr.

In the field of psychiatry, the study of behavior requires that we explore not only the treatment of its observable disorders but attempt to identify the complex events surrounding the development of normal and abnormal behavioral patterns. In addition, behavior must be viewed as a network of events in the context of genetic, sociologic, physiologic and intrapsychic factors, all in relationship to their development in time. There are limits to the investigation of many of these factors in the human subject and thus researchers have begun to explore the possibility of developing animal models of human behavioral disorders.

The analysis of behavior is aided by the use of animal models which could help clarify a human problem, pinpoint implicit assumptions and draw attention to facets of heretofore unnoticed human behavior. Work with models has shown that oversimplification of behavior has been a primary defect in understanding its human aspects. The relevance of animal models to human behavior is valid only if we remember that we seek not superficial similarities or differences in overt behavior but the underlying principles. The principles of learning and conditioning among species have led to the formulation of systematic theories of normal behavior. If normally adaptive behavioral patterns provide a foundation upon which maladaptive processes are built, we can begin to examine an environment which in its capriciousness or hostility contributes to this abnormality. Thus, we can develop systematic experimental research on the causes of subhuman pathologic behavior to endeavor to learn about the etiology of abnormal human behavior. Experimental methods, where we induce in addition to observing the natural occurrence of pathologic behavior, are coupled with the study of abnormal behavior. A deliberate manipulation of independent variables is most related to this definition. Deviant states are seen to result directly from the experiment rather than being unexpected variants.

Recognition of biologic affinities between man and the non-human primates led to consideration of phylogenetic and behavioral similarities between the species. As a resource for constructing and testing conceptual models and as a perspective on comparative evolution, the study of the behavior of primates has the potential for improving upon and enriching our understanding of that of humans.

The study of animal behavior involves a multitude of disciplines and a number of species. Social, biological, environmental and genetic factors have been and are being explored in dogs, cats and rats.

Because of the limitations of space, this chapter will focus only on the development of the field of experimental primatology and its importance in contributing to developmental theories of behavior. We will discuss the utilization of specific social and biological induction techniques to produce syndromes of abnormal behavior in primates, which can be objectively documented and evaluated. Occasional reference will be made to work in other species because of the issue of species variation. Some criticisms of the field will be followed by the delineation of criteria necessary for valid research. The areas of importance for an understanding of the development of abnormal behavior will include variables important in the development of a reciprocal mother-infant attachment bond, short- and long-term effects of varying conditions of rearing on the social behavior of primates, the role of separation in the production of abnormal behavior on short- and long-term behavior, the interactional nature between social and biological factors in the production of abnormal behavior and the rehabilitative approaches effective in ameliorating the syndromes of abnormal behavior in primates. Concluding the chapter will be a summary of those concepts most important to the field of psychiatry and a consideration of perspectives for the future.

Criteria for Animal Models of Psychopathology

There have been a number of difficulties in accepting the conclusion that phenomena observed in non-human animals are analogous to those found in human behavioral disorders.

Skepticism of the relevance of animal behavior models of psychopathology to human disorders is voiced by workers in many disciplines. Kubie (1939), a leading spokesman for those psychiatrists who refuse to accept animal models, states, "Thus, the imitation in animals of the emotional states which attend neurosis in man is not the experimental production of the essence of neuroses itself." For Kubie, behavior that is observable is only to be interpreted as "sign language" of an underlying symbolic disorder which is the real core of psychopathology. He stresses that animals do not have symbolic capacity and, therefore, it is not possible to produce a true neurotic or psychotic state in non-humans. This criticism, if true, would preclude the use of any non-human subjects for the study of human psychopathology. However, the assumption that higher-order primates do not have symbolic capacities is being seriously questioned, as evidenced by the work of Premack in the area of language in nonhumans. Also, the concept that behavior is only important as a superficial indicator of a "real" symbolic disorder is now not a generally accepted viewpoint.

Most early studies in animal psychopathology suffered from lack of preciseness in the descriptions of methodology as well as of resultant observable behaviors. Therefore, a key advance in this field has been the recognition of the need to rigorously define the criteria of behavior that would be considered applicable to animals. This was, perhaps, first done by Hebb (1954), when he defined human neurosis in behavioral non-verbal terms which permitted the definition to be used at the animal level.

In 1966, the concept of an animal model which would reflect human depression was put forth by Senay. Using dogs and separation from the experimenter as the precipitating incident, he noted depressive symptomatology that lasted for two months until the puppies were reunited with the investigator. Seligman et al. (1968) then presented an analysis of the response of dogs to electric shock. They worked on two premises of learning and the relationships that produced learning, acquisition and extinction. A third relationship was proposed, that of independence between events. The term they used was "learned helplessness" defined as the perception (or learning) of independence between the animal's responses and the aversive event, whether it was withdrawal or presentation. A later paper by this group reported that the pathological behavior which resulted from inescapable trauma

was alleviated by having the animals repeatedly respond to the event which terminated the shock. They speculated that, like dogs, humans also become passive in situations where they can neither mitigate nor control future traumatic events.

The 1950's and 1960's saw a greater number of publications concerning loss of a previous affectional bond. Lorenz noted that geese and jackdaw birds separated from their families showed decreased appetite and "acute grief," with the animals searching almost compulsively for lost partners. Saul observed that, for three months following the death of the last of her litter in an accident, a dog became classically depressed with a spontaneous remission. In the African parrot, being excluded in the presence of an observable bond formation led to decreased activity and, often, death within six months.

In 1959, Harlow and Zimmerman presented their work with cloth and wire surrogate mothers and the development of affectional responses in rhesus monkeys which will be described later. This classic work has often been keynoted as the beginning of the era of primate behavior studies more directly relevant to psychiatry. Many authors began reporting on experimental mother-infant separations or disruption of affectional bonds.

The need for animal models of depression in which we can systematically manipulate the interactional and social variables thought to be relevant to this disorder was described by McKinney and Bunney (1969). These authors outlined criteria for evaluating animal models. The five requirements to be met in an animal model of depression were: (1) the symptoms of the depression so induced should be reasonably analogous to those seen in the human syndrome, (2) there should be observable behavioral changes which can be objectively evaluated, (3) independent observers should agree on objective criteria

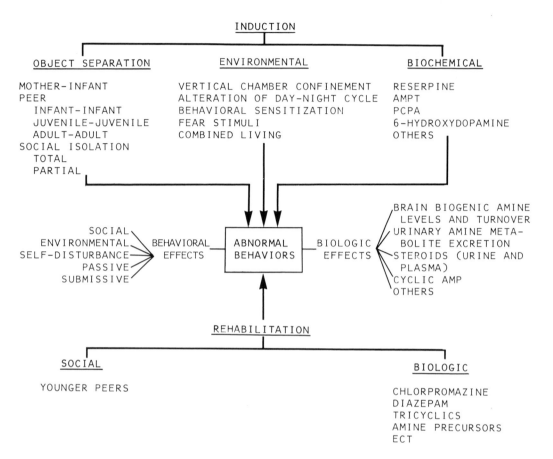

Fig. 1. **Experimental psychopathology research system illustrating techniques of induction and rehabilitation with attendant behavioral and biological changes.**

for drawing conclusions about the subjective state, (4) the treatment modalities effective in reversing depression in humans should reverse the changes seen in animals and (5) the system should be reproducible by other investigators. Also, mechanisms found to be important concomitants of the syndrome in animals should be comparable to those felt to be important in the syndrome in man. This system would then permit further elucidation of the variables mentioned above and would also allow for greater diversity in further biochemical and behavioral studies.

Fig. 1 shows an outline of the experimental system where social, biologic and environmental factors are presented that are considered important in the production of behavioral changes in animals and that are commonly associated with depression in human beings. In the remainder of this chapter, we will discuss both induction and rehabilitation techniques with associated biological and behavioral changes which accompany them. We will present in detail several induction techniques of social or object separation, and of biochemical and environmental paradigms. The rehabilitative methods using both social and bio-logical approaches to a stable experimental animal model add to our ability to evaluate a variety of treatment techniques.

Induction of Abnormal Behavior in Primates: Variable Rearing Conditions

There are two principle techniques used to produce behavioral abnormalities in primates—*social isolation* and *separation*. In social isolation, one does not permit normal attachment bonds to develop, whereas separation involves the disruption of such a previously developed bond. The technique of social isolation can be utilized to demonstrate the importance of early social rearing environments on subsequent development in the primate. In contrast, the separation technique is sometimes considered an object-loss model. The attachment of one human being to another, be that child-adult or peer-peer, is a powerful reinforcer of behavior; its loss can lead to serious separation reactions. There is abundant evidence that the disruption of significant attachment bonds may represent some of the most traumatic kinds of withdrawal of reinforcement in primate species, including man. Separation techniques with primates, then, allows further study of multiple variables thought to be important in the development of separation reactions.

Total Social Isolation

The relationship between social competency and development and the early social rearing environment is best exemplified by the primate social isolation syndromes.

Isolate animals show deficiencies in behavior that are related to the impoverishment of the social environment whereas primates raised in more complex social environments develop into social beings of greater complexity. Total social isolation denies the animal any visual, tactile or social contacts and minimal physical restrictions as to food, water and milk. If isolated for the first three months of life, monkeys often exhibit severe behavioral abnormalities, with refusal to drink which often necessitates force feeding for survival. However, placement of these three-month isolates in an environment of adult females and peers eventually sees a relatively normal development of social behaviors.

Six-month isolates develop a behavioral repertoire of self-directed idiosyncratic behavior during isolation. These behavioral abnormalities reflect variations of normal monkey behavior. Newborns are born with a suckling reflex and if unable to find a surrogate, they develop patterns of self-orality which is abnormal in its excessiveness. A clinging reflex, also denied without a surrogate, leads to self-clasping behavior. Kinesthetic stimulation, to which monkeys respond, if also denied from an external source, is provided by the isolate in stereotypic rocking. All of these activities of stereotypy, self-clasping and self-mouthing are seldom seen in primates raised in socially complex environments. Removal from isolation into a social environment sees a maintenance of these abnormal behaviors at the same or higher levels as seen in isolation rather than a decrease or their disappearance. With placement into social situations where there are age-mates who are socially competent or incompetent, there is an absence of appropriate social initiations. The behaviors seen are mostly inappro-

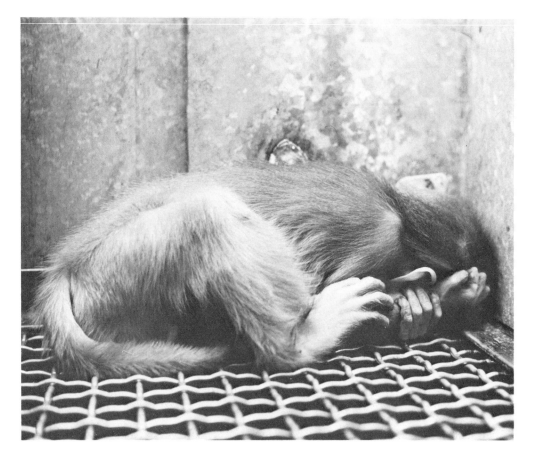

Fig. 2. Withdrawal, huddling and self-clasping behaviors typical of an animal isolated for six months.

priate ones, characterized by withdrawal, stereotypic huddling and rocking, and self-clasping.

Gross deficits are seen in the inappropriateness of aggressive activity, both in form and target of aggression. Normally, a seven-month-old monkey is capable of aggression, as is true of the isolates. The inappropriateness of the isolate is seen in attacking the self if a social other is unavailable, often leading to severe self injury. The isolate also will repeatedly attack a neonate, rare in occurrence in normally-socialized monkeys. Often, more serious injury can result to the isolate who repeatedly attacks the dominant adult male of the troop, a foolish and potentially fatal

mistake in judgment. Sexual behavior is inappropriate for both sexes in isolates, with males showing typical thrusting behavior most often directed to all but the appropriate end of the female. Presents are not held for sufficient time. Techniques of artificial insemination for the female isolates, or as Harlow terms them "motherless mothers," are used for impregnation but mothering is usually deficient. Either they are abusive to their infants with physical attacks and occasional fatal injuries or they ignore and avoid the contacts of their infants.

There is a direct correlation between the severity of impairment and the duration of the isolation with nine-month isolates, often being characterized as "social vegetables." The theoretical position in respect to these results is to view the behavior induced by isolation as reflecting a learning deficit in the social sphere.

Chronological variations have proved to be important variables in terms of outcome in isolation studies, with placement in isolation at later ages and stages of development resulting in less severe behavioral deviations. Placement at six months for the next six months of life results in neither the intensity nor range of self-directed, idiosyncratic behaviors of monkeys isolated at birth but rather a tendency to be hyperaggressive. Isolated subjects at three and six months of age essentially showed hyperaggressiveness with an indication that the behavior persists regardless of exposure to varied social environments. Feral (wild) born and raised monkeys, isolated during second or later years of life, seem relatively unaffected and, if adequate social behaviors have developed prior to isolation, few gross deficits are seen after removal from it.

Many terms have been applied to the behavioral manifestations of these isolate monkeys. Labels such as anxiety, phobia, autism, chronic emotional disorder, behavioral disorder, and experimental neurasthenia have been too often utilized without adequate behavioral description. This laxity has contributed to the alienation of those clinicians who fail to see similarities between conditions used to produce abnormal behavior in animals and those thought to predispose to human psychopathology.

While observable behavioral similarities between animal and man need not imply similarities in the etiology of these behavioral states, they do at least allow the detailed investigation of the mechanisms underlying these behaviors. The disorders observed in animals may not equate wholly with human psychiatric illnesses, but they may well represent important components of these syndromes.

Separation Experiences

Another social induction technique involves the experimental use of separation experiences. In human children, separation-induced depression has been studied by several investigators since Spitz (1946) first described the syndrome of "anaclitic depression." Robertson and Bowlby postulated that the reaction of children and infants to maternal separation occurred in distinct stages. Initially, the "protest" stage was characterized by high agitation and attempts to return to the mother; a subsequent "despair" stage with weeping and reduced activity, and a final "detachment" phase by withdrawal from any activity in the environment and rejection of initial attempts on the part of mother to re-establish the relationship when she returned. Several authors reported similar responses in infant Rhesus monkeys following separation from their mothers and this work suggested the possible existence of behavioral parallels which might provide a model of human depression in monkeys.

This work, however, required the careful description and experimental documentation of the various stages of attachment of "affectional systems" that are important for the developing organism. The affectional systems which have been described in the Rhesus monkey include:
1. Infant-mother affectional system
2. Mother-infant affectional system
3. Peer affectional system
4. Heterosexual affectional system
5. Paternal affectional system

The baseline data was needed prior to experimental approaches to abnormal behavior in young monkeys. Both the description of normal behavior characteristics of each of these systems and the sequence in which they mature needed to be established before there could be any scientific understanding of the failure of the development of any affectional system or its disruption once active.

In the description of many mother-infant studies, the responses of these infants roughly fit the model of protest and despair, usually within six days of the separation. Jensen and Tolman concluded that brief separation from mother at five and seven months of age with reunions produced the following effects: (1) mother-directed behaviors are increased in the infant, (2) "own infant" directed behavior on the part of the mothers was higher than "other infant" directed behaviors, (3) learned "own mother" specificity occurs after several separations, (4) separations increased interactive behavior between mother and infant. Senay, Hanson and Harlow, after separating four mother-infant pairs for a three-week period, interpreted their data as supporting the Bowlby formulation of protest, despair and withdrawal. Hinde, Spencer-Booth and Bruce separated infants for six days at eight months of age with the infants showing similar responses to the studies noted above. Kaufman and Rosenblum investigated separation in pig-tailed Macacques with separations occurring at different times and concluded that their data were consistent with a probable primate model of Spitz' "anaclitic depression."

However, not all investigators have found these clear-cut stages following separation. For example, Kaufman and Rosenblum found that *bonnet Macacques* subjected to similar separations showed less severe reactions than did the *pig-tailed* subjects. The authors ascribed the differences between the monkey sub-subjects to basic differences in social patterns. Pig-tail Macacques have lower levels of "passive-contact" behaviors and, therefore, young bonnet Macacques have a greater chance in early life to form relationships with monkeys other than their own mothers. In fact, during separations, the bonnet Macacques established mother-like substitute relationships with other adults. Hinde and Spencer-Booth (1971) removed the mothers from eight-month-old infants with no evidence of the "detachment" phase but noted that mother-infant contact increased during the reunion phase. In another study, they separated Rhesus monkey infants at ages 18, 21, 25 and 30 weeks for six-day periods. In comparing the date across age of separation they found no significant differences in the response to separation. In addition, they observed a high degree of variability in infant behavior. Lewis and coworkers (1976) presented summary data on 20 Rhesus monkeys from five studies of mother-infant separations. They concluded that caution must be exercised in using protest-despair type responses as an animal model for depression in neurobiological investigations and for rehabilitative studies, since the changes produced may not be sufficiently predictable nor stable.

Peer separation has been presented as a possible model for depression. This technique involves rearing groups of monkeys together from early in life and then separating individuals from the groups. Animals so separated show behaviors consistent with the protest-despair sequence. Data from studies performed so far indicate a more reliable, stable and predictable separation response. The latter also has the advantage of being more efficient and powerful in terms of subjects. Repetitive peer separations offer methodological advantages of repeated treatments and a potential for crossover designs, both important considerations for drug treatment studies.

Induction of Abnormal Behavior in Primates: Biological Techniques

The basic methodology involves selective depletion of one or more amines, combined with observation of resultant alterations in behavior. McKinney and Bunney (1969) reported the first use of depletion techniques in monkeys by the administration of reserpine. At a dosage of 4 mg/kg, given daily by intubation for 81 days to three monkeys, significant decreases in locomotion and visual exploration, and increased huddling and posturing were noted. The behavioral patterns have many similarities to those seen in the despair stage which may follow mother-infant separation. Agents more specific than reserpine which depletes both indolealkylamines and catecholamines in the brain and periphery, have been used in a somewhat limited way. Alphamethyl-paratyrosine (AMPT) blocks norepinephrine synthesis by inhibiting tyrosine hydroxylase. Monkeys treated with AMPT became inactive as seen by decreased initiated social behaviors, reduced locomotion, huddling and passivity.

Parachlorophenylalanine (PCPA), a serotonin synthesis inhibitor, has been reported to increase aggression in cats and rats, which contrasts with the findings of Redmond and McKinney who have reported that despite dose levels of up to 800 mg/kg there is little or no effect on monkey social behavior.

Because of the peripheral and central effects of both PCPA and AMPT, several investigators began to search for more refined methods of studying the relationship between the depletion of brain amines and behavior.

Breese reported on the neuropharmacology of 6-hydroxydopamine (6-OHDA) which, given centrally by intraventricular injection, selectively destroyed central noradrenergic neurons without affecting the serotoninergic or peripheral noradrenergic system. Since central noradrenergic depletions are postulated as one of the defects in human depressions, work has continued toward producing this depletion experimentally and studying its effects on urinary metabolites of norepinephrine and on social behaviors.

Using stereotaxic implantation of a guide cannula into the lateral cerebral ventricles, injections of 6-OHDA were

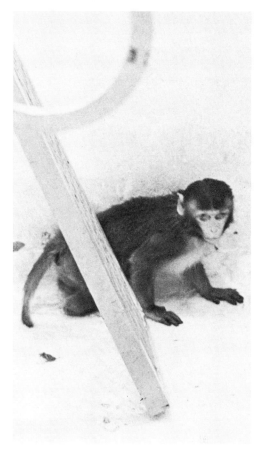

Fig. 3. Two-year-old Rhesus monkey showing ptosis and posturing following administration of reserpine, 5.0 mg/kg.

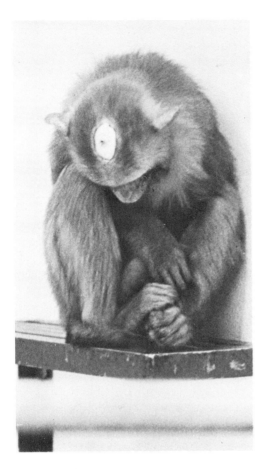

Fig. 4. Withdrawal and huddling of Rhesus monkey after receiving intraventricular 6-hydroxydopamine.

given to deplete central amines. Behavioral changes were characterized, on a chronic basis, by a shift away from the social environment to a seemingly compensatory exploration of the inanimate environment. Assays for brain norepinephrine showed an average whole brain depletion of 45% of the controls, with significant depletions found in the hippocampus, frontal, and parietal cortex. Brain dopamine was significantly depleted in the hippocampus and significantly increased in the medulla and pons. In contrast, neither urinary MHPG (3 methoxy-4-hydroxyphenylglycol) or VMA levels were found to be abnormally changed. Finding normal levels of urinary VMA or MHPG does not rule out the possibility that depletions of central amines may be sufficient to adversely affect behavior but not of a magnitude to alter urinary metabolites.

A fair statement might be that in primates, catecholamine depletion is accompanied by some of the behaviors seen in clinical depression, or the "despair" stage of anaclitic depression. However, many other of the signs and symptoms of depression are not observed in primates with central biogenic amine depletion.

In some current theories relating biogenic amines to depression, it has been speculated that an amine deficiency, of and by itself, is not sufficient to produce full-blown depressive symptomatology, but can when coupled with other factors (e.g., precipitating stresses). A great strength of animal modeling lies in its ability to critically evaluate such ideas. For example, a major area of concern has been the association between precipitating stresses and psychopathology. Among precipitating stresses, separation has been studied by several workers. With regard to depressive symptomatology, the data would suggest that separation events figure prominently among the possible precipitating stresses of depressive illness; however, they are probably not specific in eliciting depressive symptomatology. Furthermore, separation alone need not be a sufficient cause of depression, because many individuals who have apparently suffered it do not develop depression.

What would happen, though, if separation were coupled with a pre-existing amine depletion? This type of controlled experiment can be done with primates, and such experiments are now underway. Preliminary results indicate that there is an interaction between separation and amine-depletion, in that amine-depletion tends to intensify the behavioral effects of separation.

It is possible, then, in the case of animals to experimentally manipulate, under controlled conditions, several variables to study their interactional effects. In this way, the multicomponent nature of much human psychopathology (Fig. 1) can be studied experimentally in animals.

Rehabilitation of Abnormal Behavior in Primates

Social Techniques

Attempts to reverse these behavioral syndromes until recently have been relatively unsuccessful. Aversive conditioning used by Sackett saw little generalization of increased social contact. Adaptation to social playrooms prior to testing with social animals resulted in no change in the incompetent social behavior patterns. The potential responsiveness of these isolates was first noted when infants who continued to cling to the "motherless monkeys" were eventually able to have the mothers accept them for feeding. Following the second impregnation some of these isolate mothers showed appropriate maternal behavior, related to learning acceptability of contact. This observation led to the design of a study which employed the social stimuli of "monkey therapists," chosen from younger, normal monkeys. This first

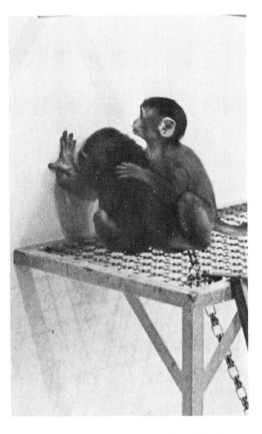

Fig. 5. Initial playroom behavior of isolate monkey on left and monkey therapist on right.

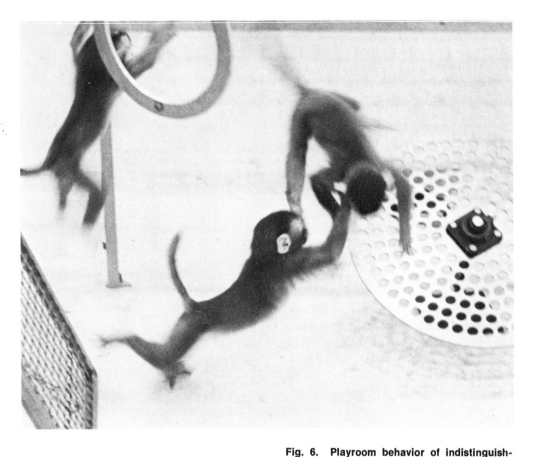

Fig. 6. Playroom behavior of indistinguishable isolate and therapist monkey after rehabilitation.

successful rehabilitation utilized three-month-old female animals as "therapists" for six-month isolates, all males.

The "therapy" consisted of isolates interacting with therapists on a one-to-one basis two hours per day at a frequency of three days a week and in groups of two isolates and two therapists in the playroom two days a week. Initially, the isolates showed high levels of stereotypic rocking disturbances, huddling, self-clasping and self-mouthing. Gradually, the isolates began reciprocating play behaviors and initiating play behaviors. Correlating with these changes were decreases in disturbance behaviors to insignificant levels, and by one year of age the isolates and therapists were equivalent in levels of non-social and social behaviors. Twelve-month isolates were also treated with this paradigm and showed similar results, with a follow-up at age three-and-a-half showing no regression in behavior, the formation of dominance hierarchies, nearly uniform acts of appropriate sexual behavior and minimum inappropriate aggression.

Biological Techniques

Social treatment has been successful and, in addition, rehabilitation has been effective with the use of pharmacological compounds. Chlorpromazine was given at two-and-a-half years of age to monkeys raised in partial social isolation for the first year of life. The dosage schedule of 7.5 mg/kg per day by intubation significantly decreased self-disturbance behaviors, with some social exploration and play seen within four to eight weeks of the regimen.

Pharmacological rehabilitation paradigms for reversal of deficits produced by social isolation led to work using diazepam, an antianxiety agent, following the premise of Novak and Harlow that reduction of anxiety would effect some degree of rehabilitation. Although only four subjects were used, the data showed that diazepam, like chlorpromazine, reduced disturbance behaviors. In comparison with chlorpromazine, diazepam more consistently led to increases in environmental exploration, and social and aggressive behaviors. These data argue against the conclusion that social isolation syndromes in primates are a model for human psychosis, though not necessarily ruling it out entirely. This follows from the recognition that chlorpromazine is not the only agent which can ameliorate abnormal behaviors of isolate Rhesus monkeys. Its effectiveness in producing therapeutic change in these monkeys may be due to its "non-specific" rather than its antipsychotic properties.

These data serve to illustrate that until comprehensive mechanism and rehabilitation studies are completed, the application of clinical labels to the abnormal behavior of animals is premature.

Aside from pharmacological agents used for the treatment of affective disorders, electrically induced convulsions (EIC) remain important in the treatment of serious depression. A pilot study in monkeys was undertaken by Lewis and McKinney to investigate two related issues. Those were whether EIC treatments would result in a change of the social interactions of the monkeys and would a therapeutic effect be seen on the abnormal behaviors shown by chamber-confined monkeys. To summarize, the control group which received sham EIC consisting of administration of anesthetic and neuromuscular blocking agents by themselves had a general lessening of activity. The experimental group showed a general activation effect with decreases noted in self-disturbance behaviors. Thus, this approach offers promise of helping to validate the usefulness of the social isolation model and may also be of value in studying the mechanisms associated with electroconvulsive therapy in humans.

The Task of the Future

This chapter has dealt with the contributions of animal models and experimental primatology to the behavioral and clinical sciences, particularly in the context of development. The major areas of special interest for scientists and clinicians in regard to primate behavioral research include: (1) the development of attachment behaviors; (2) the effects of social isolation and separation on the disruption of attachment bonds; (3) the long-term consequences of separation and isolation; and (4) the use of primate models to study the interactions between and consequences of social, biological

and environmental determinants of behavior.

Careful knowledge of the baseline behavior of the species being used is necessary in creating an experimental animal model. Key concepts involve an understanding of the definitions for those terms used in this chapter that are often erroneously equated with clinical definitions employed in psychiatry today. Depression is used here in the operational sense to refer to observable behavioral changes commonly associated with depressive syndromes in humans. In animals, these behaviors include changes in play activity, motor activity, sleep, and in the animal's responsiveness to its environment. Separation requires careful delineation of its attendant variables, with the understanding that it is more than just an event and needs definition in terms of the many parameters discussed earlier in the chapter.

In essence, the value of animal model systems are that: (1) they lend themselves to more direct control and manipulation of biological and social variables, this not being often possible in humans because of ethical or practical considerations; (2) the life span of the Rhesus monkey is greatly telescoped in comparison to the human one, thus enabling the more direct evaluation of early experiences and their contributions to development of behavior in later life; (3) the opportunity to study more directly the amine systems in the brain, without depending only on peripheral measures of their activity is another advantage of animal models; (4) giving drugs to produce experimental lesions postulated to be important in depression in man, and giving drugs to a species with wide repertoires of social behaviors, permits the controlled study of their effects on both biological and behavioral parameters; (5) continual re-evaluation of the nature of the relationship between biology and behavior will provide data to disallow either a deterministic or simplistic explanation of this relationship.

The induction methods for producing psychopathology merit reiteration. In object separation, infants are removed from mothers or from peers with the eliciting of a protest-despair reaction, similar to that seen in human infants in "anaclitic depression." Variation of the living situation with the infant permitted visual but not physical access to others intensifies the reaction in both protest and despair, with a greater intensification of the despair reaction. Age at separation is a critical variable for determining the reaction to separation. Peer-only reared monkeys under one year of age exhibit the biphasic reaction of protest and despair. Adolescent Rhesus monkeys show a uniphasic reaction of the protest stage with no observable emergence of the despair stage. If previously separated, animals show a significant increase in self-disturbance behaviors if separated again, whereas non-separated peer-reared monkeys respond with increases in locomotion and hyperactive type behaviors.

Biological induction methods involve the experimental alteration of brain and/or peripheral amine levels and the study of the changes in the behavior of the animal after these alterations. Reserpine produces behaviors similar to those seen in separated animals in the despair stage. However, once the drug is stopped, the behavior returns to normal. Alpha-methyl-para-tyrosine (AMPT), a norepinephrine blocker, produces a syndrome similar to that of a reserpinized animal. Parachlorophenylalanine, an inhibitor of serotonin synthesis, produces no major behavioral changes. Intraventricular 6-hydroxy-dopamine is currently thought to specifically destroy noradrenergic nerve terminals in the brain but not in the periphery. This tool is being explored to evaluate the contribution of peripheral and central amines in regulating social behavior.

Rehabilitation studies, social and biological, are being used alone and in combination to investigate not only the reversal of the abnormal syndromes produced but also for clarification of the possible facilitative and interactive effects of combined therapeutic approaches.

What of the question of "relevance" of the animal model in the study of behavior and its applicability to the human? The amusement or wonder used in reporting anecdotes of animal behavior lead to these theories being rarely incorporated into a process of theorizing about human psychology. On the other hand, excessive anthropomorphism has often alienated thoughtful students of human psychopathology and animal behavior. However, there exists little doubt that the ability to experimentally manipulate behavior is a tool of considerable significance for the clinician. The special advantages of experimentation over isolated clinical observations in the study of psychopathology have been amply described.

Future studies need to focus on social and neurobiological mechanisms underlying the syndromes of abnormal behavior produced in the laboratory. Basic studies of neurobiochemical and genetic components can eventually yield theories more fundamental to the understanding of human behavior. Animal models provide for an open systems approach in these and other areas relevant to human psychopathology.

Selected References

Harlow, H.F., and Harlow, M.K.: Psychopathology in monkeys. In *Experimental Psychopathology: Recent Research and Theory,* H.D. Kimmel, ed. Academic Press, Inc., New York, 1971, pp. 203-229.

Hebb, D.O., and Thompson, W.R.: The social significance of animal studies. In *Handbook of Social Psychology,* Vol. 1, Theory and Method, G. Lindzey, ed. Addison-Wesley, Cambridge, 1954, pp. 532-561.

Hinde, R.H., and Spencer-Booth, Y.: Effects of brief separation from mother on Rhesus monkeys. *Science* 173:111-118, 1971.

Kubie, L.A.: The experimental induction of neurotic reactions in man. *Yale J. Biol. Med.* 11:541-545, 1939.

Lewis, J.K., McKinney, W.T., Young, L.D., and Kramer, G.W.: Rhesus monkeys as a model of human depression: A reconsideration. *Arch. Gen. Psychiat.* 33:699-705, 1976.

McKinney, W.T.: Primate social isolation: Psychiatric implications. *Arch. Gen. Psychiat.* 31:422-426, 1974.

McKinney, W.T., and Bunney, W.E.: Animal model of depression: Review of evidence, implications for research. *Arch. Gen. Psychiat.* 21:240-248, 1969.

Redmond, D.E., Maas, J.W., Kling, A., Graham, C.W., and Dekirmenjian, H.: Social behavior of monkeys selectively depleted of monoamines. *Science* 174:428-431, 1971.

Seligman, M.E.P., Maier, S.F., and Geer, J.: The alleviation of learned helplessness in dogs. *J. Abnorm. Soc. Psychol.* 73:256-262, 1968.

Senay, E.C.: Toward an animal model of depression: A study of separation behavior in dogs. *J. Psychiat. Res.* 4:65-71, 1966.

Spitz, R.A.: Anaclitic depression: An inquiry into the genesis of psychiatric conditions in early childhood II. *Psychoanal. Study Child* 2:313-342, 1946.

Chapter 8

Clinical Studies of Brain Organization and Behavior

Raquel E. Gur
Jerre Levy and
Ruben C. Gur

Introduction

The conception of the brain as the organ of the mind goes back to at least classical Greece. Hippocrates (460–377 B.C.) was struck by the apparent unity of mind emerging from a brain whose structures constitute two symmetrical organs, one on the left and one on the right. The problem of correlating cerebral anatomy with psychological pro-cesses has been, for over two millennia, and still is of major concern to those who seek to understand the biological bases of behavior. Descartes (1596–1650), in attempting to resolve the paradox of a unity of mental function and a duality of brain anatomy, concluded that the single monomorphic structure of the brain, the pineal gland, was the seat of the mind. Apart from the host of philosophical difficulties entailed by a mind-body dualism, this conception has no scientific utility. Neuroscientists have been increasingly successful at identifying the relationship which exists between cerebral and cognitive organizations. It has even been shown that the

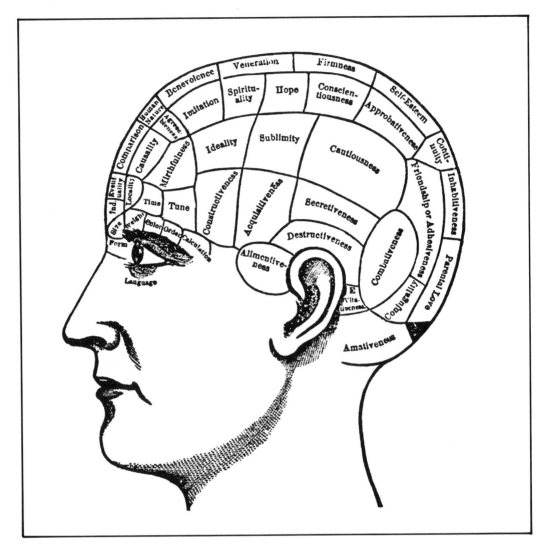

Fig. 1. Functional localization according to the theory of phrenology (from Davis, 1955).

left and right cerebral hemispheres generate two different cognitive and conative modes of mentation, thus questioning the view of consciousness as unitary and substantiating the value of a biological approach to problems of human psychology.

Although the relationship between brain organization and behavior has been acknowledged for over a hundred years, there has been a wide discrepancy in views over the nature of the relationship. On the one hand, there have been

those who conceived of the bain as acting holistically, no part dominating over any other in the control of any function. On the other hand, the brain has been seen as consisting of many distinctive parts, each responsible for subserving a particular function. Early neurologists sought the localization of specific sensations, perceptions, memories, and ideas. An extreme position was held by Henschen, a 19th Century neurologist, who postulated that single ideas were located in single neurons. A more prevalent, and hardly less radical position, was represented by Gall's phrenology (Fig. 1). This theory claimed that the personality of people could be inferred from the conformation of the skull, which reflected underlying expansions of the brain.

For example, people who had a slight protrusion of the anterior portion of the temporal bone were said to be attracted to wine. It became clear, however, from a number of clinical observations, that while the basic sensory modalities were integrated in different regions of the cortex, higher level functions seemed to be affected by lesions occurring almost anywhere in the brain. Such findings led Kurt Goldstein, over half a century ago, to the conclusion that it was invalid to attempt localization of function, that when any region of the brain was damaged, there was an entire reorganization of the personality as an adaptive reaction to the insult. Simultaneously, Karl Lashley, a neuropsychologist, in his investigations of the effects of experimental brain lesions in rats, was suggesting the principle of mass-action by which the severity of behavioral deficits were said to be a function of the amount, rather than the location of cerebral damage. The holistic, mass-action view of brain function held sway over neurological thinking until the middle of the 20th Century. However, throughout all these developments, there was a consensus that regardless of the generality of the mass-action principle for most functions, language processes, as Paul Broca had postulated in 1861, were integrated entirely in the left cerebral hemisphere of right-handers.

During the last 25–30 years, a new synthesis has been emerging, in which it is recognized that although functions and faculties can not be said to reside in particular regions of the brain, nevertheless, quite specific functional defects arise from disruption of particular brain regions. It is established that certain neural pathways, and certain groups of neurons, play a particularly critical role in the integration of processes such as the interpretation of complex spatial relations. At the same time, electrophysiological investigations strongly suggest that wide-spread changes occur all over the brain during the anticipation and processing of sensory input and motor output. The various regions of the central nervous system are mutually interdependent for the integrity of their functions. The emergence of any neurological syndrome is as likely to be due to the release from inhibition of an intact part of the brain, as it is to the destruction of regions whose excitation is necessary for maintaining the function. As an example, certain symptoms of Parkinson's disease can be alleviated by destructive neurosurgery which removes overactive non-inhibited portions of the basal ganglia.

In the sections to follow, we shall first review the methods which scientists utilize in their attempts to understand the neurological mechanisms underlying behavior. Secondly, we shall present current evidence relating to the neurological bases of intellectual and emotional functioning. Finally, findings pertaining to inter-individual variability in brain functioning will be discussed.

Methods of Investigation

There are two fundamental methods available for assessing the functional relations among variables under investigation. The first can be described as *correlative*, while the second is *experimental or manipulative*. In the correlative method, an attempt is made to deduce the structure of interrelations in naturally occurring variations in two or more variables. As an example, one might wish to determine the nature of electroencephalographic (EEG) pattern as a function of state of arousal. With the correlative method, one would measure the EEG during naturally occurring changes in state of arousal. In the experimental method, the investigator produces variation in the independent variable and observes the consequent changes in the dependent variable. Thus, in the above example, the experimentalist would artificially manipulate states of arousal (e.g., by drug injection), and observe the resulting EEG changes. It is often asserted by certain neuroscientists, particularly by animal experimentalists, that the experimental method is far more powerful than the correlative method, and is the only one which allows conclusions to be drawn regarding causal control of one variable over another. This, however, is an oversimplification. On many occasions, causal relations can be inferred with a high degree of confidence from correlational data (as, for example, Darwin's principle of Natural Selection). Conversely, one may arrive at erroneous statements about causality from experimental procedures (e.g., the theory of spontaneous generation). It should be kept in mind, that in some of the more advanced sciences, such as physics and astrophysics, major theoretical breakthroughs have been based on correlational observations. In the study of brain-behavior relations, both methods have been essential in guiding us to our present state of knowledge.

Measures of Brain Activity and Organization

Although a refined picture of the organization of the brain can only be gained *post mortem* via histological techniques, this method is of little value to the clinician who may require neuroanatomical knowledge for both diagnosis and treatment. For the basic scientist, likewise, progress in neuropsychological understanding could be retarded for 50 years if the researcher could draw no conclusions regarding a patient's neurological condition until after his death. Fortunately, neurologists, and, recently, psychologists have devised various tools which allow them to draw inferences regarding cerebral organization in the living human subject.

Electroencephalography — One of the most widely used measures of brain activity is the electroencephalographic recording obtained when electrodes are attached to various points on the skull and voltage differences between a reference and recording electrodes are monitored for amplitude and frequency. Although, as of yet, there is no understanding of the detailed neurophysiological events underlying the EEG, it is known that certain patterns of activity are generally present during certain behavioral states.

Conjugate lateral eye movements — That eye movements are a behavioral consequence of cerebral activation may be inferred from the fact that stimulation of one side of the brain with cortical electrodes induces contralateral eye deviations because of the asymmetry of activation of the two sides of the brain. Such asymmetry also follows brain lesions, the intact side usually being more active, with the result, on some occasions, that the eyes continuously sweep toward the side of space ipsilateral to the lesion. Recently it has been demonstrated that the direction of lateral eye movements in neurologically normal populations is an indicant of asymmetric cerebral activation. As will be discussed in later sections, this index is correlated with a number of personality and cognitive factors. Consequently, eye movements have become an increasingly important tool in assessing neuropsychological relationships.

Sensory and motoric losses — Another approach available for the student of brain-behavior relationships utilizes neuroanatomical knowledge in order to make inferences regarding the location of neurological lesions from sensory, motor, affective, or cognitive defects. Since most of the afferent and efferent pathways from one side of the body decussate and lead to the contralateral hemisphere, it is possible to infer the side of brain damage by knowledge of the side of the body which is paralyzed or numb. If consistent cognitive deficits are then found to be associated with the malfunctioning side of the body, inferences can be drawn as to the cognitive aspect subserved by the contralateral hemisphere. As associations between psychological disorders and localized cerebral damage are repeatedly confirmed, the psychological disorders themselves become localizing symptoms.

Radiology — One of the methods for localizing lesions is known as arteriography. This method involves the injection of a radiopaque substance into the internal carotid arteries, thus enabling the detection of abnormalities in the chief cerebral blood vessels by radiography. Other procedures for detecting abnormalities are the ventriculogram and the encephalogram. In the first, spinal fluid is withdrawn and then oxygen is injected into the lumbar subarachnoid space. In the second procedure, oxygen is introduced by tapping the posterior horn of the lateral ventricle after the removal of a small area of bone.

Tachistoscopic and dichotic listening procedures — For a number of years, psychologists have been utilizing certain behavioral measurement techniques wthout realizing their pertinence for assessing aspects of brain organization. It is only in the past few years that these techniques have been applied to the study of the functional organization of the brain. *Tachistoscopic presentation* involves very rapid visual presentation of

stimuli, in the right and left visual fields, while the subject maintains fixation on a central point. The visual presentations last no longer than 200 milliseconds, which is too brief a period for eye movements to occur. Subjects are either required to indicate the stimulus seen and accuracy rates are determined, or they are required to respond as rapidly as possible in a discrimination test and reaction time constitutes the measure of interest. Since the human brain is laterally differentiated in function, and since the left and right visual fields project to the contralateral hemispheres, depending on the nature of the visual discrimination test, either the left or right visual field (and, by inference, the contralateral hemisphere) will be superior on task performance. By measuring the performance level of the superior hemisphere on some tasks, and by determining the differential performances of the two sides of the brain, it is possible to learn a great deal about functional brain organization.

The *dichotic listening* procedure, based on similar principles, utilizes simultaneous input of two different auditory stimuli to the two ears. Although the auditory pathways project bilaterally, it appears that *the ispilateral channel is subordinate to the contralateral channel.* Consequently, a right ear discrimination superiority indicates left hemisphere specialization for a listening task and vice versa.

Both the visual field and dichotic listening techniques have been predominantly used for measuring lateral organization of the brain in normal populations, and have rarely been applied to clinical groups. However, psychiatrists and neurologists are increasingly coming to realize the potential value of these behavioral tests.

Measures of Psychological Function

An enormous variety of psychological tests are currently available for assessing characteristics ranging from intelligence

and personality to hypnotic susceptibility and psychopathology. There are
literally thousands of tests described in
the *Yearbook of Mental Measurements*,
designed to measure almost any conceivable trait. In addition to these
standardized tests, it is possible to learn
a great deal about behavior from infor-
mal interviews. A clinician can determine the general memory function,
orientation of the patient in time and
place, his emotional state, insight into his
problems, etc.

Most of the tests used in an attempt
to understand the relation between neurological and psychological functions,
have concentrated on the assessment of
cognitive structure. Probably the single
most widely used test is the *Wechsler
Adult Intelligence Scale (WAIS)*. This
test is divided into 11 subtests designated
as follows: Information, Comprehension,
Similarities, Arithmetic, Digit Span, Vo-
cabulary Digit Symbol, Picture Completion, Picture Arrangement, Block Design
and Object Assembly. The sum of scores
on the first six of these yields the so-
called Verbal I.Q., while that of the
latter five yields the so-called Performance I.Q. The total score on all 11

tests represents the full-scale I.Q. measure. The pattern of scores on the various
subtests, as well as the comparative
ability on the verbal and performance
scales, can provide much information
about cognitive structure.

Another test frequently used by neuropsychologists is the *Bender-Gestalt*, in
which the patient is asked to *copy a
series of simple designs*. The nature and
extent of deviations from the standard
reflect various kinds of cognitive disintegration. For example, if a patient is required to copy a wavy line with three
peaks and three troughs and he produces
a wavy line which continues all the way
across the page and which contains as
many waves as space will permit, this is
indicative of the loss of inhibitory function. It is a regressive characteristic in
that it is often seen in very young children.

Other widely used tests include the
Street Figure Completion Test (Fig. 2),
the *Witkin Embedded Figure Test*, the
Benton Revised Visual Retention Test,
the *Reitan Neuropsychological Battery*,
and tests of *left-right orientation and
map reading*.

Psychological Manifestations of Neurological Lesions

For a number of years, clinicians had
made an attempt to differentiate those
cases of behavioral pathology which were
said to be functional from those which
were thought to have an organic basis.
It is coming to be recognized, however,
that ultimately *all behavior has its origins in the functioning of the nervous
system* and that all behavioral pathologies are, therefore, reflections of cerebral
dysfunction. This does not mean that
the psychological environment has no
effect. To the contrary, cerebral dysfunction itself can be a direct consequence of psychological stress and many
times can be alleviated by psychother-

apy. It should also be kept in mind that
biochemical and sometimes even surgical interventions are the most effective
and, in certain instances, the only means
of treatment. Since all behavior is a
reflection of the patterns of activity in
the brain, and this holds equally for
normal, psychiatric, and neurological
populations, it follows that variations
in behavioral patterns are manifestations
of the state of equilibrium of the brain.
Even in cases of extreme neurospychiat-
ric syndromes, whether due to psychological stress, toxicity, or gross brain
lesions, the symptoms stem from extreme
disequilibrium of the brain in which

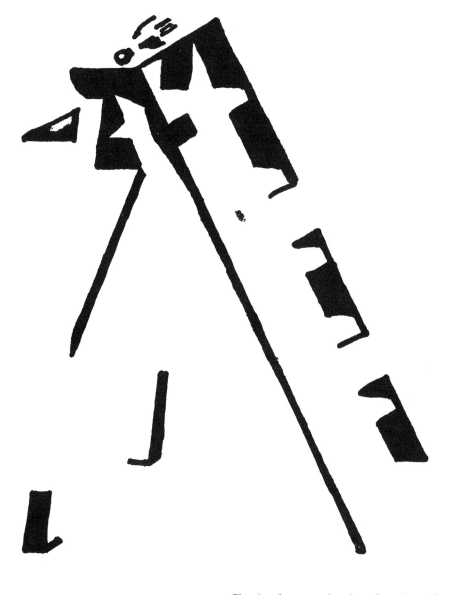

Fig. 2. An example of an item from the Street Figure Completion Test (from Street, 1931).

there is either over-excitation or pro-found inhibition of regions which are normally in dynamic equilibrium. In fact, these syndromes seem to be marked deviations along the continuum of normal behavioral variations.

For the following sections, in which the major neuropathological syndromes

will be presented, the reader may wish to refer to Fig. 3 to remind himself of the major cortical regions.

The Aphasias

Prior to 1836, it was thought that the human brain, like the animal brain, was

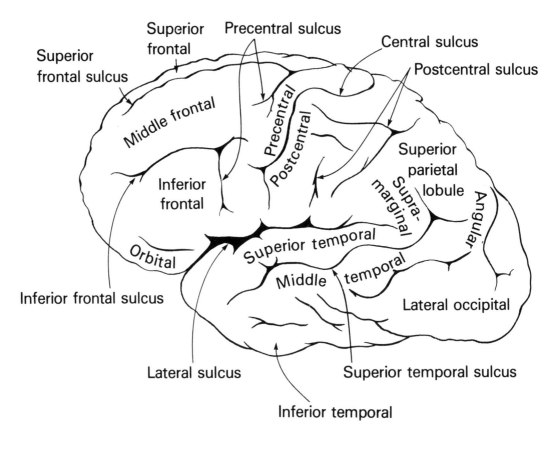

Fig. 3.   Major divisions of the cerebral cortex (from Gardner, 1975).

bilaterally symmetric in function, reflecting the apparent symmetry of structure. In that year, Marc Dax presented a paper in which he claimed that speech disorders were associated with right hemiplegia and left cerebral lesions. It was not until 1861, when Paul Broca reported two cases of aphasia with post mortem examination, that the association between speech disorders and left hemisphere lesions became generally accepted. Broca maintained that: "the integrity of the third gyrus (and possibly of the second) appears to be indispensible for the use of the faculty of articulated speech". The word, aphasia", in reference to speech disorders, was proposed by Trousseau in 1864. It

should be noted that the various aphasic symptoms are exaggerations of the occasional linguistic dysfunctions to which all people are susceptible at times. In particular, expressive aphasia often involves phonetic distortions, distortions which are also observed during the development of speech in the child and under conditions of cortical inhibition in adults produced by extreme fatigue, alcohol, or any other de-encephalizing conditions. The inability to think of an appropriate word has been experienced by all of us, and psychologists have even labeled this frustrating experience as the "tip-of-the-tongue phenomenon." In receptive aphasia, one of the most salient characteristics is the patient's utterance of a meaningless string of words, which he insists makes perfect sense. When the physician quotes back to him what he has said, the patient vigorously denies that he was responsible for such a meaningless statement. Again, we see a mild form of this phenomenon in normal people when they occasionally substitute one word for another which they intended, and deny having made the substitution. The resemblance between aphasic symptoms and the language misusages of neurologically intact individuals underlines the fact that in both cases there is a disequilibrium of inhibition and excitation among various brain regions.

The Apraxias

The apraxias refer to disorders of gestures and action. There are a variety of different apraxias, such as ideomotor apraxia, ideational apraxia and constructional apraxia.

In *constructional apraxia,* for example, there is a defect in the representation of Euclidean space. Great deficiencies are seen in drawing, where there is a disappearance of perspective in mild cases, and the total absence of a recognizable configuration in severe cases. There are two kinds of defects, both of which are referred to as constructional apraxia, one arising from lesions of the right cerebral hemisphere, and the other from lesions of the left cerebral hemisphere in right-handers. In the right hemisphere, form disturbances are generally more severe. Drawings are lacking in configuration and are constituted of many separate parts of the object to be represented, the parts being without a structural relation to each other. Furthermore, the left side of the page is

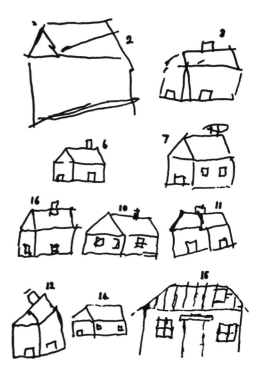

Right Hemisphere Lesions
(Left Hemisphere Intact)

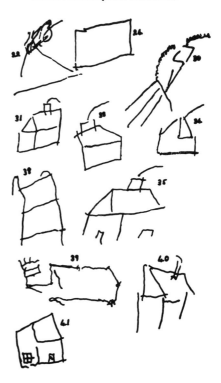

Fig. 4. Copies of a house drawn by patients with lesions of the left or right hemisphere (from Piercy et al., 1960).

neglected, and there is a gross disturbance of the axes of the figures. In the left hemisphere form neither side of the page is neglected, the axes of the figures are correctly represented, and the main defect is a profound absence of details in the drawing, while good configuration is preserved (Fig. 4).

Constructional apraxias usually result from lesions of the parietal lobe, particularly in the region of the angular gyrus and sometimes extending to the posterior part of the first temporal convolution. As in the case of the aphasias, the apraxias seem to be an extreme manifestation of normal behavioral variants.

The Agnosias

The agnosias consist of an *impaired recognition of an object* in which sensory defects, mental deterioration, or nonfamiliarity with the object is not responsible for the impairment; also, typically, but not always, an object which is not recognized through one sensory modality can be recognized through another. Many different types of agnosias exist. Among them are: (1) *spatial agnosia,* a unilateral neglect of the left half of space and, at times, the left side of the patient's body. This syndrome is due to *lesions of the parieto-occipital area of the right hemisphere in right-handers.* (2) *Facial agnosia,* another defect due to right hemispheric lesions, in which the patient, although able to identify his friends and relatives through their voices, or by various items of clothing, cannot recognize them by their facial features. (3) *Anosognosia,* a denial of illness. In this syndrome, the patient denies completely that he displays any defects of function deriving from his lesion. The attempt to demonstrate the various dysfunctions to the patient can lead to a great display of anger. The anosognostic syndrome often occurs in conjunction with other neurologically caused disorders and it is almost always present in cases of aphasia resulting from lesions to Wernicke's area. Anosognosia possibly demonstrates, better than any other neurological syndrome that, in the presence of neurological insult, the patient undergoes a readjustment in his entire cognitive and personality structure. A lesion in the cortex of the brain, thus, not only produces a direct consequence, but triggers in the patient a compensatory reorganization which allows him to deal with the fact that the very organ of his mind has been partly destroyed.

The Amnesias

The amnesic syndrome is characterized by a severe disorder of memory in spite of normal intelligence, perceptual skills, or other cognitive functions. It can result from *temporal lobe surgery, electroconvulsive shock, alcoholism, encephalitis,* or any form of *trauma to the brain.* There are two basic types of amnesia, referred to as retrograde and anterograde.

In *retrograde amnesia* memories are lost for events antedating the onset of illness by months or even years. The closer in time are the events to the beginning of the illness, the more profound the memory loss. Remote memories are usually well preserved, while recently experienced events are not remembered. On many occasions, memory function recovers, first for the more distant past, and moving up in time toward events just preceding the beginning of illness. Recovery of memories means, of course, that the memories had not been erased during the amnesia, but had become inaccessible to retrieval.

In *anterograde amnesia,* defective learning and retention of ongoing events is the central component. Patients with the severest form of this disorder are totally incapable of retaining anything they have learned more than a few seconds previously. As one patient with this disorder says, "Every moment is like waking from a dream." This form of amnesia results from bilateral hippo-campectomies, senility, alcoholism and any other disease which produces lesions of the medial thalamus. Its specificity of effects is quite remarkable. The first patient ever described with anterograde amnesia, in a report published in 1889 by S. S. Korsakoff, was able to play a good game of chess (learned, of course, prior to the disease) despite being unable to remember the course of moves which had brought about the current position on the board.

Anterograde amnesia appears to be a disorder of consolidation in which short-term memories (of a few seconds) are intact and remote memories are intact, but the contents of short-term memory cannot be transferred into a long-term store, so that nothing new can be learned.

In summary, the neurological syndromes just described clearly indicate that pathology of the brain results in major behavioral changes. The most dramatic example of the relation between brain function and observed behavior is the case of the commissurotomized patients described below.

The Commissurotomy Syndrome

Until the early part of the 1960's, such symptoms as alexia, agraphia, ideomotor apraxia, apathy, and amnesia, as well as various personality changes had been ascribed to lesions of the corpus callosum. Typically, however, such lesions resulted from tumors or cerebral vascular accidents, and it is likely that the symptoms observed were caused by extracallosal damage. During the 1940's, a series of 25 patients underwent complete surgical division of the corpus callosum for the control of intractable epilepsy. Psychological investigations of these patients revealed no symptoms which could be attributed to division of the corpus callosum, leading a famous neuropsychologist, Carl Lashley, to suggest jokingly that the sole function of

this massive bridge of fibers was to support the cerebral hemispheres. However, during the 1960's, Philip Vogel and Josept Bogen performed complete neo-commisurotomies, sectioning the *corpus callosum, the anterior and posterior commisures, and in some cases, the massa intermedia*, all in a single operation. Their patients, like the earlier group, were all epileptics and the surgery proved to be quite effective in controlling generalized convulsions. A long series of studies of their psychological functioning has been continued since that time, for the most part in the psychobiology laboratory of Roger Sperry (1964) at the California Institute of Technology. In normal everyday behavior, the patients exhibit no obvious changes in personality, intellect, mannerisms, conversation, strength, vigor, or even bimanual coordination. They seem, to all outward appearances, to be perfectly normal and it would seem quite impossible for a casual observer to detect that the most massive tract of fibers in the brain had been completely severed. However, careful laboratory investigation conducted by Sperry and Gazzaniga, revealed that these patients have two sets of perceptions, two sets of memories, two motivational systems. In other words, two streams of consciousness, each proceeding independently of and totally unaware of the other, one in each side of the brain. Objects which are placed in one hand of a patient, the hand hidden from view, cannot be cross-matched by the other hand. A picture shown in one visual half-field, and therefore to the contralateral cerebral hemisphere, is not known or recognized by the other half of the brain. Because only the left hemisphere is capable of expressive language, objects placed in the patient's right hand or right visual field can be easily named, while those placed in his left hand or left visual field cannot be verbally described. Nevertheless, it has been repeatedly demonstrated that, in spite of its

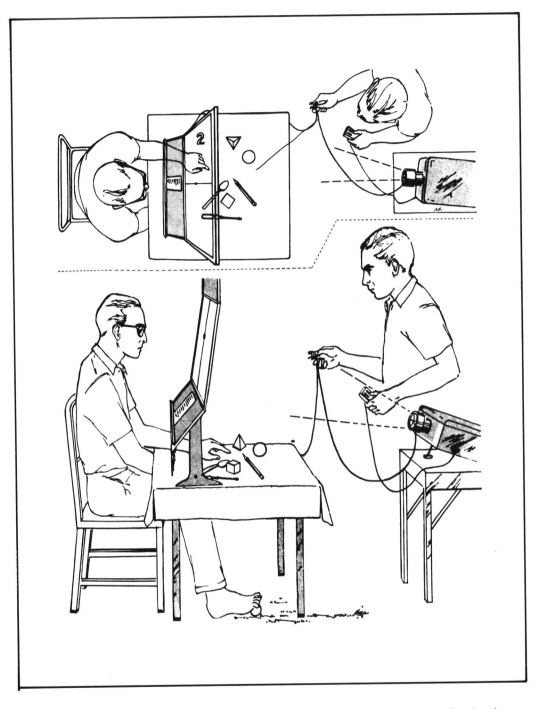

Fig. 5. Typical method of testing hemispheric function in commissurotomy patients (from Sperry et al., 1969).

total expressive aphasia, the right hemisphere is fully aware of what it has seen or felt. If the commissurotomy patient is told to fixate on some central point and a picture of some object such as a toothbrush, is briefly flashed into the left visual field (right hemisphere), though the patient is unable to say what he saw, he can easily point with his left hand to a matching picture, or can retrieve by touch from a large array of objects the tothbrush he saw. If so directed, he can even pick out by touch some object which has some categorical relationship with the perceived object (e.g., a tube of toothpaste) (see Fig. 5 for an illustration of the basic experimental setup). Note that the right hemisphere is capable of following verbal test instructions, and is thus competent at *understanding* language, in spite of its inability to speak. The sensory projections appear to be bilateral for every simple tactual or visual information. A touch or a flash of light, occurring in the left or right sensory fields, is detected by both hemispheres. However, tactual or visual pattern information is only accessible to the contralateral half-brain. The patient's left and right hands are hidden from his view by a screen, and two different pictures are simultaneously flashed to the left and right visual half fields. The patient is then directed to select by touch, from a large set of objects the stimulus he had seen. Under these conditions, each hand will tactually explore the various objects hidden behind the streen, continuing its exploration, totally ignoring the object for which the other hand is searching, until it identifies the simulus presented in the ipsilateral field. One might wonder how one hemisphere reacts to behavior which is under control of the other. In one experiment a series of pictures were flashed to the right hemisphere of a female patient in order to ascertain the emotional reaction which would occur when a pictue of a nude was inserted into the series of slides. Immediately af-

ter this picture was shown the patient blushed, giggled, and said: "Oh, Dr. Sperry, that's some machine!" When asked what she had seen, she replied that she didn't know, but, again, indicated that it had been something funny. We interpret this sequence of behavior to mean that the right hemisphere became embarrassed at seeing the nude and was responsible for the blushing, grinning and giggling, and that the left hemisphere, confronted by behavior for which it could not account, inferred that whatever had been seen justified the behavior. The verbalization which it produced we interpret as a rationalization.

The foregoing examples clearly show that both hemispheres are capable of sensory understanding, of carrying out task instructions, of making mental associations, and of emotional reactions. However, as the reader may have inferred from the differing apraxic, agnostic and amnestic disorders following upon lesions to one or the other cerebral hemispheres, the left and right sides of the brain are laterally differentiated not only for language functions, but in a number of other ways as well. Although it is possible to gain some notion of the nature of this asymmetry from patients having unilateral lesions, in order to do so one must make a series of assumptions which may or may not hold. In addition, even if these assumptions are valid, the picture that can be developed could, at best, be vague and incomplete. In support of this claim, as late as 1962 most neurologists, in spite of their knowledge of the various unilateral syndromes discussed, still believed that the only asymmetric function in the hemispheres was language. With the availability of the split-brained patients for psychological testing, it has been possible to gain a far deeper understanding of cerebral lateralization which has led to a radically new conception of human brain function.

Evidence gathered through careful testing of the commissurotomy patients,

Choice Stimuli

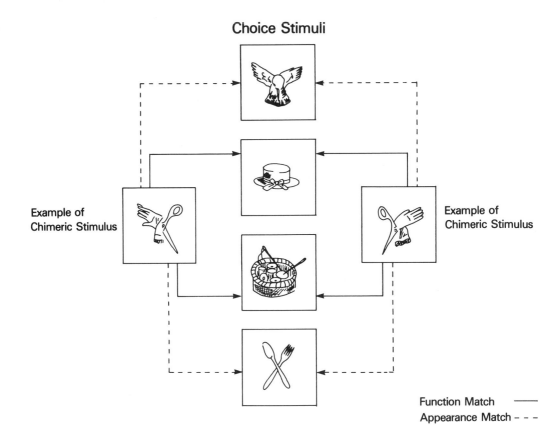

Example of
Chimeric Stimulus

Example of
Chimeric Stimulus

Function Match ———
Appearance Match – – –

Fig. 6. An example of a double stimulus shown to split-brain patients and the choices available to them. When patients were making a function choice they matched the stimulus to a choice which was functionally related to it. When patients were making an appearance match, they made their choice on the basis of physical resemblance (from Levy, 1977).

accumulating over the last ten years, proves beyond any doubt that the right cerebral hemisphere is just as specialized in its own set of cognitive functions as is the left. The first observations giving any indication of the double specialization of the brain were made by Bogen. During the first few months after surgery, when patients were asked to copy figures using their left or right hand, a profound dyscopia was apparent with right hand copying. This was

so in spite of the fact that these patients were right-handed. Furthermore, although the left hand performed adequately on the Block Design subtest of the WAIS, the right hand manifested almost total incapacity. In other words, the right hand, but not the left, suffered from constructional apraxia. Since, during the recovery period following surgery, motor control of the hands is strictly contralateral, these findings mean that the left hemisphere was defective in those capacities mediating constructional apraxia. Fortunately for the patients, but unfortunately for the investigator, bilateral motor control develops with recovery from surgery. Consequently, assessment of right hemisphere specializations cannot be obtained via dependence on lateralization of the motor system following full recovery. Presumably, this bilateral control is mediated by the ipsilateral pyramidal tracts. In the absence of motor lateralization, the separate functions of the two hemispheres can be tested through unilateral sensory input. Using this technique, Jerre Levy and Roger Sperry found that when patients must tactually explore a three dimensional form and match it with an "opened-up," two dimensional visual representation, they were greatly superior when using their left hands to feel the stimulus form. This finding reveals that, in addition to the praxic advantage shown previously for the right hemisphere, it also excells in spatial gnosis. A recent technique developed by Levy, Trevarthan and Sperry (Fig. 6) has allowed investigators to look at the differing "intentional" specializations of the two hemispheres, that is, at the conditions under which each hemisphere becomes activated and takes control over behavior. With this procedure two different stimuli are simultaneously projected, one to each hemisphere, and the patient is asked to point to one of an array of pictures, displayed in free vision in front of him, which matches in some way the stimulus he has perceived. Although each hemisphere has received its own stimulus input, it has been found that patients select only one of the two possible matches. It is as if sensory input has only been processed up to the level of consciousness in a single hemisphere. If the matching task involves selection of a choice which is identical in every way to the stimulus, these patients invariably select the picture which was seen by the right hemisphere. Apparently, when visual identity matches must be made, it is the right hemisphere which becomes activated and takes control of behavior. When matches between stimulus and choice require semantic decoding of the stimulus, or the formulation of phonetic images of stimuli and choices, or the catergorization of stimuli and choices into a superordinate class, then it is the left hemisphere which becomes activated and which takes control of behavior.

In summary, deductions from many experiments converge to produce the following picture of hemispheric specialization. *The left hemisphere may be described as symbolic, categorical, logical, analytic, propositional, a serial processor*, all of which might account for its superiority in linguistic functions. *The right hemisphere, by contrast, may be described as concrete, holistic, intuitive, synthetic, appositional, a parallel processor*, all of which might account for its superiority in visuo-spatial and imagistic functions.

Implications for Human Psychology

As should be apparent from the nature of the various symptoms which follow neurological damage, a state of disequilibrium in dynamic interactions among portions of the brain is an invariant characteristic of all neuropsychological syndromes. As emphasized earlier, other factors ranging from pathological to adaptive produce changes in the inhibitory-excitatory relationships of the nervous system. It is for this reason that the neurological syndromes have such relevance for the understanding of the neural basis of the whole spectrum of behavior. Not surprisingly, therefore, studies of normal populations, using some of the techniques described earlier, have confirmed and extended deductions drawn from neurological patients. In the sections to follow, we shall discuss the empirical findings and the new theoretical insights which they have produced over the last twenty years.

The Basic Pattern of Organization

Tachistoscopic studies — During the 1950's, a series of tachistoscopic studies were conducted on normal populations, in which words or letters were briefly flashed in the left or right visual fields. It was found that subjects were consistently more accurate in reporting stimuli which had appeared on the right. At the time, various interpretations of this phenomenon were offered, e.g., selective training to read material in the left hemiretinae, superiority of crossed optic fibers in transmitting information from the dominant eye (usually right), direction of the perceptual scan, etc. In 1959, it was discovered, however, that the majority of people were better at recognizing nonverbal forms which appeared in the left visual field. Clearly, then, the explanations offered for the right field superiority for words would not be correct, for if they were, a right-field superiority should emerge for forms as well. It was not until the sixties that the etiology of these effects was finally understood and accepted by most researchers. A wealth of data is now available giving proof that the asymmetries in perception under tachistoscopic conditions derive from the fact that the human brain is laterally differentiated in function. *When any form of verbal material is displayed briefly, a right field recognition superiority almost always emerges, reflecting the language specialization of the left cerebral hemisphere.* It has been shown by Kimura

and others that a left-field superiority occurs for recognition of patterns, dot localization, binocular depth perception, dot and form enumeration, discrimination of line slopes, and other nonverbal material, reflecting the specialization of the right cerebral hemisphere for visuospatial functions.

Recent findings demonstrate that the capacities of the two cerebral hemispheres undergo a dynamic fluctuation because of shifts in attention, presumably under control of brain-stem activation centers. As Levy and Trevarthen deduced from work with split-brained patients, there appears to be an asymmetric allocation of activation into the left or right hemisphere, in accordance with the adaptive demands confronting the person. Problems necessitating the specialized capacities of one or the other half brain usually result in the selective arousal of the appropriate hemisphere. Such asymmetric arousal can produce an orientation reflex, or its covert homologue, an attentional bias, toward the contralateral half of space. Thus, a verbal problem will selectively activate the left hemisphere and an attentional bias toward the left.

Dichotic listening studies — Lateralization of the brain is also reflected in accuracy measures in response to auditory input to the left and right ears. It will be recalled that the dichotic listening technique involves the simultaneous input of two different messages to the two ears. If the messages are verbal, i.e., words, digits, or syllables, subjects give more accurate reports to the right ear stimuli. If on the other hand, the auditory input consists of environmental sounds, laughs, musical chords, or musical melodies, there is a left-ear advantage. It has been postulated by Kimura that although the auditory pathways from each ear are bilaterally projected, under dichotic conditions the ipsilateral input is inhibited by the simultaneously arriving contralateral input. However, it has been recently found that ear asymmetries emerge even under monaural listening conditions. It is now believed that the contralateral auditory pathway is a more efficient channel for information transmission and suffers from a smaller loss than the ipsilateral pathway.

These techniques, and others similar to them, using the tactile modality, may eventually be of great value in the diagnosis of clinical populations and in planning therapeutic programs.

Perceptual asymmetries under normal viewing conditions — The fact that manifestations of cerebral asymmetry appear in normal populations under laboratory conditions suggests that there may also be reflections of this asymmetry in daily life. Three recent studies have shown that during the act of visual perception of nonverbal pictorial material, there is, apparently, an asymmetric activation of the right hemisphere which results in a perceptual bias toward the left half of space. This bias results in a greater awareness of visual features on the left. Gilbert and Bakan found that subjects reported, when looking at photographs of human faces, a greater resemblance between the whole face and the part of the face which is on the viewer's left compared to that part on the viewer's right. Nelson and MacDonald showed that when asked to select titles for paintings, subjects selected titles which better describe the content in the left half of the painting than in the right. Finally, Levy found that when viewing natural scenery photographs which have been judged asymmetric to the left or right, right-handed, but not left-handed subjects, prefer those which are right asymmetric. This has been interpreted to mean that the perceptual asymmetry induced by brain lateralization operates conjointly with an opposite stimulus asymmetry to produce a balanced and aesthetically preferred precept.

Variations in Neuropsychological Organization

It is widely accepted that human beings vary enormously in psychological functioning. It is less well known that they also display measurable variations in neurological organization. These variations in neurological organizations are extremely important for understanding the relation betwen cerebral and psychological functions in normal people. Until recently, inferences regarding the brain-behavior relations derived solely from studies of patients with neurological pathology. Fortunately for the progress of neuropsychology we are no longer forced to rely entirely on the accidents of nature to give us insight into the neurological foundations of psychological processes. There are a number of normal, naturally occurring variations in brain organization which allow us to examine their relationship to variation in psychological functioning. A number of easily observable characteristics are found to indicate particular kinds of cerebral patterns, among them handedness, sex, conjugate lateral eye movements, and hand positioning in writing.

Handedness — There has been much controversy surrounding the question of brain organization in left-handers. From the time it was first deduced that the left hemisphere was the integrative organ for language, there have been two opposing views regarding cerebral asymmetry in sinistrals. One maintained that the brain of the left-hander was a mirror version of that of the right-handers, while the other maintained that all people had language functions organized in the left hemisphere. Over the years, dozens of clinical reports of left-handers with unilateral cerebral lesions have appeared, some supporting one view and some supporting the other. Luria (1966) published a series of observations on the frequency of occurrence of and recovery from aphasia in left-handers, right-handers with left-handed relatives, and right-handers, following lesions to the language areas of the left hemisphere. While a majority of right-handers never recovered fully from their aphasic symptoms, a much smaller percentage of lefthanders and righthanders with sinistral relatives became and remained permanently aphasic. Some never became aphasic at all and others were transiently aphasic, but recovered. Evidence which has been accumulating over the years suggests very strongly that a significant portion of sinistrals are only weakly lateralized for cerebral functions and that approximately 40% have language functions in the right hemisphere and visuo-spatial functions in the left, while about 60% are lateralized in the same direction as dextrals.

Levy (1969) postulated that since, on the average, left-handers were less well lateralized than right-handers, there should be cognitive consequences. A bilateralized brain may be bilateralized in both verbal and spatial function or in either alone. If both functions are bilateralized, then either hemisphere is specialized for either function and performance on both should be depressed. This expectation has been confirmed in several studies of left-handed students with adequate verbal functions. In left-handed architects, however, spatial ability is enhanced relative to their right-handed colleagues.

Variability in organization as a function of sex — That the brain organization of males and females differs is a conclusion derived mainly from work with normal people, using dichotic or tachistoscopic techniques. Recent studies investigating sex differences can leave little doubt that differences in lateral sensory fields are smaller for females than males. Specifically, females are superior to males in measures of verbal fluency and are inferior in spatial-visualization abilities. These differences have been related to differences in brain organization: It has

been postulated that the right hemisphere of females is incompletely organized for spatial-visualization and is partly organized for linguistic functions. The etiology of male-female differences in brain organization is unknown, possibly resulting from different maturational rates of boys and girls, from sex-linked genetic effects, from sex-limited hormonal effects, from socio-cultural differences, or from an interaction or joint contribution of any or all of the above.

Hand position in writing — In a very recent study of Levy and Reid, highly reliable tachistoscopic tests were given to dextrals and sinistrals. It was found that, in both handedness groups, the hand position used in writing was an excellent predictor of side of language dominance. Specifically, in those subjects who held the hand in the normal writing position, i.e., the hand held below the line of writing and the pencil pointing toward the top of the page, the language hemisphere was contralateral to the writing hand. In those subjects who used the inverted hand position, i.e., the hand held above the line of writing and the pencil pointing toward the bottom of the page, the language dominant hemisphere was ipsilateral to the writing hand. Only one right-handed subject was found who had an inverted hand position, and her language functions were located in the right hemisphere, while her visuo-spatial functions were located in the left. The various groups of subjects differed on a number of dimensions. Left-handers with the normal hand position displayed good overall performance on the test and were lateralized as strongly as right-handers. Left-handers with the inverted hand position showed poor overall performance, but with a great deal of variability across subjects, over 16% exceeding the performance of all right-handers, and the group being only very weakly lateralized. The performance of the one right-handed subject with the inverted hand position was unusual also. On the test measuring lateralization, her performance was below the average of right-handers, but on the test measuring visuo-spatial lateralization, her performance surpassed that of other dextral females. These findings suggest rather strongly that the degree and direction of cerebral lateralization, indexed by hand position, has profound consequences for cognitive function.

Eye movement asymmetries arising from cerebral lateralization — A series of experiments, conducted during the past two decades, has discovered that conjugate lateral eye movements are another index of cerebral organization. It has been found that, when a subject is faced by a questioner, he usually breaks eye contact following presentation of a question and moves his eyes either to the right or to the left. The direction in which the eyes move is fairly consistent for a given individual. There are various differences between "left-movers" and "right-movers", primarily in the experience of anxiety, in verbal and cognitive style, and in a number of personality measures. It has been concluded that eye movement directionality reflects the relative tendency of a person to rely consistently on one of the hemispheres during problem solving. Other investigators have found that subjects show a significant tendency to move their eyes to the right for verbal problems, to the left for spatial problems, and to no consistent direction for numerical problems. Gur, Gur and Harris have amplified these findings by demonstrating that the direction of eye movements during problem solving can be influenced by the amount of stress under which the subject is operating. When the stress is minimal, eye movements are related to problem type. When stress is increased, the subjects tend to move their eyes consistently in one direction, either right or left, regardless of problem type. In this situation, the quality of their performance deteriorates, as they use the "wrong" hemisphere for a given problem type. The investigators reasoned that problem saliency decreased under stress and subjects resort to a stereotypic response mode, which reflects their "hemisphericity."

In a number of subsequent studies, they found that hemisphericity is a good predictor for a wide range of personality traits, including hypnotic susceptibility, type of defense mechanisms employed, and self-reports of psychopathological symptoms. The nature of personality correlates revealed is consistent with our knowledge of right and left hemisphere functioning. Thus, for example, left hemisphericity subjects (right-movers) tend to intellectualize, and use defense mechanisms such as projection, while right hemisphericity subjects (left-movers) are more emotional and tend to use holistic defense mechanisms such as repression. These differences in conative aspects of personality functioning would lead one to expect hemisphericity to affect the nature of psychopathology. Indeed, the study of the association between psychiatric disorders and functional brain asymmetry can potentially shed some light both on the neurological basis of psychiatry and on the way in which conceptualizations of normal behavior ought to be revised in light of the discovery of the nonunitary nature of human consciousness.

Functional Brain Asymmetry and Psychiatric Disorders

There has been a growing body of evidence suggesting that left and right hemispheric specialization has implications for psychiatric populations. Schizophrenia has been linked to left hemisphere dysfunction whereas affective disorders have been related to right hemisphere dysfunction. Gruzelier and Venables have hypothesized that schizophrenia is related to a temporal-limbic dysfunction of the left hemisphere. In their studies, the skin conductance orienting responses to auditory stimuli with and without attentional significance were examined in left and right hands of schizophrenics and controls. A marked imbalance in responsivity was seen in the schizophrenic patients, indicating minimal reaction in the left compared to the right hand. It was found that, in the majority of cases, the schizophrenics' response features resembled those reported by Luria (1966) for patients with brain-damage in loci outside the frontal lobe. Studies of unilaterally brain-damaged patients report absence of skin conductance responsiveness in the hand ipsilateral to the lesion. This suggests that the laterality imbalance in skin conductance found in schizophrenics, with less response in the left hand, is related to pathology in the left hemisphere. Flor-Henry described an association between pathology of the left temporal lobe and schizophrenia. Examination of the location of epileptic foci in temporal lobe epileptics revealed that patients who manifested schizophrenic-like symptoms had a high incidence of foci lateralized to, or involving, the temporal lobe of the left hemisphere, whereas foci in the right hemisphere were associated with manic-depressive symptoms of mood change. The literature on unilateral electro-convulsive therapy in the treatment of depression supports these impressions and suggests further that the two hemispheres differ in their response to treatment. Right hemisphere ECT tends to produce better results, while left hemisphere ECT worsens the condition. Rosenthal and Bigelow studied brain specimens of ten chronic schizophrenic and ten control patients and found that in the schizophrenic group the corpus callosum was significantly wider than in the control groups. Beaumont and Diamond investigated transfer between the two hemispheres in schizophrenics, compared to other psychiatric and normal control groups. The subjects were asked to cross-match two stimuli flashed simultaneously to the two hemispheres, and this was compared to the presentation of both stimuli to the same hemisphere, either the left or right. The results indicated that the schizophrenic group responded like normals in matching within a hemisphere, with the exception of a significant deficit in matching letters presented to the left hemisphere. In addition, schizophrenics exhibited poor performance on the inter-hemispheric matching tasks of letters and shapes, compared to both control groups. The investigators concluded that in schizophrenia the two cerebral hemispheres are partially disconnected, and that some left hemisphere deficiency might be manifested as well. This conclusion, however, seems premature in view of the fact that if there is a left hemisphere dysfunction, the ability of this hemisphere to either transmit information to the other or to decode callosally received information from the other, would be greatly depressed.

The relationship between cerebral and motoric dominance, which has been discussed earlier, has led Raquel Gur to the hypothesis that the left hemisphere dysfunction found in schizophrenics should result in a concomitant shift in motoric lateralization and should produce a relative increase in left-sidedness in this psychiatric population. She tested 200 schizophrenic patients, compared them to 200 control subjects, and found that, indeed, schizophrenics manifested a higher degree of left sidedness, as measured by handedness, footedness and eye dominance. The motoric imbalance of schizophrenics suggests a concomitant imbalance. Specifically, the relative leftward motoric imbalance shown by schizophrenics lends further support to the hypothesized disturbance in the left hemisphere attributed to this psychiatric disorder. Schizophrenics seem to evidence some attenuation in left hemisphere functions. The thought disorder prevalent in schizophrenia, which is primarily manifested in a reduced ability for logico-linguistic processing, can be linked to this attenuation since these are the kinds of processes which have been shown to characterize left hemisphere functioning. Laterality imbalance in schizophrenia has been primarily studied by physiological measures, such as skin conductance. Very little, however, is known about the cognitive and conative functional brain asymmetries in this group as well as in other clinical populations. Hemispheric specialization for cognitive functions can be studied through a variety of techniques which were discussed earlier. Applying these techniques to the schizophrenic population may provide insight into the specific nature of the hemispheric disturbances associated with the disorder and clarify the effect of this disturbance on more refined measures of cognitive and conative functions.

A very recent study by Boklage gives further support to the view that schizophrenic symptoms are associated with left hemisphere dysfunction and affective psychoses with right hemisphere dysfunction. Specifically, when a population of monozygotic twins, at least one of whom was schizophrenic, was divided into those concordant for right-handedness versus those either discordant for handedness or concordant for left-handedness, the first group was 96% concordant for schizophrenia and had nuclear schizophrenic symptoms, while the latter was only 40% concordant for schizophrenia and manifested schizo-affective symptoms.

The findings of this line of investigation are also congruent with recent theoretical formulations and empirical studies which link hemispheric asymmetry to emotions and to various forms of psychopathology. The studies which looked into correlates of individual differences in hemisphericity have shown differences between right hemisphericity and left hemisphericity people on defensive styles, manner of handling emotions and characteristic psychopathology. The association between right hemisphere activation and emotions was also reported by Schwartz and discussed by Galin, who has called attention to the implications of left and right cerebral specialization for psychiatry, particularly with regard to affective disorders. The increasing body of knowledge on the effect of functional brain asymmetry on human behavior suggests that further research on brain organization will contribute a new dimension to the understanding of cognitive and conative processes in a wide range of psychiatric disorders.

Conclusion

This chapter has attempted to convey the enormous gains in the understanding of the relationships between cerebral and cognitive organization which have been achieved over the last century. Yet, what has been presented here is but the roughest outline of a picture which is becoming increasingly defined. We have reviewed some of the classical and some of the most recent techniques for investigating brain organization, and have tried to point out the kinds of studies which these procedures make possible. An attempt was also made to show the intimate association between neurological syndromes and the functioning of the non-pathological brain. Evidence from clinical observations and laboratory investigations is shown to converge into a coherent conception of the neurological

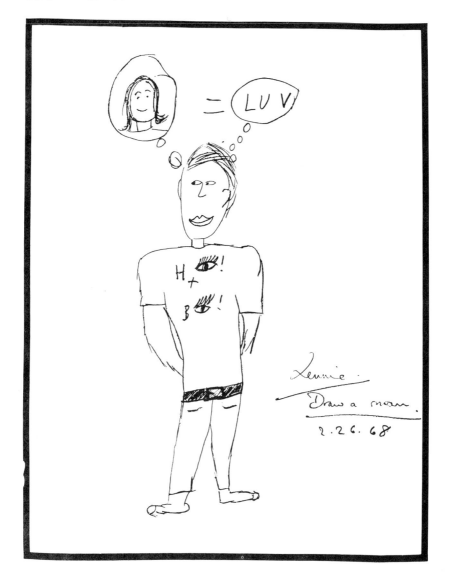

Fig. 7. A drawing by a young commissurotomy patient when he was instructed to draw a man (from Levy, 1974).

foundations of cognition and behavior. One of the most central elements in this new conception has been the realization of the pervasive psychological consequences of cerebral asymmetry. In retrospect it could hardly have been otherwise (Fig. 7).

Selected References

Davis, J.D.: *Phrenology Fad and Science, a 19th Century American Crusade.* Yale University Press, New Haven, 1955, p. 6.

Diamond, S.J., and Beaumont, J.G. (Eds.): *Hemisphere Function in the Human Brain.* John Wiley & Sons, New York, 1974.

Gardner, E.: *Fundamentals of Neurology. A Psychophysiological Approach.* W.B. Saunders Co., Philadelphia, 1975, p. 130 (Fig. 7-4).

Harnard, S.R., Doty, R.W., Goldstein, L., Jaynes, J., and Krauthamer, G.: *Lateralization in the Nervous System.* Academic Press, New York, 1976.

Kinsbourne, M., and Smith, W.L. (Eds.): *Hemispheric Disconnection and Cerebral Function.* Charles C. Thomas, Springfield, Ill., 1974.

Levy, J.: Cerebral asymmetries as manifested in split-brain man. In *Hemispheric Disconnection and Cerebral Function,* M. Kinsbourne and L.W. Smith, eds. Charles C. Thomas, Springfield, Ill., 1974.

Levy, J.: Shifting hemi-inattention in split brain patients. In *Hemi-Inattention and Hemisphere Interaction,* E.A. Weinstein and R.P. Friedland, eds. Raven Press, New York, 1977.

Luria, A.R.: *Higher Cortical Functions in Man.* Basic Books, New York, 1966.

Piercy, M., Hecaen, H., and De Ajuriaguerra, J.: Constructional apraxia associated with unilateral cerebral lesions—left and right sided cases compared. *Brain* 83 (Part 2):234-235, 1960.

Schmitt, F.O., and Worden, F.G. (Eds.): *The Neurosciences Third Study Program.* The M.I.T. Press, Cambridge, Mass., 1974.

Sperry, R.W.: The great cerebral commissure. *Sci. Am.* 210:42-52, 1964.

Vinken, P.J., and Bruyn, G.W. (Eds.): *Handbook of Clinical Neurology,* Vol. 4. North-Holland Publishing Co., Amsterdam, 1969.

Part III

Psychotropic Drugs

PROBABLY *no other psychiatric treatment modality has had as beneficial an effect in so great a number of patients as chemotherapy. The introduction of psychotropic drugs during the 1950's opened the way to progressive changes in the treatment of psychiatric patients. Physical restraints for the acutely agitated psychotic patient became less necessary, and a greater number of patients could be treated successfully without hospitalization. It has been estimated that the advent of psychopharmacology reduced the number of patients that would have been in state mental hospitals by 650,000 over the past two decades and made possible immeasurable gains in the personal well-being and productivity of countless thousands of patients.*

In this section, both therapeutic and pharmacological aspects of various classes of psychotropic drugs are described. The first chapter outlines the techniques and strategies used to demonstrate properly the behavioral effects of psychotropic drugs. Factors such as patient selection, evaluation of response and placebo influences are emphasized. Furthermore, the strengths and weaknesses of both open and controlled clinical trials are discussed.

The second chapter provides an overview of drugs used in the treatment of schizophrenia, depression, mania, and anxiety. Evidence summarizing their effectiveness is reviewed, and their major therapeutic uses and important side effects are outlined. Particular attention is focused on effects these drugs have on central biogenic amine systems (discussed in Chapter 3), as such pharmacological effects may be responsible for their clinical efficacy.

We hope that this section will provide an understanding of both the value of drugs in psychiatric practice and also of the existing limitations of chemotherapy. Such information may initiate more rational use of existing psychotropic drugs and stimulate the search for new and improved medications.

Chapter 9

Clinical Evaluation of Psychotropic Drugs

Andrew Winokur and
Karl Rickels

The fact that certain drugs can markedly alter human behavior has been known for centuries. Many societies have used mind-altering drugs for pleasure, meditation and as a central part of religious ceremonies. In the 1950's, a remarkable series of events led to the discovery of all of the major types of psychotropic drugs that are in current use (see Chapter 10). These agents have brought about striking changes in the treatment and management of a number of the psychiatric disorders (e.g., schizophrenia, depression, mania,

anxiety states). In addition to their role as therapeutic agents, *the psychotropic drugs are also of importance in providing clues to understanding the biological bases of psychiatric disorders.* Thus, by studying the effects on brain function of drugs that alter behavior, it may be possible to obtain clues about the neurochemical regulation of behavior.

Many of the chapters in this book are devoted to a discussion of the effects of psychotropic drugs on neurotransmitters, and what the implications of this are for theories regarding the biological bases of behavior. Before considering such approaches, however, it is necessary to discuss the manner in which the behavioral effects of psychotropic drugs can be demonstrated and evaluated.

In any research investigation, the validity and relevance of the data obtained depends upon the soundness of the experimental design. Factors to be considered in planning a clinical study include: the hypothesis to be investigated, the choice of the most appropriate design to obtain an answer to the posed question, the selection and distribution of subjects to be studied, the employment of double-blind techniques (i.e., neither patients nor physicians know which of several medications the patient is receiving), the implementation of the study under stringent, controlled conditions, the mechanism for obtaining informed consent from the subject or patient, the collection and interpretation of the data obtained, the use of techniques of statistical analysis to aid in interpretation of the data, and the consideration of non-specific or non-drug factors influencing the response to the administration of a medication. Throughout the remainder of this chapter, we shall discuss the importance of each of the factors cited above in carrying out sound clinical studies of psychotropic agents.

Selection and Distribution of Subjects in Clinical Studies

In clinical investigations of psychotropic agents, two types of studies are routinely conducted, studies on normal volunteers and studies involving patients with specific psychiatric disorders. In the first case, the effects of the index drug on normal subjects are evaluated. The purpose of this type of study is to look for the presence of effects that might be therapeutic in a specific patient group, as well as to evaluate the types of undesirable side effects that may appear during administration of the drug. Subjects participating in such a study may be recruited as paid volunteers, they may be individuals who have a particular interest in or commitment to the field, or they may volunteer out of altruistic motives of contributing to scientific knowledge. Regardless of the reasons for the subject's volunteering to participate in the study, it is clear that his interests, privacy and welfare must be protected at all times by the research investigator.

In recent years, the Food and Drug Administration, along with academic institutions, has markedly tightened the regulations regarding ethical conduct in clinical studies. Moreover, pharmaceutical companies, in carrying out studies of new drugs, have insisted upon greater assurances for protection of subjects in clinical trials. It is now standard practice for an investigator to be required to obtain written *informed consent* from subjects prior to including them in a clinical study. Informed consent means that, before the subject agrees to participate in an investigation, all aspects of the clinical study are explained to him/ her, including drugs to be used, procedures to be utilized, and possible risks and side effects involved. Moreover, no pressure (either implicit or explicit) should be placed upon the subject in order to obtain his/her consent.

Studies are carried out using patients with various psychiatric disorders in order to evaluate the efficacy (effectiveness) and the severity of side effects of an index drug. It should be emphasized that the same types of rights and protections apply for patients as for normal volunteers in clinical studies. Thus, a patient has the right to informed consent, and he should not be subjected to pressure to influence his participation in a clinical study. It is imperative that the welfare of the patient be given the utmost importance during the course of the study. Not only must the patient be protected from harm by procedures used in the study, but he must also not be denied effective treatment procedures that would be available to him if he were not a participant in the study. Therefore, in any research design, one has to build in a proviso to terminate from a study a patient who does not improve or gets worse, and to treat such a patient with a marketed, clinically effective medication.

Most of the studies of psychotropic drugs will involve the use of patients who have one of the following psychiatric disorders: depression, mania, anxiety, or schizophrenia. Decisions about which patients to include in a given study can be very complicated. The diagnosis of one of these disorders cannot be made on a totally objective basis, with complete agreement between various observers. It is very important for an investigator to define, as clearly as possible, the criteria being utilized in making a diagnosis. This is important not only in assuring the consistency of patients in a given study, but also in making possible comparisons among studies conducted by different groups of investigators on patients of the same diagnostic category. Rating instruments have been developed to serve as aids in diagnosing, quantifying, and operationally defining a given disorder.

For example, in depression, the Beck Depression Inventory, the Zung Depression Scale, the Hopkins Symptom Checklist, and the Hamilton Depression Scale may all be completed by either the patient or physician to provide several indicators of the degree of depression present in a given patient. These scales provide data pertaining to the current mood state, cognitive patterns, behavioral state and physical symptoms present in an individual, complaints which are believed to reflect various aspects of depression. Similar rating scales have been developed to quantify scores for mania, anxiety and schizophrenia (psychoticism).

These scales, while certainly not infallible, have become important tools in clinical psychopharmacology research because they do make possible a degree of objectivity and quantification of the data obtained in a given study, not possible less than 20 years ago. Inter-rater reliability has been shown to be quite good for many of these scales; and the use of such scales provides data that can be compared across various studies. It should be emphasized that these scales, at best, provide only a quantification of our current understanding of the phenomenology of a given disorder.

The problem of diagnosis as an issue of patient selection does not stop at the level of major diagnosis. There may be subgroups within a major diagnostic category (see Chapters 11, 13 and 14). For example, in a clinical study of an antidepressant drug, it must be determined whether all patients with a diagnosis of depression are to be included, or whether only some more discrete subcategory of depressed patients will be utilized (e.g., unipolar or bipolar depressed patients, reactive depressed patients, agitated, or anxious depressed patients, to mention only a few subcategories of depressed patients). This is a very important issue because the outcome of antidepressant drug treatment may be very much influenced by the type of depression studied. The search for more meaningful ways to subdivide patients into diagnostic categories represents one of the important areas for advance in this field.

Once a decision has been made about the diagnostic criterion to be used for inclusion of patients in a study, there are still a number of other issues to be faced regarding the distribution of patients in the trial. In general, a clinical study involves the comparison of the effects of two or more treatment procedures on the course of a specific illness or set of symptoms. It is important that the two groups being compared be as similar as possible in a wide range of characteristics. Thus, it is important to use a process of *randomization* to distribute patients into treatment groups in order to assure that the characteristics of the two groups are similar. Without randomizing treatment groups, it may be impossible to determine whether differences between the groups in response to drug treatment are due to drug effects or simply due to differences in patient samples. The kinds of characteristics that are generally important to consider when randomizing patients include: age, sex, prior psychiatric treatment, severity and duration of illness. Depending on the type of study in question, it may be important to identify and control many other factors, such as: race, socio-economic background, weight, previous medication, family history and many others. The setting (i.e., inpatient, outpatient, charity clinic, private practice, family practice) in which the study is to be carried out should also be clearly given.

Controlled Conditions for Clinical Investigations

It has already been pointed out that the data obtained from an experiment is only as useful and open to interpretation as the experimental design allows it to be. In designing protocols for clinical investigations, extraordinary attention must be paid to controlling the conditions of the study as carefully as possible. Only by achieving careful control of the experimental conditions is it possible to determine whether or not the variations in treatment response are due to differences in therapeutic regimen.

As discussed in the previous section, one aspect of control in an experiment involves adequate randomization of patient groups. In addition to this factor, it is important to make sure that as few as possible of the individuals involved in a study are aware of the nature of the treatments to which the different subject groups are exposed. A study in which the patients do not know the identity of the drug they are receiving is referred to as a *single-blind* experiment. When possible, the treating physician and the individual filling out the rating scales should also be unaware of the type of treatment a given patient is receiving. This condition may be satisfied if the different drugs being used in the study are dispensed in capsules that are identical in appearance and numbered successively. Moreover, if possible, and it is realized that this is frequently not feasible, drugs should not produce readily identifiable differences in side effects. When these conditions are achieved, the experiment is considered to be a *double-blind* study.

Another level of control that may be important is to ascertain that all laboratory studies are conducted under randomized and, if possible, blind conditions. The conditions of an assay may change during the course of the procedure, leading to a variation in the data. This variation could appear to represent a real, rather than artificial change if the order of the tubes is not randomized. Moreover, it is important to have the laboratory technicians be unaware of the order of the tubes to be tested so that they do not introduce an unintentional bias in the outcome of the data, i.e., unconsciously influencing the data to come out in support of a prior hypothesis.

In certain situations, a technique used to control the experimental variables is the *cross-over* design. In this approach, a patient is used as his own control. He may be started on a certain treatment procedure. After a prespecified time, without either the patient or treating physician being told, the patient is switched to a second treatment procedure or drug, and later may be switched back to the original drug treatment. This treatment schedule may be referred to as an a-b-a schedule. The study may continue through several cycles, a-b-a-b-a. Other patients may be on a schedule of b-a-b. With this design, it is possible to look at differences in the response of an individual, rather than the responses of different groups, to various drug treatments. It is a complicated study to carry out, and certain factors may make interpretation of the data difficult. For example, the nature of the patient's illness may change over time in a manner unrelated to the treatments utilized. Also, in the a-b-a protocol, treatment *a* may start to produce effects at the time that the patient is being switched over to treatment *b*, leading to confusion in interpreting the data. When a patient in a study using the cross-over design responds to a certain treatment, relapses when the treatment is withdrawn, and improves again when the treatment is reinstituted, an unequivocal drug response is said to have taken place.

A further aspect of control in experimental conditions involves the placebo factor. This is an extremely important issue in pharmacology in general, and in psychopharmacology in particular. The placebo phenomenon refers to the observation that an individual may respond to the administration of an inactive chemical or placebo (such as a sugar tablet) as if he had been given an active pharmacological agent. The subject's response to the administration of the placebo may depend upon his expectations of the "drug" he is receiving, as well as the conditions under which the placebo is administered. Moreover, there may be a placebo component to an individual's response to an active pharmacological agent. A dose of alcohol that might be mildly sedating if consumed alone in a quiet setting, may be

quite stimulating and activating in the context of a lively party.

The placebo effect must be considered in testing the efficacy of any pharmacological agent. For example, even patients suffering from severe pain may experience a real, albeit transitory relief after the injection of a saline placebo. In evaluating the effects of psychotropic drugs, it is particularly important to provide adequate controls for placebo effects. This appears to be true in particular for drugs used in the treatment of anxiety and depression, two illnesses that may fluctuate markedly in response to a number of factors. The response of schizophrenics to placebo administration is less pronounced, and patients with full-blown manic episodes or with bipolar depression show little responsiveness to placebo.

In the pharmacological treatment of anxiety, however, it can be difficult to demonstrate drug efficacy because of the large number of patients responding to placebo (up to 50%). Similarly, in studies of patients with depression, particularly if the sample also includes reactive or neurotic depression, 35 to 45% of patients receiving placebo treatment may show marked improvement. Thus, an antidepressant drug may be found to produce improvement in 70% of the patients studied, yet this may represent an improvement of only 30% of the patients who do not respond to placebo alone. Thus, it is important to test a psychotropic drug in placebo-controlled conditions in order to obtain an estimate of its true efficacy. Optimally, every placebo-controlled study should be carried out under double-blind conditions.

In conducting studies of drug efficacy, there are a variety of experimental designs that incorporate different degrees of controls. There are various problems or difficulties with each of these designs in terms of cost, numbers of patients required, logistical complexity, difficulty in carrying patients through the entire study, inconvenience to patients, etc. In general, the reliability of data obtained increases as one moves from uncontrolled clinical trials through single-blind studies to studies carried out under carefully controlled double-blind conditions. The cross-over design or a design employing sequential analysis also may be employed to obtain well-controlled data. Each of these research designs has a place in contributing data about the effects of a given drug. It is usually necessary to put together data obtained from a variety of types of studies in order to gain a complete picture of the effectiveness of the drug in question. In analyzing these studies, one must be aware of the strengths and limitations of the data, as determined by the experimental design utilized in each case.

Sample size is another important design feature, as only an adequate sample size per treatment group will allow a more definite assessment of the clinical effectiveness of the drug in question. Usually sample sizes of 30–40 patients per group are considered adequate in drug-placebo comparisons. Larger sample sizes are needed to detect possible drug-drug differences. Since many single investigators do not have the large amount of patients needed to conduct a clinical trial with an ample sample size, collaborative studies, planned and designed prior to the data collection phase of the study, are more and more frequently planned and conducted to provide sample sizes needed in psychopharmacology.

While the combining of data from several investigators has its methodological problems, usually these are outweighed by its advantages, particularly if a collaborative study is properly planned, investigators are brought together for a discussion of study protocol, intake and exclusion criteria, and for the viewing of several patient video tapes for joint rating, using the rating instruments to be employed in the study.

Collection and Interpretation of Data

It has already been pointed out that there are particular problems entailed in psychopharmacological studies concerning the type of data that can be obtained. Thus, unlike other studies which may be based on hard objective data (blood pressure, temperature, bacterial counts, etc.), all data obtained in psychopharmacological studies are, by nature, subjective. In order to attain greater objectivity, there has been a tendency to utilize a variety of rating scales to be completed by physician and patient to provide a data base for these studies. These rating scales are used not only to aid in the initial diagnosis, to operationally define each patient entering the study, and help in the evaluation of severity of illness, but also to follow the course of the illness during treatment, and to provide a numerical indication of response to treatment. Thus, data obtained in these studies depend upon the sensitivity and validity of the rating scales employed. Most clinical investigators have found that rating scales are quite useful in reflecting change in clinical condition for most of the psychiatric disorders. This is particularly true if they have participated in video tape training sessions and thus learned to use rating scales most appropriately. Nevertheless, the fact that all of the rating scales involve a degree of subjectivity, and that their sensitivity to change is, at best, limited, means that the data obtained from these studies should not be overinterpreted. In evaluating data obtained from an investigation, it is important to be familiar with the methods used for obtaining data, and to be aware of the limitations implicit with each of the rating scales used. A major area for the advance of psychopharmacological research is the development of better and more sensitive methods of obtaining, scoring and evaluating data about psychiatric disorders.

Statistical Analysis of Psychopharmacological Studies

With the myriad of problems in experimental design and data collection in psychopharmacological studies, it is important to subject the data obtained to rigorous statistical analysis. In fact, the statistician has become an important member of the psychopharmacology research team, providing advice about experimental design as well as data interpretation.

Commonly used statistical techniques in these studies include Students t-test and analysis of variance and covariance. The t-test is employed in a study of two different drugs to determine which of them produces a significantly (generally at 95% of probability or better) greater improvement in treatment response. An analysis of variance gives identical results to Students t-test when comparing two drugs, but is most frequently employed when comparing more than two drugs. Some of the most sensitive statistical methods are analysis of variance or covariance, discriminant function, and multiple regression, the latter two methods being particularly applicable for estimating the independent contribution of a number of variables to drug treatment outcome. Not forgotten, however, should be the usually simple nonparametric tests, such as chi square or the Mann-Whitney U test.

Non-specific Factors Involved in the Response to Psychotropic Drugs

Several researchers have identified a number of non-specific factors that may alter or influence the response to a psychotropic drug. These non-specific factors represent extensions and amplifications of the placebo factor that has already been discussed, and include such conditions as characteristics of the patient, various attributes of the treating physician, and certain general conditions in the treatment milieu (Fig. 1). The list of non-specific factors that may contribute to drug response is extensive, and we can offer only a few examples for purposes of illustration.

In some cases, the socio-economic background of the patient may influence his response to the drug treatment of anxiety. Thus, groups of patients from lower class populations respond relatively well to treatment with barbiturates, and these patients seem to be rather unconcerned about the sedating effects of these drugs. Conversely, upper social class patient groups are quite disturbed by treatment with anti-anxiety drugs that are notably sedating. It has been hypothesized that this difference in treatment response to the same drug in different social classes may be explained in the following manner: Lower social class patients respond positively to being "sedated out" from their unpleasant, intrusive environment, while upper social class patients tend to have jobs requiring that they remain alert (therefore, not sedated) throughout the day.

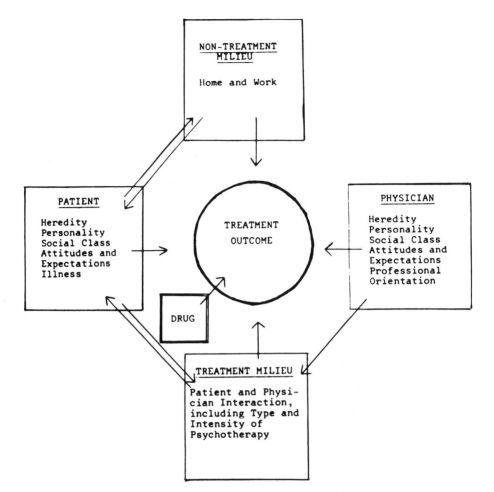

Fig. 1. Non-specific variables in drug therapy (from Rickles, 1968, with permission).

A number of factors related to characteristics of the physician have also been shown to be important in determining the response to psychotropic drugs. In particular, the physician's interest in, belief in, and knowledge of these drugs, as well as his empathy and warmth in relating to the patient have all been shown to be important factors that influence the likelihood of a favorable treatment response. The recognition of the variety of non-specific factors involved in the response to psychotropic drugs presents an additional level of complexity in addition to the elements previously discussed in this chapter. These non-specific factors are significant not only from the point of view of research investigations, but also in terms of clinical practice. The finding that the attitude and bearing of the physician may markedly influence a patient's response to a psychotropic drug has widespread clinical implications.

Conclusion

In this chapter, we have discussed a number of the *methodological factors involved in psychotropic drug studies.* It can readily be appreciated that obtaining meaningful data from such clinical investigations is a very complicated endeavor. It is important to be aware of and critically evaluate the limitations of data obtained in such studies.

As mentioned at the beginning of this chapter, a major activity in the field of biological psychiatry have been the efforts to understand the neurochemical mechanisms of action of drugs that af-fect behavior. This is an important strategy—one that merits serious elaboration. However, underlying this strategy is a basic acceptance of the behavioral effects of the psychotropic agents. It may now be appreciated that demonstrating behavioral effects of drugs is a complex undertaking that must be pursued with care and diligence. The application of sophisticated techniques of psychopharmacological investigation may provide further evidence and clarification of the behavioral effects of the psychotropic drugs.

Selected References

Efron, D.H. (Ed.): *Psychopharmacology, A Review of Progress,* 1957-1967. Public Health Service Publication No. 1836, U.S. Government Printing Office, Washington, D.C., 1968.

FDA Guidelines for Psychotropic Drugs. *Psychopharmacol. Bull.* 10:70-91, (October) 1974.

Hamilton, M.: *Lectures on the Methodology of Clinical Research.* E & S Livingstone, Ltd., Edinburgh and London, 1961.

Levine, J., Schiele, B., and Bouthilet, L. (Eds.): *Principles and Problems in Establishing the Efficacy of Psychotropic Agents.* Public Health Service Publication No. 2138, U.S. Government Printing Office, Washington, D.C., 1971.

Pichot, P. (Ed.): *Modern Problems of Pharmacopsychiatry,* Vol. 7, Psychological Measurements in Psychopharmacology. S. Karger, Basel, 1974.

Rickels, K.: *Non-Specific Factors in Drug Therapy.* Charles C. Thomas, Inc., Springfield, Ill., 1968.

Chapter 10

Therapeutic and Pharmacological Aspects of Psychotropic Drugs

A. Frazer and
A. Winokur

Psychotropic drugs are chemicals that alter mental states. Within this category of drugs are several classes of agents that are used in the treatment of psychiatric disorders. In this chapter, we shall be concerned with four major categories of psychotropic drugs: antipsychotic, antidepressant, antimanic and antianxiety agents. It is apparent that the terminology used to describe these types of psychotropic drugs is based upon their primary clinical role. However, these compounds may also be of value in a number of other conditions which are not indicated by their class name.

The psychotropic drugs did not come into clinical usage in the United States until the mid-1950's. In the past twenty years, there has been a veritable explosion in their popularity, so that these drugs are now among the most frequently prescribed medications in the United States (representing almost one-fifth of all drugs prescribed, according to one survey). The advent of the psychotropic drugs into clinical practice has had striking effects on the treatment and management of psychiatric disorders. This impact can be measured in a variety of ways: in marked reductions in the census of psychiatric hospitals, in rapid recoveries from formerly long-term, incapacitating illnesses, and in the reduction and relief from distress and suffering provided to countless numbers of individuals.

It should be pointed out immediately that these drugs are not a panacea. In no present instances is it possible to talk in terms of cures. Moreover, many of the drugs in question take a considerable period of time before they begin to work, and most are associated with a number of bothersome side effects. Recently, a number of critics have asserted that these drugs are prescribed excessively and injudiciously by physicians, and are relied on by some patients to the point of psychological or even physiological dependence. These reservations have merit and importance, but they do not detract from the enormous contributions that the psychotropic drugs have made to the treatment of psychiatric disorders; rather, they underline the need to make even greater advances in understanding the actions of these agents and developing safer and more effective drugs through psychopharmacological research.

In view of the importance of devising more effective psychotropic drugs, a brief discussion of the issues involved in the development of new drugs will be presented. The development of a new drug is a costly undertaking. Drug development is divided into two stages: (1) preclinical testing which is conducted in laboratory animals or in the test tube, and (2) clinical investigation. Initially, thousands of compounds are screened for indications of some potential therapeutic effects. To screen for such properties as antianxiety or antidepressant effects, a variety of animal test situations are employed, e.g., "conflict" tests, reversal of reserpine-induced sedation. When a compound does manifest potential promise, it is subjected to intensive laboratory investigation. The effects of the compound on all of the major organ systems are evaluated in labor-

atory animals. Studies are carried out to look for any potential toxic effects of the compound, such as the capacity to produce tumors, and the effect of the compound on the offspring of pregnant animals (teratogenic effects).

When a drug has been shown to have therapeutic promise and does not appear to have excessive toxic effects in animals, it is then examined in a series of clinical studies which are referred to as Phase I, Phase II and Phase III studies. In Phase I studies, the drug will be tested in normal human volunteers to evaluate such characteristics as toxicity, absorption, metabolism and dosage range. When the safety of the drug in humans has been established, it is then tested in Phase II studies in an *open* trial involving small numbers of patients to determine the apparent efficacy of the drug in the condition(s) for which it was developed. Finally, the drug reaches Phase III in which it is tested under controlled situations, e.g., comparison with placebo, single- or double-blind studies (see Chapter 9). In this phase, the safety and efficacy of the drug must be clearly established.

When the pharmaceutical company has amassed this extensive data from the pre-clinical and clinical trials, it then submits a report of its findings to the Food and Drug Administration (FDA). The FDA has the responsibility to evaluate all new drugs, and to approve for clinical use only those considered safe and effective. Representatives of the FDA review in detail the reports on a new drug which have been submitted by the sponsoring pharmaceutical company. They must determine whether these reports indicate adequate and reliable testing, whether the drug has been demonstrated to have clear therapeutic value, and, above all, whether it has been shown to be reasonably safe and free from toxic effects under all conceivable conditions. As can be imagined, this is a time-consuming process. It has been estimated that 7½–10 years elapse between the discovery of a new chemical and its final approval as a marketable drug by the FDA.

This brief description only begins to indicate the complexities involved in the development of new drugs. Pharmaceutical companies must undertake this process with no assurances that a given drug will turn out to be safe or effective, that it will be approved by the FDA or that it will be a well-received and commercially successful product. Yet, as has been demonstrated, particularly in the psychotropic drug area, the development of an important new drug can bring about large financial rewards, as well as providing a considerable degree of prestige and recognition to the company. Thus, with this incentive, a number of pharmaceutical companies are currently making major investments of time and money toward the development of new and more effective psychotropic agents.

The rest of this chapter will involve a discussion of the major psychotropic drugs, considering such factors as their historical development, important physicochemical properties, demonstration of efficacy, clinical uses, and theories of mechanism of action.

Antipsychotic Drugs

History

There is no doubt that the modern era of psychopharmacology began with the demonstration of the beneficial effect of chlorpromazine on psychotic behavior. The enthusiasm that this compound engendered paved the way for the development of a host of different drugs that modified abnormal behavioral states. It is interesting, then, that the development of chlorpromazine was due primarily to the efforts of the French surgeon, Laborit, and not to psychiatrists.

Laborit needed agents that would control shock, as this condition was retarding the development of surgical progress. He speculated that shock resulted from exaggerated autonomic responses to stress. To control this condition, therefore, required the inhibition of the autonomic nervous system, both peripherally and its central components. As histamine was thought to be involved in the effects produced by the autonomic nervous system, Laborit tried the phenothiazine, promethazine, a good antihistaminic agent. In 1949, he reported that patients given promethazine were calm and relaxed after major operations—they appeared to suffer less.

At this time, the "central" effects of the antihistaminics were considered *undesirable* side reactions—drowsiness and sedation. Laborit recognized these central properties as being clinically valuable and attributed it to blockade of the central components regulating activity of the autonomic nervous system. As promethazine was not a sufficiently potent agent, the search began for compounds with strong central effects, even if having weak peripheral antihistaminic action. Chlorpromazine was synthesized by Charpentier in 1950. The drug was found to have strong antiadrenergic and anticholinergic properties, but little antihistaminic activity. In the patients on whom he used chlorpromazine, Laborit found that it left consciousness unclouded and induced a lack of interest in the environment. As a consequence, chlorpromazine seemed to counteract anxiety, excitement and other stress reactions.

Laborit persuaded French psychiatrists to use the drug, and in 1952 it was used by Delay and his associates in the treatment of patients with acute psychoses at St. Anne's psychiatric hospital; the

Anti Psychotic Drugs

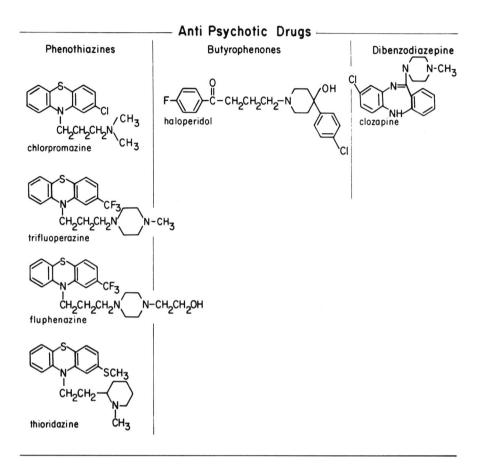

Fig. 1. The structures of representative antipsychotic drugs.

results were excellent. The drug then began to be promoted with enthusiasm initially in Europe and then in the rest of the world. Chlorpromazine became, and still is, the test drug to which all subsequent antipsychotic drugs were compared. These drugs, taken as a group, have had a more significant impact in the beneficial treatment of schizophrenic patients than any other form of therapy.

Chemistry

There are primarily two major classes of antipsychotic drugs used clinically: (1) phenothiazines like chlorpromazine, trifluoperazine and fluphenazine; and (2)

butyrophenones like haloperidol. Thioxanthene derivatives like thiothixene have also been demonstrated to have antipsychotic properties. In addition, the dibenzodiazepine compound clozapine is becoming increasingly important clinically due to its reported lower incidence of extrapyramidal side effects. The structures of these and related compounds are shown in Fig. 1.

Phenothiazines are three-ring structures in which two benzene rings are linked by a sulfur and a nitrogen atom. Substitutions are usually made at positions two and ten. All phenothiazines used in psychiatry have a three-carbon bridge between the nitrogen atom found in the side chain and that present in the middle ring. The three-dimensional conformation of these drugs appears to be critical for their antipsychotic effects.

Clinical Efficacy

While there is little general agreement as to what symptoms are necessary to make the diagnosis of schizophrenia, these drugs do seem to modify what many have chosen as the core symptoms of the schizophrenic syndrome. For example, what Bleuler referred to as the fundamental symptoms of schizophrenia (thought disorder; flat affect; autism) respond very well to phenothiazine treatment. Other symptoms, such as hallucinations, paranoid ideation, hostility and uncooperativeness are also lessened by phenothiazines. In contrast, symptoms not specific to schizophrenia, like grandiosity, anxiety, and tension and agitation are less responsive to treatment. These drugs, then, are not merely sedatives, but act on the most marked symptoms of schizophrenia.

As reviewed by Klein and Davis (1969), the over-all clinical efficacy of the antipsychotic agents in schizophrenia has been demonstrated in a relatively large number of well-designed double-blind studies. Among 100 investigations comparing any of the commonly used phenothiazines, chlorpromazine, perphenazine, trifluoperazine, fluphenazine, and thioridazine with placebo, the phenothiazines were found to be more effective than placebo in 86 of the studies. Since most of the studies finding chlorpromazine to be ineffective used rather small doses of the drug, the figures demonstrating clinical efficacy are even more impressive than those given. In contrast to this, the sedative agent, phenobarbital, was no more effective than placebo in the three studies in which it was used.

Another way of looking at the question of efficacy is to compare the percentages of responders and non-responders to active medication and to placebo in studies with large sample populations.

In the first cooperative study of the National Institute of Mental Health and the Psychopharmacology Service Center, 75% of phenothiazine-treated patients were evaluated as very much improved. Only 25% of patients receiving placebo improved to this extent. While half of the placebo-treated patients were judged as unchanged or worse, only 5% of the phenothiazine-treated group had such an outcome.

Among the phenothiazines now used in psychiatry, most have therapeutic efficacy equivalent to that of chlorpromazine. However, a number of phenothiazines, like promazine and mepazine, are no longer used in schizophrenia, as they are clearly less effective agents than chlorpromazine.

Clinical Uses

There are currently a large number of efficacious drugs available for the treatment of schizophrenia. Unfortunately, drug selection for an individual patient can only be made on an empirical basis, since studies attempting to demonstrate differential effects of various antipsychotic drugs on specific schizophrenic symptoms or syndromes have not yielded convincing results. The choice of a drug for a given patient is usually made on the basis of side effects (especially sedation, hypotension, or parkinsonian symptoms). Because of the high incidence of parkinsonian side effects associated with antipsychotic treatment, it has become a common practice to prescribe an antiparkinsonian agent, such as benztropine mesylate, at the initiation of drug therapy. However, such a practice exposes the patient to potential side effects from a drug (the antiparkinsonian agent) which may be unnecessary. Moreover, data from recent studies indicates that treatment with these drugs actually produces a lowering of plasma phenothiazine levels, therefore potentially interfering with the antipsychotic effects. Thus, it now seems advisable to withhold antiparkinsonian agents until the actual appearance of side effects.

Antipsychotic drugs are of value in the management of acutely agitated, psychotic or violent patients, and are frequently utilized in the emergency ward setting to bring such patients under rapid control. The treatment of less acute or excessively agitated psychotic patients may be initiated by the oral administration of an effective drug like chlorpromazine in doses that are gradually adjusted (usually upward) to obtain an optimal balance between therapeutic and side effects. The effective dosage range for chlorpromazine is generally between 400 and 1800 mg daily, although much higher doses have been used. In the case of a number of drugs, the upper limit of drug dosage is undergoing considerable re-evaluation. For example, haloperidol, which had been used in doses up to 20 mg daily, is sometimes used effectively in daily doses as high as 100 mg.

The management of antipsychotic drug dosage is made on the basis of clinical observation. An active area of current research involves evaluating the relationships between plasma phenothiazine levels, therapeutic response and side effects. It is anticipated that such investigations will provide a more rational and objective basis for regulating the dosage of antipsychotic drugs in the near future.

With adequate doses of antipsychotic drugs, patients may begin to show a reduction in symptoms of psychotic behavior within 48 hours of the initiation of treatment. However, full clinical recovery may often take several weeks or more. It is of interest that in most patients, tolerance develops rather rapidly to the sedative effect (usually within a few days), while the therapeutic effects become evident over a considerably longer period of time. The clear-cut temporal dissociation between the sedative effects and the antipsychotic effects of these drugs provides strong evidence that their clinical efficacy is not due merely to a sedative effect, but represents some more specific antipsychotic action.

As patients improve, they generally show markedly decreased levels of anxiety and agitation, and more coherent, organized thought patterns. Affect may become more responsive and appropriate, hallucinations may diminish, and, less frequently, paranoid delusions may dissipate. Once a satisfactory clinical response has been obtained, the dosage of the antipsychotic medication is generally tapered down over a period of time to a maintenance level. Several studies have demonstrated that patients maintained on some level of antipsychotic drug show a lower relapse rate than do untreated groups, but it is also known that some patients on careful maintenance therapy may still relapse. A frequently utilized form of maintenance therapy for chronic schizophrenic patients is fluphenazine enanthate, which is administered intramuscularly. Given in this manner, the drug is effective for a period of two weeks. Thus a patient may be treated in a clinic on an intermittent basis, with the assurance that adequate drug dosage is being maintained.

In addition to their use in schizophrenia, phenothiazines are also employed to control nausea and vomiting. This is due to their ability to depress stimulation of the chemoreceptor trigger zone (an area involved with emesis) in the brain stem. The butyrophenone, haloperidol, has been reported to be effective in the treatment of Gilles de la Tourette syndrome. This is a peculiar neurological disorder characterized by violent muscular jerks, grimacing, and explosive utterances of foul expletives.

The most dangerous side effects of these drugs are those resulting from hypersensitivity reactions, particularly blood dyscrasias. However, the extrapyramidal signs produced by the antipsychotics are probably the most disturbing side effects to the largest number of patients. Four types of extrapyramidal syndromes may be associated with antipsychotic treatment:

1. Parkinsonian syndrome, characterized by akinesia (slowing of volitional movement), rigidity, and tremor at rest.
2. Akathisia — a compelling need to be in constant movement, rather than a specific movement pattern. The patient feels that he must get up and continuously move about.
3. Acute dystonic reactions — facial grimacing and spasmodic movement of the head to one side (torticollis).
4. Tardive dyskinesias — usually occur late in therapy or when the latter is discontinued. Characterized by stereotyped involuntary movements, especially around the mouth — sucking and smacking the lips, lateral jaw movements, fly-catching dartings of the tongue.

The incidence of extrapyramidal side effects produced by the antipsychotic agents varies considerably. Fluphenazine and perphenazine produce the greatest incidence of such side reactions, chlorpromazine and haloperidol somewhat less, and thioridazine and clozapine have the least incidence.

Death from overdosage with antipsychotic drugs is a relatively infrequent occurrence. While fatalities have been reported after ingestion of only 2000 mg, patients have also been known to survive up to 17,000 mg of chlorpromazine. The concurrent intake of other drugs which cause central nervous system depression may increase the lethality of the antipsychotic agents.

Mechanisms of Action

The antipsychotic drugs produce a myriad of pharmacological effects, e.g., adrenergic and cholinergic blockade, cell membrane expansion, etc. It is difficult to ascertain which particular pharmacological effect best correlates with clinical efficacy. To do this, one needs to know that the pharmacological effect under investigation does indeed occur in patients being treated with the drug. In addition, one can make use of the fact that there is a wide range of clinical potencies among the different antipsychotic drugs. A high correlation between the varying clinical potencies and the ability of these drugs to exert a particular pharmacological effect suggests that the effect may be clinically relevant. Within such a framework, inhibition of dopaminergic transmission seems to be the most likely candidate for producing the clinical efficacy of the antipsychotic drugs.

There are several ways in which the antipsychotics could interfere with dopaminergic transmission. Two mechanisms have received the most attention. Seeman and his associates (1975) have proposed an "impulse blockade theory" for antipsychotic drug action. This theory is based upon the ability of phenothiazines to expand biological membranes, causing a "local anesthetic-like" effect. In areas of the brain contributing to schizophrenic-like symptomatology, the local anesthetic effect would lead to decreased impulse frequency and/or decreased impulse amplitude. This would produce less impulse-triggered release of neurotransmitter, in particular dopamine. Evidence has been gathered showing that the phenothiazines can inhibit impulse-triggered release of dopamine.

The evidence seems strongest, though, that the antipsychotic drugs inhibit dopaminergic transmission by blocking dopamine receptors. This mechanism of action was first suggested in 1963 by Carlsson and Lindqvist. These investigators found elevated concentrations of dopamine metabolites of animals given antipsychotic phenothiazines and haloperidol; no elevation of dopamine metabolites was observed after administration of promethazine, an antihistaminic but not antipsychotic phenothiazine. It was suggested that the elevated dopamine metabolites resulted from drug-induced blockade of dopamine receptor sites. This would cause a message to be sent back to the pre-synaptic neuron—"We need more transmitter!" The dopaminergic neuron would fire more rapidly, synthesizing and releasing more dopamine, thereby elevating dopamine metabolism. By and large, these speculations have now been confirmed.

It has been found, for example, that iontophoresis of dopamine onto neurons in the limbic area receiving a dopaminergic input results in inhibition of these neurons. Very low doses of intravenously administered phenothiazines and butyrophenones block this effect of dopamine, in proportion to their clinical potency in the treatment of schizophrenia. It should be emphasized that in this experiment, and those to be described later, the antipsychotics are blocking the effect of *exogenously* administered dopamine. In such systems, then, their effects cannot be due to inhibition of release of *endogenous* dopamine.

Other evidence favoring blockade of dopamine receptors comes from two types of experiments. As mentioned in Chapter 3, an adenylate cyclase has been isolated in homogenates of the caudate nucleus and certain areas of the limbic system that is particularly responsive to dopamine. This enzyme has many of the characteristics of the dopamine receptor. In general, it has been demonstrated that the antipsychotic drugs are good competitive inhibitors of the dopamine-induced stimulation of the enzyme isolated from caudate or limbic areas. Structurally related compounds with little antipsychotic activity were poor inhibitors of dopamine-stimulated adenylate cyclase. Some discrepancies exist, though. For example, haloperidol is only a modest inhibitor of dopamine-stimulated adenylate cyclase, whereas it is a very potent antipsychotic agent.

The approach taken by Creese, Burt, and Snyder (1976) reveals an even superior correlation between dopamine receptor blockade and clinical potency. These investigators isolated membranes from the caudate nucleus to which radioactive dopamine or radioactive haloperidol bind rather specifically. They measured the ability of a wide range of antipsychotic drugs to displace labeled haloperidol from these membranes. This provides a measure of the affinity of binding of these drugs to the dopamine receptor. A highly significant correlation was found between the clinical and pharmacological potencies of these drugs and their ability to displace radioactive haloperidol from postsynaptic dopamine receptors. This result strongly suggests that these drugs act by blocking postsynaptic dopamine receptors.

A current unitary hypothesis, then, is that the antipsychotic properties and extrapyramidal symptoms of the antischizophrenic drugs reside in their ability to block dopamine receptors in the limbic system and caudate nucleus, respectively. One fact that, on the surface, might mitigate against this idea is that the antipsychotic drugs produce varying incidences of extrapyramidal side effects. If the antipsychotics produce similar effects on all dopamine receptors, and the evidence suggests that they do, then they all should produce a similar degree of extrapyramidal symptomatology. Resolution of this paradox is possible, though, without destroying the hypothesis. Those antipsychotic agents which produce the least incidence of extrapyramidal symptoms, like clozapine and thioridazine, have the greatest anticholinergic properties, as revealed by the experiments of Snyder and his associates (1974) on the binding affinities of these drugs for the muscarinic cholinergic receptor in brain. In contrast, haloperidol has little anticholinergic properties and produces a rather high incidence of extrapyramidal effects. Thus, when giving an antipsychotic drug like thioridazine with strong anticholinergic properties, the balance between dopaminergic and cholinergic systems in the caudate nucleus is maintained in such a manner that extrapyramidal syndromes are less likely to develop.

This explanation provides an excellent example of one of the fundamental adages in pharmacology—no drug has a single effect. Quite often, these multiple effects contribute to the development of adverse reactions. More rarely, the multiple effects may interact so as to lessen the incidence of a particular unwanted response.

In summary, then, the antipsychotic drugs are very effective in the treatment of schizophrenia. They do not act as sedatives, but rather affect some of the primary manifestations of schizophrenic behavior. While these drugs produce a number of complex effects on neurotransmitter activity in brain, an impressive body of data has been gathered which suggests that their therapeutic action is the result of their interference with dopaminergic transmission. Blockade of postsynaptic dopamine receptors is the most likely mechanism whereby they produce this effect. While additional work will be needed to substantiate this hypothesis, it does appear to be one of the most promising and soundly based areas of psychopharmacological research.

Antidepressant Drugs

Iminodibenzyl (Tricyclic) Drugs

The tricyclic antidepressants are the drugs most commonly prescribed in the United States for the treatment of depression. Imipramine was the first compound of this class to be synthesized, and it will be discussed as a prototype for all of the tricyclic antidepressant agents.

History

Imipramine was synthesized in 1948 as one of a number of iminodibenzyl compounds that were being evaluated (along with chlorpromazine) for use as antihistamines, sedatives and analgesics. Because of the structural similarity between imipramine and chlorpromazine (Fig. 2), a Swedish psychiatrist named Roland Kuhn was commissioned by a pharmaceutical company to conduct a clinical study of the effects of imipramine in schizophrenic patients. Kuhn's initial findings were that imipramine did not appear to reduce the symptoms of schizophrenia, and certainly was much less effective than chlor-promazine, the drug against which it was being compared.

Some years later, in reflecting upon his observations during the clinical trial, Kuhn recognized that some patients did seem to improve with imipramine administration and that the majority of responsive patients had originally manifested significant degrees of depressive symptomatology. In further clinical studies with imipramine, Kuhn collected additional data indicating that imipramine did have antidepressant properties; and he described the clinical picture most consistent with a favorable response to imipramine: "Best responses were obtained in cases of endogenous depression showing the typical symptoms of mental and motor retardation, fatigue, feelings of heaviness, hopelessness, guilt and despair. The condition is more characterized by the aggravation of symptoms in the morning with a tendency to improve during the day."

Twenty years later, we would be hard pressed to improve upon Kuhn's description of a potential imipramine-responsive patient.

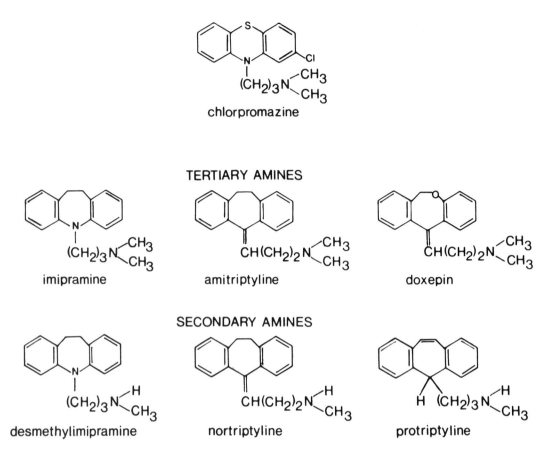

Fig. 2. The three-membered phenothiazine and dibenzazepine ring structures are presented at the top of the figure. The structures of representative tertiary and secondary amine tricyclic compounds are also shown.

Chemistry and Physiological Properties

As the name tricyclic compound indicates, imipramine contains a three-ring structure, with the middle ring being seven-membered. Fig. 2 provides a comparison of imipramine and chlorpromazine, and other representative tricyclic compounds. It can readily be appreciated that these two important psychotropic agents bear strong structural resemblances. The major difference between the molecules is the isosteric replacement of the sulfur in the pheno-thiazine ring with an ethylene bridge in the iminodibenzyl ring.

Imipramine is also similar to chlorpromazine in producing a wide range of physiological effects throughout the body. For example, imipramine causes cholinergic blocking actions resulting in such symptoms as dry mouth, blurred vision, constipation and urinary retention. Effects on the cardiovascular system may also be seen, particularly decreases in blood pressure, orthostatic hypotension, and, infrequently, cardiac arrhythmias.

Imipramine exerts a number of effects on central nervous system function that are similar to those elicited by chlorpromazine. For example, imipramine causes a slowing of EEG rhythms, and may, in high dosage, produce seizures.

It is interesting to note that imipramine, when administered to normal volunteers, does not have any mood elevating effects, but rather causes only some sedation, dry mouth, and blurred vision. Probably for these reasons, the incidence of abuse of imipramine as a street drug is extremely low.

Clinical Efficacy

After the initial studies demonstrating the antidepressant properties of imipramine by Kuhn in the 1950's, a large number of placebo-controlled single- and double-blind studies of the efficacy of the tricyclic drugs have been carried out. Klein and Davis (1969) reviewed 65 studies comparing imipramine and other tricyclic antidepressant drugs to placebo in reasonably well-controlled studies with depressed patients. In 50 of these studies (77%), the tricyclic compounds were found to be more effective than placebo. Thus there seems to be little question that these drugs do show clinical efficacy. In studies comparing imipramine with other tricyclic antidepressant drugs, no striking differences in efficacy were noted.

While depression is a disease that is clearly amenable to placebo influences (20–40% of patients responding), at least twice as many subjects will react beneficially to tricyclic compounds (60–75% of patients responding).

Clinical Uses

The tricyclic compounds have become accepted as useful and effective agents in the treatment of depression.

When administered in adequate dosages for sufficient periods of time, these drugs can produce striking changes in the various clinical symptoms of depression. Thus the patient may notice an uplifting of mood, an increase in energy, motivation and confidence, and a tendency to think more positively and hopefully. Concomitant with these changes, marked improvement in many of the vegetative signs of depression (e.g., anorexia, insomnia, loss of libido) may also be observed.

Certain limitations do exist, however, in the use of these drugs. For example, all the agents of this type take a period of time to produce their clinical actions, generally from two to four weeks or more. In the first few days of imipramine administration, a patient may experience a number of side effects and yet receive no benefit from the medication. Thus, motivation to continue taking the drug for the length of time necessary for clinical response may sharply diminish. Because of the slow onset of clinical improvement, it may be necessary to hospitalize a severely depressed and incapacitated patient while antidepressant drug therapy is initiated. This delay in therapeutic response is a particular disadvantage in such patients because of the ever-present possibility of suicide. Thus, the development of a more rapidly acting antidepressant medication would represent a most significant advance.

With the availability of numerous tricyclic antidepressant drugs, it would be a distinct therapeutic advantage if there were reliable methods for choosing the most effective drug for a specific patient. While studies are under way to explore such possibilities, methods are not currently available to make subtle distinctions among the tricyclic compounds. At the present time, the choice of a particular tricyclic drug might be based upon differences in certain secondary effects. For example, amitriptyline, which tends to be sedating, might be appropriate for a highly anxious depressed patient. In contrast, protriptyline, a more activating agent, might be of value in a depressed patient who was quite withdrawn and retarded. Such distinctions among the various tricyclic compounds represent crude empirical approximations; and it would be highly desirable to have specific and objective methods available for making therapeutic distinctions with the antidepressants. A promising correlation between a physiological parameter and drug response is the work with urinary MHPG levels. As outlined in Chapter 14, some recent reports indicate that patients who show low urinary MHPG excretion respond well to imipramine, whereas patients with normal or high MHPG excretion rates tend to respond to amitriptyline. If these observations are supported in future studies, it may provide a basis for selecting a tricyclic compound on the basis of objective data.

Decisions about dosage of the tricyclic compounds are also made on an empirical basis. The dose is often altered during the first couple of weeks of treatment in order to achieve an optimal balance for the individual patient between beneficial effects and adverse side effects. An area of active research, especially in Scandinavia, involves studies of the relationship between plasma concentrations of tricyclic antidepressants and therapeutic response. Data from such studies indicate that there are minimum levels of tricyclic antidepressant compounds in plasma that must be reached in order to obtain a therapeutic response. If this observation is substantiated in further studies, it may be possible to monitor the dose of a particular tricyclic compound by measuring the plasma concentration of the drug. Thus, decisions about dosage could be guided by objective data of plasma concentrations, as is currently the case with lithium usage.

The tricyclic antidepressants can produce a number of side effects, most of which will subside after the first few days of administration. The most commonly observed of these include sedation, dry mouth, blurred vision, urinary retention, skin rashes and orthostatic hypotension. Occasionally, one may also see such effects as congestive heart failure, tremors and hypomania or mania. Rarely are severe reactions associated with the administration of these drugs, such as hallucinations and delusions, seizures, hepatotoxic effects (liver damage) and agranulocytosis (suppression of blood cells). A few cases of arrhythmias leading to sudden death have been reported, and it is now common to exercise some caution in administering tricyclic compounds to patients with a history of cardiac disease. The tricyclic drugs have a fairly low ratio of lethal to therapeutic dose (approximately 10:1); and, as a consequence, a number of depressed patients have committed suicide by taking overdoses of these agents.

In addition to its use in depressed patients, imipramine has also become widely employed in the treatment of enuresis (bed wetting) in children. While the efficacy of imipramine in this condition is well established, the mechanism underlying this effect is not clear.

Mechanism of Action

Much of the speculation about the mechanism of action of the tricyclic antidepressant compounds has focused upon the effects of these drugs on the activity of neurotransmitters, especially norepinephrine and serotonin, in brain. Imipramine has been shown to produce a blockade of neuronal uptake of radioactively-labeled norepinephrine in the peripheral nervous system, an effect similar to that exerted by cocaine. Because of the impermeability of the blood brain barrier to the amines, it was not possible to undertake such studies in the central nervous system. However, the development of the technique of intra-ventricular and intracisternal injection made possible the administration of labeled norepinephrine directly into the ventricular system of the brain. Thus, the effects of imipramine on nor-epinephrine uptake by brain tissue could be evaluated. As was the case in the peripheral nervous system, imip-ramine was shown to block uptake of labeled norepinephrine into brain. It may be recalled that the major mecha-nism of inactivation of norepinephrine from the synaptic cleft is reuptake into the presynaptic neuron. By blocking re-uptake of norepinephrine into the pre-synaptic terminal, more norepinephrine would presumably be kept in the synap-tic cleft, available to activate the post-synaptic receptor.

It should be pointed out that several of the tricyclic antidepressant compounds have also been shown to block the pre-synaptic uptake of serotonin. In fact, a number of European investigators have focused attention primarily upon the effects of these drugs on serotonin up-take. It has become apparent that some tricyclic drugs (e.g., desmethylimipra-mine) are more potent inhibitors of norepinephrine reuptake, while others (e.g., imipramine) exert relatively stronger inhibition of serotonin uptake. It is possible that the effects of the tricyclic compounds on some balance between these two important neuro-transmitter systems may be involved in the therapeutic actions of these drugs.

As indicated in Fig. 2, the tricyclic antidepressants have a 3-carbon side chain, with a terminal nitrogen contain-ing either two or three methyl group substituents. Secondary (two substitu-ent) tricyclic compounds, like desmethyl-imipramine, are more potent inhibitors of norepinephrine uptake, whereas ter-tiary compounds, like imipramine, block serotonin uptake more effectively. Since demethylation is the primary route of metabolism of the tertiary amine tri-cyclics when these compounds are given

in vivo, they are converted to secondary amine compounds. Thus a patient treated with imipramine not only has imipramine in his body but desmethyl-imipramine as well. When administering tertiary amine compounds, then, pro-nounced effects on both serotonin and norepinephrine systems may occur. Neither secondary nor tertiary tricyclic compounds exert prominent blocking ef-fects on the presynaptic uptake of do-pamine.

The blockade of norepinephrine and serotonin uptake by the tricyclic anti-depressant agents represents an acute effect of these drugs, yet their clinical antidepressant actions are not seen for anywhere from several days to four weeks or more. For this reason, several investigators have suggested that the acute effects of the antidepressant drugs may trigger some more chronic, long-term actions of these compounds which may produce their therapeutic effects. Several studies have been conducted on the effects of chronic administration of tricyclic antidepressants on brain neuro-transmitter activity in rats. Data ob-tained from such studies have not pro-vided a clear indication of the clinically relevant effects of these drugs. For ex-ample, in one study, chronic (but not acute) administration of imipramine produced an acceleration of norepineph-rine turnover, while in another, chronic administration of desmethylimipramine resulted in a decrease in the activity of tyrosine hydroxylase in certain areas of brain tissue. It is not known how such findings are related to one another, nor to what extent they may explain the therapeutic effects of these compounds. What is important is that investigators are starting to explore the chronic ef-fects of these agents and not limiting their studies to acute effects.

Although numerous investigations have been conducted on effects of the tri-cyclic antidepressant drugs on mono-amine activity, it is still not possible to determine if these effects are wholly or partially related to the therapeutic actions of these drugs. In fact, effects on other physiological systems could well be important in their therapeutic actions. For example, all of the tricyclic compounds have marked anticholinergic properties. This observation has taken on even greater interest in light of the report by Janowsky and Davis that the administration of physostigmine (a cholinergic-potentiating drug) to manic patients produces a rapid shift in mood, with symptoms of profound depression. Clearly, much additional work is needed to establish which of the pharmacological effects of imipramine are related to its antidepressant actions.

Monoamine Oxidase Inhibitors

The second major class of drugs that have antidepressant activity are those that inhibit the enzyme, monoamine oxidase (MAO). This enzyme catalyzes the oxidative deamination of a number of naturally occurring monoamines, including neurotransmitter agents, such as dopamine, norepinephrine, and serotonin (Chapter 3). This class of drugs is not used widely now, as the tricyclic compounds are at least as efficacious and have less toxicity and dietary restrictions (see below) associated with their administration. However, the monoamine oxidase inhibitors (MAOIs) hold a prominent position in the historical development of the biology of the affective disorders—their efficacy focused attention on the role of monoamine-containing neurons in the etiology of depression, and this area of investigation continues today.

History

In the early 1950's, the compound isoniazid and its isopropyl derivative, iproniazid, were developed for use in tuberculosis. Among the side effects produced by iproniazid in some patients with tuberculosis was euphoria and elation; in contrast, isoniazid did not elicit these central stimulatory effects. Practically simultaneous with these clinical observations, Zeller and his associates showed that iproniazid was an inhibitor of MAO whereas isoniazid was not. When Nathan Kline heard that rats given iproniazid prior to reserpine became hyperalert and hyperactive in contrast to becoming somewhat sedated when given reserpine alone, this caused him to speculate that iproniazid might have antidepressant or "psychic energizing" properties. The fact that Zeller had shown the drug to be a monoamine oxidase inhibitor provided a "scientific rationale" for such an idea, and its central stimulating effect in tuberculosis patients indicated that a trial of iproniazid in depressed patients might be fruitful. In 1957, Kline and his associates reported iproniazid to be efficacious in the treatment of depressed patients. At the same time, Crane found the drug useful in the treatment of chronically fatigued tuberculosis patients with a variety of psychiatric disorders. Subsequent clinical trials indicated that iproniazid was useful in the treatment of depressed patients and the drug was widely used in the late 1950's through the mid–1960's.

Chemistry

There are currently three MAOIs marketed as antidepressants in the United States—isocarboxazid, phenelzine, and tranylcypromine. As shown in Fig. 3, isocarboxazid and phenelzine can be considered hydrazine derivatives, whereas tranylcypromine is not. Inhibition of monoamine oxidase occurs by these substances binding irreversibly to the active site of the enzyme; some differences do exist between the hydrazine and non-hydrazine derivatives in the nature of their binding to the enzyme.

Monoamine Oxidase Inhibitory Drugs

Hydrazine Derivatives   Non-Hydrazine Derivatives

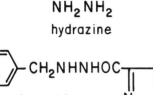

$$NH_2NH_2$$
hydrazine

isocarboxazid

tranylcypromine

phenelzine

nialamide

Fig. 3. The structures of several inhibitors of the enzyme monoamine oxidase. Note the relation of the compounds in the left panel to hydrazine.

The important point, though, is that these are "hit and run" drugs. Their effect, i.e., MAO inhibition, lasts long after they are no longer present in appreciable amounts in the body. Termination of drug effect requires the synthesis of new monoamine oxidase protein, and this can take a couple of weeks.

Clinical Efficacy and Uses

While there seems to be little doubt among many clinicians that MAOIs are useful in the treatment of depression, it has proven difficult to demonstrate conclusively their efficacy in controlled studies. Certainly, the data are not as convincing as for the tricyclic type compounds. Also, these drugs do not appear to be uniformly effective. For example, double-blind studies provide no clear evidence that either isocarboxazid or nialamide is superior to placebo. Even with tranylcypromine, there have been relatively few well designed controlled studies. Of three such investigations, tranylcypromine was found to be superior to placebo in two of the trials. When compared directly to imipramine, tranylcypromine has been found to have comparable efficacy. There have been too few studies to make any definitive statement.

While there is no doubt that the tricyclic-type drugs are the agents of choice for the average depressed patient, there are data suggesting that the MAOIs are particularly effective in certain depressed patients. For example, when tranylcypromine was withdrawn from the market, due to the hypertensive crisis it could evoke, some patients relapsed and did not respond to other types of antidepressants. However, they improved with tranylcypromine when the drug was permitted to be re-marketed. In his survey on this matter, Schiele found 603 such patients. Unfortunately, characteristics of "tranylcypromine-specific responders" that would distinguish them from other depressed patients have not been conclusively demonstrated.

Other investigators have also reported differences in the clinical response of a depressed patient to a tricyclic compound or to an MAOI. For example, Pare has found that patients tend to respond in a similar way to two different tricyclic drugs or to two different MAOIs. However, only 20% of patients improving on treatment with an MAOI showed improvement if subsequently treated with a tricyclic compound. Quite interestingly, a familial association has also been observed in drug response, in that first-degree relatives tend to respond similarly to a particular class of antidepressant drugs, i.e., MAOIs or tricyclics. However, there is no similarity of response when antidepressants of different groups are used. These results have been interpreted as evidence that there can be more than a single biochemical abnormality, determined genetically, which can lead to depressive illness. This area is certainly in need of further exploration.

A number of adverse reactions, such as insomnia, dizziness or vertigo, hypotension or hypertension and dry mouth may be caused by MAOIs. However, effects resulting from interactions with other drugs or foodstuffs are the most serious. For example, MAOIs interfere with liver enzymes responsible for the detoxication of certain other drugs, like barbiturates, alcohol, and narcotic analgesics. As a consequence, MAOIs prolong and potentiate the central depressant effects of these drugs, and this can result in very severe, life-threatening sequelae.

Certainly, the most alarming and most publicized toxic effect associated with administration of MAOIs is the hypertensive crisis they can produce. Oftentimes, the high blood pressure elicits a headache, which may be associated with sweating, pallor, nausea, vomiting, fright and muscle twitching. These painful, alarming attacks usually end after a few hours. However, much more severe or even fatal syndromes can ensue, such as the syndrome associated with severe hypertension leading to intracranial hemorrhage.

The hypertensive crisis seen with MAOI administration results from the ingestion of foodstuffs containing agents that can cause the release of endogenously stored catecholamines. Such agents are termed indirectly acting sympathomimetics, as their effects "mimic" that of stimulation of the sympathetic nervous system, e.g., a rise in blood pressure. A pharmacist, G. E. F. Rowe, noted that his wife, who was receiving an MAOI, experienced hypertensive crisis with headaches after eating cheese. Subsequent investigation of this phenomenon by Blackwell and his associates conclusively demonstrated that in the presence of an MAOI, cheese could precipitate a large rise in blood pressure, the so-called "cheese reaction." The rise in blood pressure is due to tyramine in the cheese. This amino acid is normally metabolized by MAO. In the presence of monoamine oxidase inhibition, tyramine has a longer than normal duration of action and is able to release the greater than normal amounts of norepinephrine stored in sympathetic nerve terminals. Other foodstuffs containing a variety of sympathomimetic amines include chianti wine, chicken liver, broad bean pods, certain yeast products, and chocolate. For this reason, patients placed on MAOIs are given strict diets that eliminate such foods; this constitutes a serious problem in the management of outpatients with these drugs.

Mechanism of Action — As their class name implies, the antidepressant effect of these drugs has been attributed to inhibition of monoamine oxidase. It must be emphasized that there is no conclusive evidence that this is so. Certainly, there are a number of agents that inhibit MAO which do not have antidepressant properties. However, there has been a notable dearth of investigations examining the effects of these drugs on loci other than MAO.

As a consequence of inhibition of MAO, the concentration of catecholamines and of serotonin rises in different organs, including brain. Elevations in the concentrations of dopamine, norepinephrine, and serotonin have been observed in human brain tissue obtained at autopsy from patients treated with MAOIs.

As mentioned in Chapter 3, we know now that there are several different isoenzymes of MAO. The MAOIs that are used clinically are, in general, nonspecific inhibitor drugs. It is anticipated that there may be considerable therapeutic advantage in developing compounds that would inhibit selectively the different isoenzymes of MAO.

Antimanic Drugs (Lithium Ion)

There has been a veritable explosion of interest recently in the uses of the lithium ion in psychiatry. It now seems reasonably well established that the lithium ion is effective in mania and hypomania; that it reduces the severity and frequency of affective relapses in patients with manic-depressive and probably recurrent depressive illness as well. Furthermore, evidence is accumulating that it has antidepressant effects in a subgroup of depressed patients. Its uses in other conditions (e.g., epilepsy, aggressive behavior, thyrotoxicosis; inappropriate secretion of antidiuretic hormone) are currently under investigation but are not nearly as well established as its uses in affective disorders.

History

Lithium was discovered in 1818 by Arfvedson working in Berzelius' laboratory. Perhaps the earliest mention of the use of lithium-containing solutions in medicine was made by Soranus of Ephesus in the second century, A.D. He referred to the use of alkaline waters, which contain lithium ion, in the treatment of mania.

The lithium ion was first deliberately employed for the treatment of manic patients by the Australian psychiatrist, John F. Cade, in 1949. Cade had performed experiments based on the idea that mania was due to an excess of some substance circulating in the body. He found that human urine injected into guinea pigs killed the animals, and that some specimens from manic patients killed more readily than control specimens. His investigations caused him to suspect that urea was the toxic substance and that uric acid was potentiating the toxic effects of urea. To explore this idea, he needed to inject uric acid into guinea pigs together with urea. As uric acid is quite insoluble in water, he used the most soluble urate—lithium urate—and injected it together with urea into guinea pigs. This combination did not enhance the toxic effect of urea, but rather there were less deaths than expected with injection of urea alone. Could the lithium ion be exerting a "protective" effect? Lithium carbonate was tested subsequently and also produced protection against the toxic effect of urea. Furthermore, injection of lithium carbonate alone caused the guinea pigs to become lethargic and unresponsive to stimuli, even though fully conscious. Cade reasoned that since the lithium ion "calmed" the guinea pigs, it might do the same to manic patients. After first taking the compound himself to confirm its safety, he administered the lithium ion to ten manic patients. All of them improved substantially.

In retrospect, it is probable that the "calming" effect of the lithium ion that Cade observed in guinea pigs was a sign of toxicity—due to the large doses that Cade administered. However, as Kline has pointed out, "If we were to eliminate from science all the great discoveries that had come about as the result of mistaken hypotheses or fluky experimental data, we would be lacking half of what we now know (or think we know)."

Subsequent to the publication of Cade's results in 1949, lithium began to be widely used for mania in Australia and Europe. It should be pointed out that this use of lithium in 1949 makes it the first agent in the modern era of psychopharmacology in that it preceded the introduction of chlorpromazine.

Absorption, Distribution, and Excretion

The lithium ion is only administered orally to man. It can be detected in the blood within a short time following its ingestion; peak blood levels are attained 1.5 to 3 hours after oral administration of the cation. Maximum serum levels reached upon *chronic* administration (and with fixed dosage, this usually occurs in 4 to 6 days) vary directly with the dosage and correlate negatively with both body weight and the renal clearance of the ion.

The plasma concentration of lithium that is recommended for therapeutic effectiveness varies somewhat with the clinical state for which it is being used. For mania, plasma concentrations above 1 mM are usually used, and concentrations as high as 1.5 mM may be necessary. Lower levels than these are usually used in lithium maintenance therapy and the treatment of depression, with plasma concentrations of 0.6 to 1.0 mM being employed most often. Dosages of lithium salts necessary to achieve these plasma levels vary from patient to patient. In the United States, the lithium ion is usually administered as the carbonate salt, at daily dosages raging from 600 to 2400 mg.

The lithium ion is not bound to plasma proteins. It passes from the blood into tissues so that an equilibrium is established between serum and cells. As originally shown by Schou, equilibrium occurs rapidly with organs such as liver and kidney, slower with muscle, and slowest with the brain. The slow penetration of the lithium ion into the brain is due to the retarded movement of the polar cation through the non-polar blood-brain barrier.

Most cells contain less lithium inside than outside, with the ratio of intracellular to extracellular lithium varying between 0.3 – 0.5.

The profound effects of the lithium ion on behavior, then, occur at relatively modest extracellular and intracellular concentrations of the cation. Plasma levels of lithium are less than 1% that of sodium, the monovalent cation found in highest concentration in plasma. Similarly, potassium is found in much higher concentration inside the cell than is lithium. However, plasma potassium levels are only about 4 to 8 times those of extracellular lithium ion, and intracellular sodium ion levels are not nearly as high as those of intracellular potassium. One might speculate, then, that if lithium exerts its effects by modifying sodium- or potassium-dependent systems, it affects an extracellular potassium site

Table 1. Physicochemical properties of some alkali and alkaline-earth elements

	K	Na	Li	Mg	Ca
Atomic radius (Å)	2.03	1.57	1.33	1.36	1.74
Crystal ionic radius (Å)	1.33	0.95	0.60	0.65	0.99
Corrected hydrated radius (Å)	2.32	2.76	3.40	4.65	3.21
Electronegativity	0.8	0.9	1.0	1.2	1.0
Polarizing power (z/r^2)	0.56	1.12	2.8	4.7	2.05

and/or an intracellular sodium site.

Alternatively, interactions of lithium with systems regulated by divalent cations, such as magnesium and calcium, might be important. These divalent cations are present in the body at concentrations only several fold higher than those of lithium found clinically; they are involved in neuronal function (see Chater 2); the lithium ion has certain physicochemical properties similar to magnesium ion or calcium ion (Table 1). A promising area of research is the effect of the lithium ion on both monovalent and divalent cation-dependent systems.

The main route of lithium excretion is through the kidneys. Over 90% of ingested lithium ion can be accounted for in the urine. Its elimination half-life, which is roughly equivalent to its plasma half-life (the time for the plasma concentration to be reduced in half), is about 14 to 24 hours. There is a competition between sodium and lithium ions for kidney re-absorption, so that care must be taken when administering lithium ion concurrently with certain diuretic agents that promote sodium loss.

Clinical Efficacy and Uses

Mania — Since Cade's original study, there have been more than 1,000 patients with mania treated with lithium re-ported on in the literature. The results of both open and "blind" studies indicate that it is very effective in the control of mania and hypomania. It is a more specific antimanic agent than chlorpromazine in that it dissipates the core symptoms of mania, e.g., euphoria, grandiosity, without causing the overt sedation characteristic of the phenothiazines. Its clinical effect in mania is often not observed for 10 to 14 days; for this reason, phenothiazines are often recommended for initial treatment of the acutely agitated manic patient.

Prophylaxis or Maintenance Treatment — The initial observation that the lithium ion might be useful in either preventing or reducing the intensity of depressive episodes was made independently by Hartigan and by Baastrup and reported in the early 1960's. These psychiatrists noted that some of their manic patients given long-term lithium treatment did not appear at the outpatient clinic when depressive episodes might have been expected, from the pre-lithium clinical course of the illness. When contacted by the psychiatrists, the patients said that the depressions had not appeared. Subsequently, long-term maintenance chemotherapy has been evaluated in a number of placebo-controlled studies.

Most of the controlled studies involving lithium are analyzed in terms of bipolar versus unipolar illness. This classification scheme is discussed in Chapters 13 and 16.

A number of investigations involving a total of about 400 bipolar patients have been performed to evaluate the long-term efficacy of the lithium ion. Lithium has been shown to be significantly better than placebo insofar as it reduced the total number of both manic and depressive relapses. In these patients, it appears to be somewhat better in preventing manic than depressive relapses, although it is clearly effective in preventing or reducing the intensity of depressive episodes.

A smaller number of unipolar patients have been studied in comparison with the bipolar group with regard to the long-term effectiveness of lithium. In general, lithium tended to be better than placebo in either reducing the frequency or the duration or intensity of depressive episodes. The lithium ion has recently been approved for use in the long-term maintenance treatment of bipolar patients. Further evaluation of its effectiveness in unipolar illness has been recommended before any conclusive decision is reached.

Antidepressant Effect — Finally, several investigators, notably Mendels and his associates, have demonstrated that the lithium ion is an effective antidepressant in a *subgroup* of depressed patients. The precise characteristics of this subgroup of patients and the determination of whether the lithium ion by itself sufficiently resolves all of the symptoms of this group remains unresolved. In general, bipolar patients are about twice as likely as unipolar patients are to respond favorably to the antidepressant effect of lithium. However, not all bipolar patients respond and some unipolar patients do respond.

The fact that not all bipolar depressives are lithium responsive is, of course, similar to the well-established findings that not all manic patients are lithium responsive, and that lithium is not an effective prophylactic agent for all bi-polar patients. The point to be emphasized is that lithium is not a panacea with regard to affective disorders. When it works, it is very effective. However, about 25% of manic patients do not respond, prophylaxis-failure rates may be as high as 40 to 50%, and those depressives in whom it is effective (primarily bipolar patients) constitute only a modest percentage of the total number of hospitalized depressed patients.

This is not to belittle its importance in psychiatry, however. First, the fact that it is an effective agent in manic-depressive illness has increased the likelihood of this diagnosis being made by American psychiatrists. It seems clear that there has been over-diagnosing of schizophrenia in the United States and under-diagnosing of manic-depressive illness. Second, the fact that it can be effective in both mania and depression has contributed to a theoretical reassessment of the biological relationship between these two clinical states. While the manifest symptomatology of mania and depression suggest that they are opposite states, the effectiveness of lithium in both conditions, together with other biochemical and neurophysiological data, allows for the possibility that mania and depression may have certain biological similarities (see Chapter 14).

Mechanism of Action

As with all other psychotropic agents, the precise cellular mechanism of action by which the lithium ion produces its beneficial effects is unknown. Numerous investigations of its pharmacological effects on monoamine systems have been carried out, in view of the postulated roles of the monoamines in affective disorders. In addition, its general effects on nerve function have been examined, probably because of interest in its ability to substitute for either the sodium or potassium ion. To determine the efficacy with which lithium could substitute for sodium or potassium, the extra-cellular concentration of the latter two ions has often been replaced completely by lithium. It should be borne in mind that extrapolation from these type of experiments to the clinical situation (where low concentrations of lithium are used in the presence of normal sodium and potassium levels) may yield spurious conclusions.

There appears to be general agreement that Li^+ can substitute for Na^+, at least initially, in carrying the current of the action potential. However, the efficiency of the Li^+ replacement for Na^+ is reduced with time so that the nerve becomes inexcitable. The development of inexcitability upon stimulation in a solution in which Li^+ has replaced Na^+ has been attributed to the fact that Li^+ is extruded from nerve cells at a rate very much less than that of Na^+. The lithium ion accumulates in nerves so that the concentration gradient necessary to carry the current for the action potential is eliminated. Much lower levels of Li^+ are used clinically than those necessary to cause nerves to become inexcitable by such a mechanism. It is unlikely, then, that the latter contributes to the clinical efficacy of the lithium ion.

This is not to say that Li^+ cannot effect neuronal excitability at clinically relevant concentrations. Rather, the mechanism by which it may do so is different from that described above. One way, which is receiving increasing attention, is by affecting the small potentials produced by the sodium pump. If equal numbers of Na^+ and K^+ ions are transported (1:1 coupling ratio), the pump will be electrically neutral; in contrast, if more Na^+ is extruded than K^+ is absorbed (e.g., coupling ratio of 3:2), then the pump is "electrogenic" and would contribute to the membrane potential by generating a current across the membrane. The contribution of such "electrogenic potentials" to the resting membrane potential is usually quite small. However, the contribution is more important when the nerve is stimulated to an extent such that the activity of the sodium pump is increased. This would occur when nerves are stimulated very rapidly with stimuli of maximal strength—a tetanic stimulus. There is a hyperpolarization of the nerve immediately after tetanic stimuli and this hyperpolarization is due primarily to the electrogenic nature of the sodium pump. This hyperpolarization makes the nerve less excitable to subsequent stimuli.

In an elegant series of experiments, Ploeger has shown that low concentrations of the lithium ion inhibit the amplitude of neuronal hyperpolarization due to activity of the sodium pump. The inhibition produced by Li^+ appears to be due to effects of Li^+ at both the potassium and sodium sites of the pump. The inhibitory effect of Li^+ was most pronounced during periods of increased nervous activity. It was speculated that the antimanic action of the lithium ion was related to its affecting neuronal excitability by having an inhibitory effect on electrogenic potentials resulting from stimulated nerve activity. This appears to be a promising area of research.

In addition to effects on neuronal excitability, the lithium ion has also been shown to modify neurotransmitter metabolism. In particular, its actions on catecholamine and serotonin systems have been studied extensively.

The lithium ion exerts several effects that could result in an impairment of central catecholamine transmission. For example, it has been shown to (1) decrease the evoked release of NE, (2) increase the uptake of NE into pinched-off nerve ending preparations, synaptosomes (thereby making less NE available to stimulate postsynaptic receptors), and (3) inhibit the stimulation of adenylate cyclase by NE. Inhibition of central catecholamine transmission by Li^+ could account for the antimanic properties of the cation if viewed within the framework of too much central catecholamine activity leading to mania (see Chapter 14). Its antidepressant properties, though, would appear to be incompatible with such actions.

Acute administration of the lithium ion increases the turnover of brain serotonin. It may do so by increasing the uptake of the serotonin precursor, L-tryptophan, into nerve. However, with repeated administration of the lithium ion, compensatory mechanisms appear to come into play so that there is decreased activity of tryptophan hydroxylase, the rate-limiting enzyme in serotonin synthesis. As a consequence, the synthesis of serotonin becomes reduced.

The effects of acute and chronic administration of the lithium ion on amine systems can be quite different, then. We do not know yet which effect may be more important clinically. Are the chronic effects compensatory in nature and serve no useful purpose? Or, rather, are they the clinically revelant actions, considering the delay in onset of the clinical manifestations of the lithium ion. Additional research must be directed at answering this important question.

The effects of Li^+ on the adenylate cyclase-cyclic AMP system deserve emphasis, as they may account for some of the side effects of Li^+, if not for its clinical efficacy. For example, the administration of lithium carbonate to man can produce polyuria which is resistant to the administration of antidiuretic hormone (ADH). The antidiuretic effect of this hormone is thought to result from an increase in medullary adenosine 3′, 5′ monophosphate (cyclic AMP). Since ADH activation of adenylate cyclase preparations from human renal medullary tissues is decreased by lithium ions, the diuretic effect of lithium may be, in part, a consequence of this cellular effect of the ion. Recent evidence indicates that lithium may also interfere with the effects of ADH at a site distal to the formation of cyclic AMP. In a similar manner, the antithyroid effects of lithium may be related to an inhibition of the effect of thyroid-stimulating hormone (TSH) on thyroid adenylate cyclase, in addition to effects in the thyroid gland at a site subsequent to cyclic AMP formation. The inhibitory effect of the lithium ion appears to be the consequence of its activity at an intracellular site; extracellular Li^+ is ineffective in this regard.

The lithium ion, then, has complex effects on neuronal excitability and synaptic transmission. It is hoped that the unravelling of these complex effects can provide a clue as to the underlying pathobiology of manic-depressive illnesses.

Antianxiety Agents

Meprobamate (Miltown) was the first drug in this category to be utilized in treating anxiety in patients. More recently, two drugs of the benzodiazepine class, diazepam (Valium) and chlordiazepoxide (Librium) have become the most popular of the antianxiety agents, and they currently represent, respectively, the first and third most commonly prescribed medications in the United States. While it is difficult to know the exact pattern of utilization of these drugs, it has been estimated that one out of every ten adult Americans will ingest an antianxiety agent during the course of one year. The structures of these compounds are shown in Fig. 4.

History

Meprobamate was initially synthesized in 1954 as a potential muscle relaxant. In clinical studies conducted a short time later, it was found to be effective in the treatment of anxiety.

The benzodiazepines were synthesized in 1933, and were considered to be of

antianxiety agents

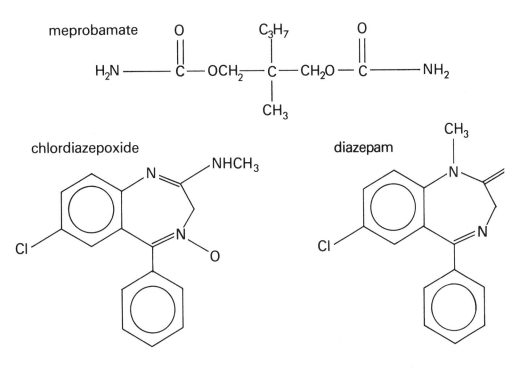

Fig. 4. **The structures of several of the commonly employed antianxiety agents.**

interest because of their muscle-relaxant properties. In 1960, Randall and co-workers reported that these agents had a "taming" effect in animals. This effect appeared at lower doses than those necessary to produce hypnotic effects in the same animals. On the basis of these results, clinical trials were conducted in humans, and the benzodiazepines were found to be effective in the treatment of anxiety, as will be discussed later.

Physiological Effects

The benzodiazepines are complicated drugs with a variety of clinical effects, including antianxiety action, sedation, muscle relaxant properties and anti-convulsant effects. It is difficult to deter-

mine whether the varied clinical effects produced by the benzodiazepines are related to one or to several of the physiological and biochemical actions exerted by these drugs. As is the case for most centrally acting agents, the benzodiazepines produce a variety of effects on several different aspects of central nervous system function, and these effects are seen at many different sites in the brain. In general, the pharmacological effects of the benzodiazepines are difficult to distinguish from those produced by sedative-hypnotic agents, such as the barbiturates. However, some studies have indicated that the benzodiazepines are less sedating, and produce less impairment of learning, coordination and motor performance than do the barbiturates.

Animal Models of Anxiety

Several animal models for anxiety states have been developed in which the antianxiety agents are capable of exerting notable effects which have been interpreted as being potentially related to their antianxiety action. In a behavioral paradigm developed by Geller and Seifter, hungry rats are trained to press a lever in order to obtain sweetened milk, which is provided at irregular intervals. Periodically, a punishment period is set up in which the rats receive an electrical shock to the feet in response to pressing the lever. During this punishment period, lever-pressing can be effectively suppressed in proportion to the intensity of the shock provided. After administration of a benzodiazepine drug, rats show a restoration of frequent lever-pressing during the punishment periods. In this conflict test, the benzodiazepines appear to *disinhibit* the suppressive effects of the punishing electrical shocks—as if the rats were no longer worried or concerned about this negative reinforcement. In contrast, a number of related drugs including barbiturates, antipsychotic agents and morphine, do not produce this type of disinhibitory effect on response during the punishment cycle. Rather, these drugs tend to produce a generalized suppression of all behavioral responses.

Clinical Efficacy

As is pointed out in Chapter 9, considerable care must be taken in evaluating the efficacy of a psychopharmacological agent. This is particularly true in the case of the antianxiety drugs, since anxiety is a difficult entity to define and measure, and since treatment outcome in anxious patients is influenced by many nonspecific, non-pharmacological factors. In spite of such limitations, there have been a number of well-controlled double-blind studies demonstrating that the antianxiety agents are clearly more effective than placebo in treating anxiety.

While the benzodiazepines are more effective than placebo, some people have argued that they are really just high-priced sedatives, and that they are no more effective or specific in treating anxiety than are barbiturates, such as phenobarbitol. Data from a limited number of double-blind studies indicates that the benzodiazepines are more effective in the treatment of anxiety than are the barbiturates, but it is difficult to know whether the dosages used for each class of drug in these studies allow a valid comparison between the two groups.

The benzodiazepines have also been compared to antipsychotic compounds in the treatment of highly anxious, non-psychotic patients. In these studies, the benzodiazepines have proven to be clearly more effective. The antipsychotic compounds, therefore, are not effective in the treatment of anxiety *per se*; similarly, the benzodiazepines are not useful antipsychotic agents. In other words, there are qualitative differences between these classes of drugs.

Clinical Uses

The widespread use of the antianxiety agents in the United States has already been pointed out. There are many critics who feel that these drugs are over-prescribed and over-utilized, that this is, in fact, the "age of tranquilization." On the other hand, data obtained by Rickels and co-workers indicates that many anxious patients receive either no treatment at all, or else too little medication for too short a period of time to achieve clinically effective results. Thus, rather than focusing on the overuse of the antianxiety agents, attention should be placed on more careful and thoughtful utilization of these drugs.

The antianxiety agents are prescribed

by both psychiatrists and general practitioners for the treatment of anxiety. They are also frequently employed in the treatment of symptoms of anxiety in patients who are suffering from depression. The antianxiety agents are not, however, an effective primary treatment for depression. These drugs are also commonly employed in the treatment of a number of other conditions. The sedative-hypnotic effects of these compounds make them valuable as mild sleeping pills, and they have the advantage, in comparison to the barbiturates, of having a very low suicide potential. In fact, there are no reported cases of death subsequent to over-dosage with benzodiazepines by themselves. This is a very important factor in treating the sleep disturbance problems of depressed patients, with whom suicide is always a concern.

In addition to the previously described uses, the benzodiazepines are also utilized in a number of other capacities. They are effective muscle relaxants, and therefore are of value in the treatment of lower back pain. Diazepam is considered to be the treatment of choice for status epilepticus, a form of epilepsy. Both diazepam and chlordiazepoxide are commonly used in the treatment of acute alcoholism, including alcohol withdrawal and *delerium tremens* (DT's). Finally, the benzodiazepines are frequently employed as an adjunct therapy in a number of medical disorders, such as hypertension. It is not known whether these agents may have any specific therapeutic value in the treatment of these disorders beyond their antianxiety properties.

Mechanism of Action
of the Benzodiazepines

The benzodiazepines exert a number of effects on neurochemical activity in brain, including a decrease in the turnover of both norepinephrine and serotonin. Administration of a benzodiazepine results in alterations in the activity of several other central nervous system neurotransmitters, including acetyl choline, glycine and gamma-aminobutyric acid (GABA). In light of the multiple physiological effects (antianxiety, sedative, muscle relaxant, anticonvulsant) of the benzodiazepines and their many complex effects on neurotransmitter activity, it has been extremely difficult to identify one "mechanism of action" for these agents. Recently, a number of research strategies have been developed to demonstrate more specific relationships between effects on neurotransmitter activity and the behavioral effects of the benzodiazepines.

Stein and co-workers have utilized the conflict test of Geller and Seifter as an animal model of anxiety. In these studies, the disinhibitory (or "antianxiety") action of the benzodiazepines appeared to be exerted through effects on serotonin activity. This conclusion was based upon data indicating that serotonin antagonists mimicked the disinhibitory actions of the benzodiazepines, whereas intraventricular administration of serotonin heightened inhibition. The effects of the benzodiazepines on norepinephrine turnover did not appear to be related to disinhibition.

Recently, much of the interest regarding the mechanism of action of the benzodiazepines has focused upon the effects of these drugs on gamma-aminobutyric acid (GABA). GABA is generally accepted to be an inhibitory neurotransmitter in both the spinal cord and brain. A number of experimental observations have pointed to an interaction between the benzodiazepines and GABA. For example, benzodiazepines antagonize convulsions elicited by pentylenetetrazole, an inhibitor of GABA synthesis. In an isolated frog spinal cord preparation, benzodiazepines produce presynaptic inhibition, an effect which is mediated by GABA in the spinal cord. Picrotoxin and other GABA inhibitors oppose the production of presynaptic inhibition elicited by the benzodiazepines. Effects of the benzodiazepines on GABA have been demonstrated at sites elsewhere in the central nervous system, including the cerebellum, cuneate nucleus and hippocampus. In the striatum, benzodiazepines produce a decrease in dopamine turnover, an effect that has been shown to be mediated by GABA. The GABA receptor antagonist, bicuculline, opposes this decrease in dopamine turnover, but the effects of bicuculline can be overcome by increasing the dose of the benzodiazepine.

Costa and co-workers have examined another aspect of benzodiazepine-GABA interactions, the involvement of a nucleotide second messenger, guanosine 3',5' monophosphate (cyclic GMP). In the cerebellum, an increase in GABA concentration was found to be associated with a decreased cyclic GMP level. Diazepam also lowers cerebellar cyclic GMP. The drug harmaline induces tremors as a result of stimulation of the nigro-striatal pathway, in association with an increase in cyclic GMP levels. Diazepam was shown to inhibit both the tremor and the increase in cyclic GMP produced by harmaline.

The effect of benzodiazepines on GABA activity could be related to the clinical actions of these drugs. For example, the enhancement of presynaptic inhibition in the isolated spinal cord preparation could be related to the muscle-relaxant properties of the benzodiazepines, while the blockade of pentylenetetrazole-induced convulsions may help to explain the anticonvulsant properties of these compounds. An explanation for the antianxiety effects of the benzodiazepines is more elusive because of the problem of developing adequate animal models of anxiety. Nevertheless, studies on the effects of benzodiazepines on GABA activity appear to offer considerable promise for advancing our understanding of the mechanism of action of the antianxiety agents.

At this time, much further data must be collected to elucidate and further clarify the neurochemical mechanisms underlying the actions of the benzodiazepines. This is an important, albeit challenging, enterprise since there is a real need for antianxiety agents that are more effective and less tied to sedative side effects.

Selected References

Asberg, M.: Plasma nortriptyline levels—Relationship to clinical effects. *Clin. Pharmacol. Exp. Ther.* 16:215-229, 1974.

Ayd, F.J., and Blackwell, B.: *Discoveries in Biological Psychiatry.* J.B. Lippincott Co., Philadelphia, 1970.

Byck, R.: Drugs and the treatment of psychiatric disorders. In *The Pharmacological Basis of Therapeutics,* 5th Ed., L.S. Goodman and A. Gilman, eds. Macmillan Publishing Co., Inc., New York, 1975, pp. 152-200.

Costa, E., and Greengard, P. (Eds.): *Advances in Biochemical Psychopharmacology,* Vol. 14, Mechanism of Action of Benzodiazepines, Raven Press, New York, 1975.

Creese, I., Burt, D.B., and Snyder, S.H.: Dopamine receptor binding predicts clinical and pharmacological potencies of antischizophrenic drugs. *Science* 192:481-483, 1976.

Gershon, S., and Shopsin, B. (Eds.): *Lithium: Its Role in Psychiatric Research and Treatment,* Plenum Press, New York, 1973.

Glowinski, J., and Axelrod, J.: Effects of drugs on the disposition of H-3-norepinephrine in the rat brain. *Pharmacol. Rev.* 18:775-785, 1966.

Klein, D.F., and Davis, J.M.: *Diagnosis and Drug Treatment of Psychiatric Disorders,* Williams and Wilkins Co., Baltimore, 1969.

Neff, N.H., and Yang, H.-Y.T.: Another look at the monoamine oxidases and the monoamine oxidase inhibitor drugs. *Life. Sci.* 14: 2061-2074, 1974.

Ploeger, E.J.: The effects of lithium on excitable cell membranes. On the mechanism of inhibition of the sodium pump of nonmyelinated nerve fibers of the rat. *Eur. J. Pharmacol.* 25:316-321, 1974.

Rickels, R., Downing, R.W., and Winokur, A.: Anti-anxiety drugs: Clinical use in psychiatry. In *Handbook of Psychopharmacology,* Section III, L.L. Iversen, S.D. Iversen, and S.H. Snyder, Eds. Plenum Publishing Co., New York, 1976.

Seeman, P., and Lee, T.: Antipsychotic drugs: Direct correlation between clinical potency and presynaptic action on dopamine neurons. *Science* 188:1217-1219, 1975.

Shader, R.E. (Ed.): *Manual of Psychiatric Therapeutics.* Little, Brown and Co., Boston, 1975.

Singer, I., and Rottenberg, D.: Mechanisms of lithium action. *N. Engl. J. Med.* 289:254-260, 1973.

Snyder, S.H., Banerjee, S.P., Yamamura, H.I., and Greenberg, D.: Drugs, neurotransmitters, and schizophrenia. *Science* 184:1243-1253, 1974.

Part IV

Clinical Considerations and Biological Investigations of Psychiatric Disorders

MENTAL *diseases are a major public health problem. The suffering experienced by the affected individuals and their families cannot be evaluated adequately; to many, it constitutes the most painful experience of their lives. It is possible, though, to estimate their financial impact. The total cost of mental illness (both direct medical and indirect social costs) in the United States is in the region of $75 billion. In the section that follows, the syndromes that contribute to a large part of this cost are described—schizophrenias, affective illnesses, opiate dependence, and alcoholism. The clinical description of these syndromes is the focus of several of these chapters, while the biological factors associated with these illnesses are emphasized in other chapters. Although our understanding of these conditions has increased considerably over the past fifteen years, careful reading of this section will illustrate that there is still a great deal to be learned.*

Thus, improvements have been made in our ability to diagnose these illnesses properly and to categorize patients having these syndromes into meaningful subgroups. Indeed, the biological approach holds great promise in this area—with diagnoses being assisted by measurement of certain biological parameters and by response to chemotherapy. However, much more research needs to be directed to this area, and we are still years away from having confirmed diagnostic tests of a biological nature for the schizophrenias and affective illnesses.

Ideas about the biological nature of these diseases seem more substantial, with emphasis being placed on abnormalities in the functioning of central biogenic amine systems. This is primarily because the drugs used to treat schizophrenia, mania, and depression modify synaptic transmission in central aminergic neurons. Unfortunately, clinical data consistent with pharmacologically-derived theories of schizophrenia and affective illness have been slow in coming forth. As is illustrated in this section, this remains an exciting and vigorously pursued research area.

The final two chapters describe the syndromes of opiate dependence and alcoholism. Current pharmacological theories of physical dependence and tolerance are discussed, with ideas centering around drug-induced changes in the functioning of central monoaminergic neurons. It appears that the establishment of drug-induced changes in the sensitivity of aminergic receptors may be an important breakthrough in this field. The current status of the therapy of opiate dependence and alcoholism is characterized, and it becomes evident that chemotherapy must co-exist with psychotherapy, social counseling and behavior modification to achieve beneficial results in these disorders.

Chapter 11

Schizophrenia: Clinical Aspects

Robert Cancro

Approximately 50% of the mental hospital beds and more than 25% of all hospital beds in the United States are filled by patients labeled schizophrenic. There is about one chance in 100 that any given individual will be hospitalized during his or her life time with this diagnosis. The total world population of these patients is estimated at 10 million. Clearly, this disorder represents a major public health problem.

Efforts at classification have reflected the various scientific and social forces operating at that particular time. The disorder has been seen as everything from a specific disease entity to a tran-scending of the mundane limits of reality. There has been no scientific classification of schizophrenia which has led to an improved understanding of the disorder and few clinical classifications which have proven to be generally acceptable. While these controversies create obvious problems for the student, many of the difficulties can be avoided by a clear delineation of the assumptions used by a particular author.

Prior to discussing diagnostic considerations, it is useful to specify the conceptualization of schizophrenia which will be utilized in this chapter. Schizophrenia is being thought of as a biobehavioral disorder which manifests itself in characteristic aberrations of thought, affect, and behavior. Conceptualizing it as a biobehavioral disorder means that there must be a number of alternative genetic pathways to the same end state. Utilizing this approach necessitates a syndrome conception of the disorder in which different patients can arrive at the same diagnostic end state from different initial conditions through a variety of pathways. The schizophrenias represent, in other words, a heterogeneous group of disorders which share certain clinical features to varying degrees. In the absence of an independent, biologic diagnostic test for this disorder, reliance on criteria which are based on the clinical phenomena will of necessity be arbitrary. At the present time, schizophrenia represents a *clinical* syndrome as opposed, for example, to diabetes mellitus which represents a *biochemical* syndrome. There are biological tests for diabetes mellitus which identify the final metabolic pathway of the disorder independent of the different genetic mechanisms for arriving at it. We have no such diagnostic procedure for the group of the schizophrenias. This leads to an inherent within and between sample heterogeneity that interferes not only with biological but with all research efforts on the syndrome. Having recognized the inevitability of utilizing arbitrary diagnostic criteria, we can still avoid the danger of making them capricious in nature.

This chapter will follow, in a slightly modified fashion, Eugen Bleuler's reliance on the altered fundamental signs for the diagnosis of a schizophrenic disorder. The advantage of using this modified approach is that it is likely to reduce population heterogeneity. Many of the ,other approaches which utilize a large number of different signs and symptoms tend to increase heterogeneity. It is, therefore, a worthwhile strategy to use those criteria which are likely to result in a more narrow and hopefully more homogeneous population.

Bleuler suggested *four fundamental altered signs of schizophrenia*. These were autism, ambivalence, affective disorder, and thought disorder. *Autism* is defined as the pathologic predominance of fantasy life over reality. Autism is not unique to the schizophrenias but is found in all people at some time. Bleuler argued there was a quantitative difference in the schizophrenias since reality was abandoned and replaced by fantasy life. This abandonment of reality is, however, characteristic of a number of mental disorders and is not specific for schizophrenia.

If autism is not pathognomonic of schizophrenia, certainly ambivalence is even less so. *Ambivalence* is a characteristic of the human condition. Nevertheless, it is true that extreme examples of ambivalence occur in schizophrenia and are not restricted exclusively to the feeling life of the individual but may invade speech and motor patterns as well. When seen in the motor system, it is referred to as ambitendence. A common example of ambitendence is the patient's offering and withdrawing his hand in response to the examiner's proffered handshake.

Affect can be described in terms of range, lability, and appropriateness. The affective range can be thought of as the difference between the peaks and the valleys of a sinusoid curve. People normally show a considerable range in their affective display and, characteristically, this range is narrowed in schizophrenia. This is described clinically as a constriction or narrowing of the affect. At times, the narrowing is so severe that the affect can be described as flat instead of constricted. The rate and frequency with which the affective display changes in character can be described as its lability. Characteristically, this lability is diminished in schizophrenia, particularly in chronic patients. The appropriateness of the affect is determined on the basis of the "correctness" of its correspondence to the ideational content. If the affect shown is not appropriate to the associated ideas, it is considered a characteristic sign of schizophrenia.

If there is any single diagnostic criterion which promises to be relatively specific for the schizophrenic syndrome, it is the *thought disorder*. The cognitive disturbance can be usefully divided into disorders of the word and disorders of the sentence. In the former category we find desymbolization of words or clang association in which words are treated as sounds and not as consensually defined representations of reality. A second type of disorder of the word is semantic shift. Most words have two or more meanings. Semantic shift is demonstrated when the patient fails to suppress the inappropriate meaning in that context and responds to the word in terms of an alternative meaning. A clinical example is the patient who saw a sign labeled "Admitting Office" and asked if that was the place where one went to admit the bad things he had done. Another type involves the use of words in an approximate sense. This sign has been called metonymic distortion. An example is the patient who referred to his half-sister as a part-sister. The final type in this category is the neologism in which the patient makes up new words. The mechanism for the neologism is often through the condensation of two or more real words.

Loosening of associations is the classical example of the disorder of the sentence. It is manifested by a break in the sequence of speech so that the observer cannot understand how the patient got from one to the next association. An example is the patient who responded to the sentence completion test statement: "The man fell on the street . . . ," with the answer "because of World War I." Another example of a disorder of the sentence is system shifting where the paitient is unable to maintain the sentence in its appropriate system of meaning. The patient was asked: "Where is your husband?" She replied: "In the photograph on the mantelpiece." The final example of disorders of the sentence is sham language or word salad where

speech becomes incomprehensible because words are scrambled together in a patternless way that does not convey meaning.

Other formal signs of thought disorder include blocking or thought withdrawal where the subject has the experience of his mind suddenly becoming empty. Thought insertion is often cited as a disorder of thought processes but is best conceived of as a delusion, since it involves the fixed, false belief that ideas are being put into the patient's mind. *Gedankenlautwerden* is also described frequently as an example of thought disorder. This term is translated into English as auditorization of thought and involves the misperception of one's thoughts becoming audible.. It is best conceived of as an auditory hallucination.

Impairment of the ability to abstract has often been described as an essential feature of the cognitive disturbance seen in schizophrenia. It is more accurate to say that impairment of the abstract attitude in the direction of literalness or concreteness is characteristic of organic brain syndromes rather than of schizophrenia. There is a contamination of abstraction seen in schizophrenia, often in the direction of overinclusiveness, but the origin of this disturbance of the thought processes is unclear. The mechanism of predicative identifications is also commonly seen in the schizophrenic thought disorder. It is characterized by two or more things being equated on the basis of a predicate rather than on the basis of an essential similarity.

The accessory symptoms seen in schizophrenia include *hallucinations* which are most commonly demonstrated in the auditory sphere. Visual hallucinations are more common in organic psychoses. There is no day/night relationship in schizophrenic hallucinations whereas in organic psychoses visual hallucinations are more common in darkness. A *delusion*, as mentioned earlier, is a fixed, false belief and it is not uncommon in schizophrenia. Delusions can be divided on the basis of their form into persecutory, nihilistic, grandiose, ideas of influence, etc. Illusions or pseudohallucinations are not common in schizophrenia and are more likely to be seen in organic psychoses.

The traditional categories of schizophrenia are: *simple, paranoid, hebephrenic,* and *catatonic*. A *simple schizophrenia* is one which shows no accessory symptoms such as delusions or hallucinations. A *paranoid schizophrenia* is one which shows a preponderance of paranoid symptomatology including but not restricted to persecutory and grandiose delusions. Paranoid schizophrenics usually show greater intactness of their cognitive and personality functioning and less of a tendency towards social deterioration. *Catatonic schizophrenia* is characterized by an involvement of the motor system. It may take the form of excitement or stupor. Patients will occasionally show dramatic swings between excitement and stupor. The *hebephrenic form* of schizophrenia which is characterized by a marked tendency towards deterioration, posturing, grimacing, mirror gazing, etc., is not seen frequently today and its former prevalence may reflect some of the poor hospital practices of the past. There are other categories of schizophrenia which are commonly utilized, including the schizoaffective which represents a variation of schizophrenia with some admixture of signs of an affective disorder.

It has been demonstrated in a number of studies that the individual signs and symptoms on which the diagnosis of schizophrenia can be based are quite reliable. Psychiatrists tend to disagree on the personal criteria they use in making the diagnosis. There is good agreement concerning the presence of a given sign but marginal agreement as to its utility as a diagnostic criterion. This curious situation produces good reliability for signs but modest reliability for diagnosis. Obviously, increasing the re-

liability of a diagnosis in no way addresses the issue of its validity.

The etiology of the schizophrenic syndrome is extremely complex. Genetic, biochemical, physiological, intrapsychic, interpersonal, and social factors undoubtedly play variable but critical roles in the onset of this disorder. The evidence for a *genetic factor* in the prevalence rate is compelling and beyond reasonable doubt (see Chapter 5). Unfortunately, that fact does not clarify the nature of the mechanisms involved. The demonstration of "genetic" transmission in a relatively constant environment can be used as evidence for the operation of an environmental factor which activates particular structural genes and not other ones. It is clear from the identical twin studies that initial isogeneticity is not enough to produce schizophrenia since at least 60% of these cases are discordant. We can only assume in the identical twins that subtle environmental differences during early development led to different effective genotypes in the pair. The mode of transmission of the schizophrenic syndrome is also unclear. This author prefers a polygenic model involving a small number of genes, in the range of 2–5, which control and regulate the flow of sensory information into the central nervous system. At a biochemical level, this model might involve a different, but not necessarily abnormal balance, between neurotransmitter substances.

The social class studies reveal *more schizophrenia amongst the poor*. Obviously, a correlation does not identify causal relationships. It is unclear whether schizophrenics become poor because of their inability to compete effectively or whether the stresses of poverty are more likely to mobilize the schizophrenic potential in a given population. Other explanations can be imposed with equal ease upon the correlation.

The family studies are not compelling in terms of explaining the prevalence rate, especially in light of the genetic loading demonstrated in the "adopted away" studies (see Chapter 5). Nevertheless, they certainly suggest the importance of family interaction in determining a variety of clinical parameters that are important in the treatment of the disorder. This author leans towards the view that the personality characteristics which are necessary but not sufficient for the form of the schizophrenic illness, should the individual become psychotic, represent normal, but atypical, variants of these characteristics rather than abnormal traits. These same variants can lead to a range of outcomes including creativity and good adaptation and not necessarily to schizophrenia and marginal adaptation.

There are a number of prognostic signs which can be helpful to the clinician in predicting outcome. The more intact the affect during the acute illness, the more likely the patient is to recover. Patients who show a very florid picture with a relatively rapid onset have a better prognosis than those who show an insidious development with marked disintegration of the thought processes. The establishment and maintenance of a marital relationship is a good prognostic sign in males but has little or no predictive value in females. The quality of the premorbid social adjustment is also useful as a prognostic variable. Patients who have been withdrawn have a much worse prognosis.

A syndrome as heterogeneous as schizophrenia cannot be treated by any exclusive method. It is equally foolish to speak of the preferred or standard treatment of this disorder. The treatment regimen must show as much of a range as the clinical phenomenon to be treated. Equally important is the fact of intra-individual variability. Patients differ dramatically over time, and treatment interventions which are useful at one point in the illness are harmful or ineffective at other periods.

The vast majority of patients who are categorized as schizophrenic will require psychopharmacologic management, even if only briefly. The *phenothiazine derivatives* are the most commonly used psychopharmacologic agents in the treatment of this disorder. It is useful for the clinician to become familiar with only a small number of these drugs in depth rather than to have superficial experience with many of them. It is also useful to include one drug from each of the major groups, including the aliphatics, piperidines, piperazines, thioxanthenes, and butyrophenones. There is no evidence at this time that any one of these drugs is inherently superior and their use in a given case remains empirical. This leads to the conclusion that polypharmacy or the simultaneous use of two or more antipsychotic neuroleptics is poor clinical practice. It exposes the patient to an increased risk of an idiosyncratic reaction, without any increased likelihood of benefit. Extrapyramidal signs are quite commonly found in individuals receiving these drugs. However, the use of antiparkinsonian agents is not a routine matter. Antiparkinsonian drugs should not be used as a prophylactic measure in the absence of extrapyramidal signs. After several months of receiving such medication, it is wise to reduce the dosage and discontinue the drug over a period of approximately a week. Of the patients who formerly showed extrapyramidal signs, about 90% will now be free of them. The remaining 10% will have to be put back on antiparkinsonian agents. It is rare to have a clinical indication for the simultaneous use of an antidepressant and an antipsychotic agent, particularly in schizophrenia. There is no evidence at this time that megavitamins or acupuncture are of any use in the treatment of this disorder. Additional details on psychopharmacologic management can be found in Chapter 10 and in more specialized volumes.

It is necessary to identify the goals of a particular treatment intervention in order to assess its efficacy. Often the goal is nothing more than symptom suppression. At other times, it is to enhance the personality development so that the patient can function at a more differentiated level. In the case of the former, medication is the most effective route. In the case of the latter, social interventions of a psychotherapeutic nature would be essential.

The use of *family therapy* can be quite helpful, particularly in reducing the family's expectation concerning the patient. It is also useful to identify and attempt to alter modes of interacting within a particular family that can be harmful to the patient's adaptation. It is important that the family treatment not be an effort to find a scapegoat for the patient's illness. Group therapy can be an effective way of mobilizing patients through peer pressure. It also can represent an opportunity to learn social and interpersonal skills which may have been inadequately learned in the past.

Individual psychotherapy remains extremely useful for selected cases and during certain phases of the illness. For many patients, it is an opportunity to enter into an intense but safe relationship in which there can be social learning and which can be generalized to other relationships as well. The individual psychotherapy of schizophrenia is a highly specialized activity and requires a major commitment of time on the part of both the therapist and the patient.

The major future direction in the treatment of schizophrenia lies in the rehabilitation of those patients who are left with a significant social deficit. The NIMH has estimated the economic cost of schizophrenia in the United States to be approximately $18 billion a year. There is a compelling need to develop rehabilitative programs which will restore these individuals to adequate vocational and social competence.

Selected References

Arieti, S. *Interpretation of Schizophrenia.* R. Brunner, New York, 1955.

Bleuler, E. *Dementia Praecox or the Group of Schizophrenias.* International University Press, New York, 1950.

Cancro, R. (Ed.) *The Schizophrenic Reactions.* Brunner/Mazel Publishers, New York, 1970.

Grinspoon, L., Ewalt, J.R., and Shader, R.I. *Schizophrenia: Pharmacotherapy and Psychotherapy.* Williams and Wilkins Company, Baltimore, 1972.

Oppenheimer, H. *Clincal Psychatry: Issues and Challenges.* Harper and Row, New York, 1971.

Chapter 12

Biological Theories of Schizophrenia

Joseph Lipinski and
Steven Matthysse

Introduction

The concept that insanity is caused by some abnormality in the functioning of the brain has existed since the time of Hippocrates. However, the present-day approach of seeking biochemical causes for mental diseases has its tap-root in the ideas of Thudichum, the "Father of Neurochemistry". In the latter part of the 19th Century, he postulated that insanity was caused by chemical toxins affecting the brain; and further, that these substances were produced by the body itself. The notion was given additional significance by the landmark discovery in 1903 that a microorganism, *treponema pallidum*, was the etiological agent in syphilis and responsible for the then widely prevalent psychosis associated with neurosyphilis, general paresis of the insane. The cause for general paresis having been found, in this case an exogenous substance, a microorganism, then could not the causes for other psychotic disorders be identified, and might they not be due to some endogenous toxin, as had been suggested?

Unfortunately, the biochemical approach to the investigation of the causes of psychotic disorders, though never quite extinguished, went into a period of eclipse shortly after the turn of the century, one from which it has only relatively recently begun to emerge. This was due partially to the disheartening failures of investigators to demonstrate conclusive changes in the brains of patients with the psychosis, *dementia praecox* (later called *schizophrenia*) and manic-depressive illness, which had been characterized in the early part of this century. It was also partially due to the emergence of the attractive psychological theories of psychosis propounded by Freud and his adherents, which had become dominant in America and much of European psychiatry by the 1930's and which continue to be promi-nent today.

In the past 25 years, biochemical theories and investigations of psychosis have again come to the fore along with studies demonstrating that genetic factors operate in the etiology of psychosis, particularly schizophrenia, and increasingly sophisticated neurochemical methodology. Not unexpectedly with these advances, there has been a resultant outpouring of reports dealing with biochemical theories of schizophrenia; and these have been the subject of several comprehensive reviews (Kety, 1967; Weil-Malherbe and Szara, 1971; Wyatt et al., 1971).

Biochemical Theories of Schizophrenia

In this chapter we will selectively discuss a number of lines of investigation which have attracted considerable recent interest. Research on the biochemistry of schizophrenia may, broadly speaking, be divided into two schools of thought: the *"inborn errors of metabolism"* model and the *pharmacological* model. The first derives from the strong evidence for genetic factors in the predisposition to schizophrenia and the large number of genetic diseases in which a generalized metabolic disturbance or circulating toxic factor can now be identified. The pharmacological model, on the other hand, starts from the premise that understanding the mechanism of action of antipsychotic drugs (drugs which are effective in the treatment of psychotic disorders such as schizophrenia and mania; see Chapter 10) may be expected to shed light on the pathophysiology of schizophrenia. The underlying assumption that these antipsychotic drugs, such as the phenothiazines, thioxanthines and butyrophenones, are not merely sedatives or simple "tranquilizers" but act on what are thought to be the most prominent symp-toms of schizophrenia, is well supported by a number of clinical studies. For example, one large-scale study conducted by the National Institute of Mental Health demonstrated that approximately two-thirds of schizophrenics treated with phenothiazines showed significant improvement, none worsened, and only one-tenth derived no benefit at all. The same study revealed that of patients treated with a placebo, only one-fourth showed significant improvement while one-half became worse or did not improve.

On the whole, the search for metabolic abnormalities or circulating toxins has been disappointing. While many abnormalities have been reported, typically they have not been confirmed by other investigators or appear to be artifacts of drug therapy, diet, stress, inactivity, or chronic infection. Several of the more intriguing hypotheses concerning abnormalities detectable in peripheral fluids will be discussed: the autoimmunity theory, "S-protein", creatine phosphokinase, histamine, and platelet monoamine oxidase.

The Autoimmunity Theory

In 1967, Robert Heath advanced the hypothesis that schizophrenia is an autoimmune disease; that is, a disease caused by the body producing antibodies directed against its own tissue(s). The theory rested on three experiments. In the first, fluorescent tagged anti-human gamma globulin was used to allow the investigators to examine visually, through microscopes, whether there were antibodies bound to post mortem brain sections. Fluorescence was observed on neural cell nuclei of the septal region (a part of the limbic system thought to be important in the regulation of thinking and emotion) and on a part of the caudate nucleus in brain specimens from schizophrenics, whereas no antibody was detected on tissues of non-schizophrenic patients. In the second experiment, serum gamma globulins of schizophrenic patients, injected intraventricularly in monkeys, caused the animals to become "dazed and out-of-contact", and the EEG's showed abnormalities in the septal region. In the third, antibodies prepared against monkey septal region and caudate nucleus produced similar behavioral and EEG changes when introduced intraventricularly in other monkeys, suggesting that lesions in this area were responsible for the abnormal behavior.

As yet there has been no confirmation of the presence of anti-brain antibodies in brain tissue from schizophrenics. It is worth noting that three separate groups of investigators, using different but standard immunological techniques have been unable to find any evidence of autoimmune disease in the brains of schizophrenics. Also, the absence of conspicuous tissue reaction in the nervous system in schizophrenics does not seem favorable to an autoimmune origin.

"S-Protein"

Frohman and Gottlieb have proposed that a low-density serum lipoprotein (the "S-protein", an alpha-2 globulin) is fundamentally involved in the etiology of schizophrenia. This protein is said to have a tertiary structure different in schizophrenics and normals. When it is in an alpha-helical configuration, it promotes the uptake of tryptophan into cells, where the tryptophan is postulated to be converted into the hallucinogenic substance N, N-dimethyltryptamine. However, in a careful study Nicol, Seal and Gottesman (1973) found that: (1) the low-density serum lipoprotein fraction does not increase tryptophan uptake into red blood cells; (2) other substances, such as hemolysins, likely to be present in sera do have this property; and (3) enhancement of tryptophan uptake was negatively, rather than positively, correlated with the diagnosis of schizophrenia among psychiatric patients. The S-protein hypothesis must be regarded as dubious on the basis of the presently available evidence.

Creatine Phosphokinase

In a careful series of studies by Herbert Meltzer (1974), the activity of serum creatine phosphokinase was investigated in acute psychotic patients.

(CPK, is an enzyme found in three distinct forms and located in three specific areas—brain, heart, and skeletal muscle. It catalyzes the reaction of adenosine diphosphate and creatine phosphate to produce adenosine triphosphate and creatine.) Meltzer has consistently found the activity of this enzyme to be elevated in acute psychoses of both manic and schizophrenic types. CPK has three isoenzymes: it is the muscle isoenzyme, not the brain variety that is elevated. Cerebrospinal fluid CPK was found to be normal in acute psychotic patients who had elevated serum CPK. Exercise, and even the muscular trauma of a single injection of chlorpromazine, can increase serum CPK, but Meltzer's studies appear to have adequately controlled these factors. It is, rather, the lack of specificity of these changes that leads one to question their significance. In the first place, they occur as well in other acute psychoses, such as maniac and depressive psychoses, rather than in schizophrenia alone. Secondly, CPK elevations have also been reported in a variety of other diseases: muscular dystrophy, myocardial infarction, tetanus, stroke, cerebral infarction, head injury, meningitis, and psychomotor epilepsy.

More recently, Meltzer and his collaborators have reported histological abnormalities in skeletal muscle biopsies from acute schizophrenics, such as "Z-band spreading". They interpret the alterations as secondary ("neurogenic") consequences of an abnormality in nervous system function. Although biopsy samples from schizophrenics can be distinguished from normals using these histological criteria, a sufficiently wide variety of other diseases has not been examined to demonstrate that the abnormality is specific for psychosis.

Histamine

Studies of histamine in schizophrenia have centered around two main areas, blood histamine levels and response to intradermally injected histamine. A number of investigators have reported that schizophrenics have abnormal (some reporting elevated and others, lowered) histamine levels in whole blood, plasma or serum. Others have noted that schizophrenics manifest extraordinary resistance to intradermal injections of histamine, responding with a much smaller wheal than non-schizophrenic patients or normal controls. There have also been several studies suggesting that schizophrenics may be less likely to have allergies or to show allergic phenomena than normals, and that occasionally preexisting allergic states may remit during an acute psychosis. Since histamine is known to be involved in allergic responses, it has been proposed that the latter findings may indicate an abnormality of histamine metabolism in schizophrenics. These reports have been made more interesting by the findings that histamine occurs in the mammalian nervous system, including that of man. It has recently been suggested that histamine may act as a central neurotransmitter.

It is difficult to interpret these observations. For example, only two of the intradermal histamine studies were conducted in the absence of drugs while in none of the studies of blood histamine levels was there control for drug effect. These are potentially critical omissions since several of the antipsychotic drugs, including chlorpromazine, are known to increase tissue and blood levels of histamine, probably by blocking its catabolism by the enzyme histamine methyltransferase (HMT). This might account for the reports of abnormally high blood levels. Also, the diminished response to intradermal histamine might be the result of the antihistaminic effects of phenothiazines or, since phenothiazines increase tissue levels of histamine by inhibiting the activity of HMT, this diminished response might be due to tachyphylaxis. To determine if there are abnormalities of histamine metabo- lism in schizophrenia, sensitive and spe- cific methods of assay for blood levels must be used and strict control of medi- cations must be exercised to insure that one is not simply finding drug artifacts.

Platelet Monoamine Oxidase

The first biochemical alteration in schizophrenia which has promise as a genetic marker is the reduction of mono- amine oxidase (MAO) in platelets, first found by Murphy, Belmaker and Wyatt (1974) and confirmed by Meltzer. The decrease does not appear to be an effect of drugs or hospitalization. Manic- depressives had MAO values interme- diate between chronic schizophrenics and normals, at approximately the same levels as patients with acute schizo- phrenic-like psychoses. The fact that this reduction was also observed in identical twins of schizophrenics, whether or not they had the illness, indicates that it may be valuable as a gentic marker. These intriguing differences prompted Wyatt and his collaborators to measure MAO in *post mortem* brain specimens from schizophrenic patients. Two forms of MAO in brain were differentiated by inhibitor and substrate specificities. No significant differences between schizo- phrenics and controls were found in either form. Also, it must be noted that it has been reported that patients with manic-depressive disease also have de- creased levels of activity, further cloud- ing the significance of the finding. The pathogenic significance of the platelet MAO decrease thus remains obscure, but the phenomenon is certainly inter- esting and worthy of further study. One interesting but still *very* much hypotheti- cal use of the finding would be to use it to diagnose the illness or to use it as a "marker" for genetic studies. The pitfalls of such premature jumps are obvious, however, from the above observations about manic-depressive illness.

The Transmethylation Theory

This productive hypothesis, which has stimulated nearly two decades of re- search on the biochemistry of schizo- phrenia, stands halfway between the inborn error of metabolism and pharma- cological models. The initial impetus for the theory was pharmacological. There is a striking similarity in molecular structure between mescaline and the catecholamines, dopamine and norepi- nephrine, and also between N,N-di- methyltryptamine and the indoleamine, serotonin. The resemblance between psychotomimetics and naturally occur- ring neurotransmitters led Harley-Mason to propose that transfer of methyl groups to neurotransmitters along pathways not usually utilized in the body might cause autointoxicating substances to be formed. The postulated process was all the more intriguing because transmethylation is not only a widely occurring biochemical process, but is important specifically in the natural transformations of catechola- mines and indoleamines. Originally, the hypothesis focused on methylation of catecholamines—dimethylphenethyla- mine (DMPEA) was the supposed path- ogenic agent—but a parallel line of investigation developed in connection with the indoleamines.

Shortly after Harley-Mason's theoreti- cal proposal, the postulated compound, DMPEA, was reported to be present in the urine of schizophrenics and not in normal controls. Subsequently, a voluminous and contradictory literature emerged. One group failed to find DMPEA at all; one found it too often—both in schizophrenics and normals; one claimed it was an artifact which disappeared when vegetable foods were removed from the diet; another group agreed that DMPEA was an artifact, but claimed that animal foods had to be omitted in order to eliminate it.

More recent investigations have shown, using the unambiguous identification made possible by mass spectrometry, that DMPEA is a constituent of at least some human urine samples, but it is only one of *several* substances which probably had been found in the original studies. DMPEA excretion has also been shown to increase after drinking tea. A decisive study, where this definitive chemical analysis is matched by equally careful clinical design, remains to be carried out.

There are a number of findings which suggest a possible association between the methylated indoleamine, N,N-dimethyltryptamine (DMT), and schizophrenia. DMT is a very potent hallucinogen, and when administered to schizophrenics can cause an intensification of their symptoms. The enzyme indoleamine N-methyltransferase is capable of synthesizing DMT from tryptamine, a natural constituent of human brain. This enzyme, originally discovered in rabbit lung, has now been reported to be present in a variety of mammalian tissues, including human lung, blood and brain.

Wyatt, Saavedra and Axelrod found that schizophrenics and patients with psychotic depression had higher activity of the tryptamine-methylating enzyme in blood platelets than did alcoholics or normal controls, perhaps because of an inhibitor found in the non-psychotic group. In studies of monozygotic twins discordant for schizophrenia, it was found that schizophrenic twins had higher platelet tryptamine-methylating enzyme activities than the discordant twins and that the latter had mean enzyme activities which were not different from 22 normal subjects. The higher enzyme activity does not appear, therefore, to be genetically determined. On the negative side, it must also be noted that several studies have attempted to measure DMT levels in whole blood, plasma and/or urine without finding significant differences between controls and schizophrenics, although it is not possible to rule out rapid metabolism of DMT in the body.

Most biological transmethylations utilize S-adenosylmethionine as a methyl donor, this activated intermediate, in turn, being formed from methionine by the action of methionine adenosyltransferase. N_5-methyltetrahydrofolate has recently been reported to be the methyl donor for the methylation of dopamine to epinine, and has been postulated to be active in the methylation of indoleamines via indolethylamine N-methyltransferase, but its role is controversial. Measurements of blood levels of S-adenosylmethionine and methionine adenosyltransferase have not revealed any abnormalities in schizophrenic patients.

The inconclusive results with DMPEA and the methylated indoleamines, and the negative conclusions regarding methyl donors, would have caused interest to wane in the transmethylation theory, were it not for the observation of Pollin, Cardon and Kety that methionine loading causes exacerbation of schizophrenic psychoses. Methionine loading is relevant because, as mentioned above, it is the ultimate source of methyl groups for transmethylation reactions. The effect is unusual among observations on schizophrenia in that it has been confirmed by a number of research groups and disproven by none. Kakimoto concluded that the symptoms resembled a superimposed toxic psychosis more than an exacerbation of schizophrenia. In another study, however, only two of the seven reactions were described as toxic, the other five as more like exacerbations of the psychotic process. Methionine has many metabolic and pharmacological actions in addition to methyl group donation, which could account for its psychotogenic effect: it reduces seizure threshold, and its metabolites include homocysteine and cystathionine, both of which have been found in some instances to be associated with psychosis (in homocystinuria and cystathionuria). The effects of methionine loading cannot, therefore, be taken as conclusive evidence for the transmethylation theory.

If a methyl donor made schizophrenics worse, it seemed possible that a methyl acceptor might make them better: hence a trial was carried out of nicotinamide, a substance which is capable of accepting methyl groups to become N^1-methylnicotinamide. Hoffer described successful treatment of 13 out of 17 schizophrenics in 3 to 5 days with daily oral nicotinamide, but several groups have not been able to replicate his claim. Indeed, in one study, nicotinamide had a harmful effect: "increased hostility, aggressiveness, and irritability". There is little doubt that the treatment does not work. On the other hand, Baldessarini observed that nicotinamide does not effectively lower rat liver or brain S-adenosylmethionine, so its failure as a therapeutic agent may not militate against the transmethylation theory. Also, L-dihydroxyphenylalanine (L-dopa) is an excellent methyl acceptor but does not help schizophrenia and often makes the illness worse. The main explanation for this phenomenon is that despite the above quality, L-dopa is very rapidly converted into dopamine in the brain and in the body generally, and that the marked increase in dopamine concentration in the brain produces the exacerbation of the illness (see DOPAMINE HYPOTHESIS, below).

Megavitamin Therapy

In view of the absence of *scientific* evidence for the efficacy of "megavitamin therapy", it is surprising that the treatment is still widely practiced. Four factors may account for its continued usage: (1) nicotinamide of the B-vitamin complex is presumed to be harmless, although in the large doses that are prescribed there may be a danger to patients with ulcer, gout, diabetes or liver disease. Lesions of the skin have also been reported. (2) Advocates of nicotinamide therapy have generally avoided double-blind design on the grounds that the vitamin treatment has to be individualized for each patient. (3) The treatment plan usually consists of adding large doses of vitamins to the medically recognized standard therapy, but favorable results are often attributed to the vitamins. (4) Vitamin therapy was also proposed by Pauling for a different reason, namely, that schizophrenics might be vitamin-deficient in the brain, even though dietary intake was normal. The rationale was that loss or partial reduction of the capacity to synthesize vitamins would have a selective advantage in an environment where they were abundant; mutation to restore the synthetic machinery would be rare. At the present time the vitamin deficiency theory is highly conjectural.

Dopamine Hypothesis

The pharmacological approach to schizophrenia has been dominated, in the past few years, by interest in the hypothesis that the antipsychotic phenothiazines and butyrophenones block dopamine receptions in the brain. The evidence is necessarily indirect, since the "dopamine receptor" has not been isolated and characterized as a molecule. Closest to a direct demonstration of receptor blockade is the work of Greengard's laboratory on dopamine-stimulated adenylate cyclase. This enzyme, present in homogenates of rat caudate nucleus and limbic forebrain increases in activity in the presence of dopamine. The facilitatory effect is blocked by chlorpromazine and haloperidol. Direct neurophysiological evidence of dopamine blockade is difficult to demonstrate, because when phenothiazines are introduced into the vicinity of a neuron they have an anesthetic action. Responses of striatal neurons to iontophoretic dopamine, however, are blocked by local application of chlorpromazine, even after the anesthetic effect wears off.

The remaining evidence for blockade of dopamine synapses by antipsychotic phenothiazines and butyrophenones is more indirect than the adenylate cyclase and iontophoretic studies, but taken as a whole it is compelling. The rate of turnover of dopamine in the brain (synthesis and destruction, which are equal in the steady state) is increased by antipsychotic drugs. Turnover is thought to rise because dopaminergic systems (at least the nigrostriatal tract) increase in activity to compensate for the synaptic blockade. There is evidence for a descending inhibitory pathway from the striatum to the substantia nigra, which could function in this way as a feedback control mechanism. Feedback control within the synapse, mediated by *presynaptic* receptors that inhibit the release of dopamine, may operate in the same direction. There is also some interesting neurophysiological evidence in support of the hypothesis. Systemic administration of amphetamine causes a reduction in the firing rate of neurons in the substantia nigra, presumably by stimulating the negative feedback control system;

chlorpromazine restores the firing rate to normal.

Clinical observations also support the hypothesis of dopamine blockade. Motor side effects reminiscent of the symptoms of Parkinson's disease are a major complication of antipsychotic drugs; and in Parkinson's disease there is a deficiency of brain dopamine. Conversely, L-dopa cannot be used to counteract the extrapyramidal side effects because it makes the psychosis more florid. It is interesting that anticholinergic agents can be used to treat the parkinsonian side effects of antipsychotic drugs without making the psychosis worse (although not all agree); this fact is important in the development of the theory (see below).

Another important source of evidence for the dopamine blockade hypothesis is the action of several drugs which although not specific for dopamine, inhibit or facilitate dopaminergic transmission. Reserpine, alpha-methyltyrosine, methylphenidate, and amphetamine are in this category. Reserpine, which interferes with vesicular storage of biogenic amines, was the first effective substance used in the chemotherapy of schizophrenia, and alpha-methyltyrosine, which inhibits catecholamine synthesis, is reported to decrease substantially the dose of phenothiazines required for treatment. Methylphenidate and amphetamine, which facilitate catecholamine transmission, are both psychotomimetic under certain conditions: methylphenidate exacerbates existing psychotic states and amphetamine is capable of eliciting a paranoid psychosis in non-psychotic individuals.

Starting from the blockade of dopamine transmission by antipsychotic drugs, it is possible to formulate hypotheses of the etiology of schizophrenia in a number of ways. The most obvious is that too much dopamine is released at synapses in the central nervous system. Alternatively, dopamine receptors may be hypersensitive and react excessively to a normal quantity of released dopamine. An antagonistic system (perhaps cholinergic) may be underactive. The conversion of dopamine to noradrenaline could be impaired, causing a relative dopaminergic excess and noradrenergic deficiency. There might be a defect in a feedback pathway controlling a branch of the dopamine system. Thus, there are several "dopamine hypotheses" of the etiology of schizophrenia, corresponding to the premise that antipsychotic drugs block dopamine synapses.

There is a subtle shift of emphasis in passing from the pharmacological to the etiological level, which poses a logical problem, more serious than the fact that there are several alternative formulations. There is not much doubt that dopamine blockade is *an* action of phenothiazines; the question is whether it is *the* action of phenothiazines; that is, whether of the many actions of these drugs dopamine blockade is the one which underlies their antipsychotic properties.

There is some reason to think the logical step can be made. In the first place, the dopamine-blocking effects occur *in vivo* at clinically relevant doses and *in vitro* at reasonable concentrations. Secondly, non-antipsychotic phenothiazines (closely related chemically, but used as antihistaminics, anticholinergics, or sedative) generally do not share the dopamine turnover enhancing action of the antipsychotics or block DA-stimulated adenylate cyclase in caudate or limbic forebrain. Thiethylperazine, an antiemetic phenothiazine, is an exception, because it does have a marked effect on dopamine turnover, although it is not used in the treatment of schizophrenia. It is possible, however, that its antipsychotic properties have not been thoroughly tested; and one recent but unconfirmed pilot study indicates that it does act as an antipsychotic.

Thioridazine is generally agreed to have a lower incidence of parkinsonian side effects, and also to have a weaker effect on dopamine turnover, than its therapeutic efficacy would predict. It appears that this discrepancy may be accounted for, however, by the interaction of the cholinergic system. As mentioned before, anticholinergic agents can be used to counteract the extrapyramidal side effects of antipsychotic drugs without destroying their antipsychotic action. This is one of several lines of evidence that led to the hypothesis of a cholinergic-dopaminergic balance in the corpus striatum. According to recent experiments by Snyder (1974), thioridazine has a much stronger anticholinergic action in the central nervous system than other phenothiazines of similar antipsychotic potency. To complete this formulation, it is necessary to assume that in those regions of the brain involved in the pathophysiology of schizophrenia, a dopaminergic-cholinergic balance does *not* prevail. Actually there is some evidence that this is the case. The reduction in firing rate of substantia nigra neurons by amphetamine (see above) is antagonized by chlorpromazine but not by thioridazine, whereas when the same experiment is carried out in the region which contains the cells of origin of the dopaminergic tract innervating the limbic system, the two drugs have an equivalent action. Antichlorinergic agents antagonize the dopamine turnover enhancing effect of haloperidol in the striatum but apparently not in the limbic system. Clozapine, a drug which like thioridazine has antipsychotic actions without strong extrapyramidal side effects, causes a greater increase in dopamine turnover in the limbic system than in the caudate.

A question which remains to be clarified is whether tolerance develops to the dopamine-blocking effects of antipsychotic drugs. The antipsychotic actions of phenothiazines do not diminish after repeated dosage, whereas tolerance formation is characteristic of many of their other pharmacological actions. One would expect, therefore, that if dopamine blockade accounts for the antipsychotic properties of phenothiazines, it ought not to decrease after chronic administration. Some authors find tolerance; others do not.

The most direct formulation of the dopamine hypothesis referred to above, excessive release of dopamine at central synapses, is not supported by the clinical studies that have been performed. The major metabolite of dopamine, homovanillic acid, is not elevated in the cerebrospinal fluid of schizophrenics. Prolactin release is under inhibitory control by dopaminergic neurons (see Chapter 4) so that serum prolactin might be expected to be lower than normal if dopamine release is abnormally high; but no significant difference in schizophrenia was found. It is, of course, conceivable that dopaminergic systems other than those of the striatum and hypothalamus, which are primarily reflected by these two measurements, are the ones affected.

The formulation of the dopamine hypothesis in terms of diminished conversion of dopamine to noradrenaline is given some support by studies of Wise, Baden and Stein, who reported a pro-

found decrease in dopamine beta-hydroxylase in brains of schizophrenics as compared with controls. This observation could not be confirmed by Wyatt and his collaborators, who concluded that the results (they observed a nonsignificant trend in the expected direction) could be accounted for by differential *post mortem* degeneration. Dopamine beta-hydroxylase is not decreased in the plasma of schizophrenic patients.

Even though the experimental evidence for these two formulations of the dopamine hypothesis is not convincing, it is well to recall that there are other possibilities, such as hypersensitivity of dopamine receptors or underactivity of an antagonistic system. It is also conceivable that the regional extent of the neurochemical abnormality is too small for it to be detectable in peripheral fluids or by gross *post mortem* analysis. The indirect evidence from the blocking action of antipsychotic drugs is not sufficient in itself to establish the etiological significance of dopamine, but as one of the first good clues to the pathophysiology of the baffling disease it is not likely to be abandoned easily.

Conclusions

When one reviews the lines of biological investigations of schizophrenia touched upon in this chapter, it is quite apparent that, perhaps excepting parts of the dopamine hypothesis and parts of the transmethylation hypothesis, most of them do not stand up terribly well. Also, most biological theories of schizophrenia have not been included in this review, only those that are attracting active investigation. Thus with some reason, one could develop quite a pessimistic attitude toward such biological research of schizophrenia. However, before doing so it would be well to consider additional factors: Much of the research in this area took place in the years prior to 1955. In those times, bio-

logically oriented psychiatrists lacked specific clues as to where to begin their investigations. The illness was poorly defined. There were no medicines (or any treatments really) that helped the illness. Research methodologies and equipment were extremely crude compared to those of today. Investigators were often forced to conduct "screening" tests, measuring one substance or another depending upon what the state of technology would allow, in the hope that by chance "the" abnormality might be found. Considering the bewilderingly vast numbers of body chemicals and states/substances that can alter their metabolism it is not terribly surprising that most of the older work produced inconclusive or even misleading results, e.g., a 'positive' result being due to an artifact. Also, it was not even clear whether schizophrenia had any biological (genetic) basis. Most claims supporting a genetic component until recently could be as easily explained by environmental factors.

The investigator of present times has marked advantages over those of earlier periods. As has been mentioned in Chapter 5, there is now *very* strong evidence that genetic factors exert a powerful influence in the development of schizophrenia; and these factors must necessarily express themselves through biochemical processes. Also, there have been enormous advances in the understanding of central nervous system function in the past 25 years and today's

technology is formidable compared to that of the 1930's or 40's, or even the 50's. Also, the investigator has available a host of pharmacological agents which have been found to produce significant improvement in patients with schizophrenia. These substances at last give scientists something solid upon which to base their research. The antipsychotic drugs have a dismayingly large number of biochemical actions, but one of them or a particular combination of actions must be responsible for their beneficial effects. They probably are our best clue as to what biochemical processes describe schizophrenia. The biological answer or answers to the riddle of schizophrenia may not be immediately forthcoming, but at least one now can say that the search has begun in earnest.

Selected References

Boehme, D.H., Cattrell, J.C., Dohan, C., and Hillegass, L.M.; Fluorescent antibody studies of immunoglobulin binding by brain tissue. *Arch. Gen. Psychiat.* 28:202-207, 1973.

Iversen, L.L.: Dopamine receptors in the brain, *Science* 188:1084-1089, 1975.

Kety, S.S.: Current biochemical approaches to Schizophrenia. *N. Engl. J. Med.* 276:325-331, 1967.

Matthysse, S.: Implications of the catecholamine systems of the brain in schizophrenia, In *Brain Dysfunction in Metabolic Disorders*, F. Plum, ed. Assoc. for Research in Nervous and Mental Disease, Res. Publ., Vol. 53. Raven Press, New York, 1974, pp. 304-314.

Matthysse, S., and Lipinski, J.: Biochemical aspects of schizophrenia, *Ann. Rev. Med.* 26:551-565, 1975.

Meltzer, H.Y., and Crayton, J.W. Subterminal motor nerve abnormalities in psychotic patients. *Nature* 249:373-375, 1974.

Murphy, D.L., Belmaker, R., and Wyatt, R.J.: Monoamine oxidase in schizophrenia and other behavioral disorders. In *Catecholamines and their Enzymes in the Neuropathology of Schizophrenia*, S. Matthysse and S.S. Kety, eds. Pergamon Press, Oxford, 1974, pp. 221-247.

Nicol, S., Seal, U.S., and Gottesman, I.I.: Serum from schizophrenia patients: effect on cellular lactate stimulation and tryptophane uptake. *Arch. Gen. Psychiat.* 29:744-751, 1973.

Snyder, S.H., Banerjee, S.P., Yamamura, H.I., and Greenberg, D.: Drugs, neurotransmitters and schizophrenia. *Science* 184: 1243-1253, 1974.

Task Force Report 7: *Megavitamin and Orthomolecular Therapy in Psychiatry*. American Psychiatric Association, Washington, D.C., 1973.

Weil-Malherbe, H., and Szara, S.I.: *The Biochemistry of Functional and Experimental Psychoses*. Charles C. Thomas, Springfield, Ill., 1971.

Wyatt, R.J., Saavedra, J.M., Belmaker, R., Cohen, S., and Pollin, W.: The dimethyltryptamine forming enzyme in blood platelets: A study of monozygotic twins discordant for schizophrenia. *Am. J. Psychiat.* 130:1359-1361, 1973.

Wyatt, R.J., Termini, B.A., and Davis, J.: Biochemical and sleep studies of schizophrenia: a review of the literature—1960-1970. Part I. Biochemical studies. *Schizophrenia Bull.* 10-66, 1971.

Chapter 13

Depression: Clinical Aspects

*Aaron T. Beck and
Ruth L. Greenberg*

From earliest times, writers have been strikingly consistent in their descriptions of the depressed person. Hippocrates, Aretaeus, Plutarch would have agreed with modern professionals that the depressed person is morose, gloomy, and taciturn; hopeless and inactive; preoccupied with a vision of reality that is not congruent with the views of people around him. And the early writers, impressed by the profound changes which people undergo when they are depressed, were as convinced as many moderns that the cause must lie in biochemical changes or physiology, or in spiritual influences far removed from current, everyday experiences.

Today, depression is recognized as a major public health problem. A national survey has suggested that of a random sample of American adults ages 18–74, 15% may have "significant depressive features" at any one time. While most depressions probably go untreated, each year 200,000 people receive outpatient therapy for depressive symptoms and another 125,000 are hospitalized for depression.

Depression is a factor in such social problems as alcoholism and drug addiction, and it is the type of mental disorder most frequently associated with suicide. In fact, suicide has been viewed as the mortality of depressive illness.

There are more than 23,000 reported deaths by suicide yearly in the United States, or about 10 per 100,000 population, and the actual number of suicides is almost certainly much higher. In addition, there are probably 8 to 10 times that number of suicide attempts.

Symptomatology

Change is a key factor in recognizing depression. In fact, the depressed patient may bewilder his family and friends by seeming to be a wholly different person from the way he was before he became ill. Clinicians have observed that he more often resembles other depressed patients than his own premorbid personality. While the most noticeable change is in mood, depression also manifests itself in changes in motivation, thinking, physiological function, and behavior.

Changes in Mood

The depressed person describes his feelings as "blue," "sad," "low," "desperate." He may complain of loneliness or boredom or a sense of loss or disappointment. He may be apathetic about activities and responsibilities that formerly elicited enthusiasm, involvement, and pleasure. His emotional ties to other people seem to have become flat and dull, and his sense of humor has deserted him. He may experience lengthy crying spells.

Highly characteristic of the depressed person's emotional life are his *negative feelings about himself*. These range from mild disappointment in himself to extreme self-hatred and self-loathing. He may also feel guilty, humiliated, or anxious.

Changes in Thinking

Cognitive changes are also apparent. The depressed patient devalues himself, underestimates his abilities, and over-estimates the extent of his problems. He is persistently self-critical and pessimistic and has great *difficulty in making decisions*. Although his troubles may not be of his own making, he tends to *blame himself for them*. Frequently, he experiences a distortion in body image. Female patients in particular may believe they have become ugly or unattractive, or become excessively concerned with minor flaws in their appearance. In severe cases, delusions and hallucinations may be present. Like the cognitive distortions noted above, these experiences also tend to reflect the patient's belief in his own worthlessness, guilt, or deprivation. Somatic and nihilistic delusions are common in psychotically depressed patients.

Motivational Changes

The cognitive components of depression are invariably tied in with motivational changes. Since the depressed person believes he is doomed to failure and misery no matter what he does, he is unlikely to make a real effort to solve his problems; he resists the ploys and suggestions of family and friends. At the same time he is *increasingly dependent, wishing to be cared for and guided by others*. He withdraws from work and social engagements, may pass up recreational possibilities since he sees even these as burdensome chores. While he sometimes blames his inactivity on fatigue or illness, the depressed person is able to mobilize adequate energy to escape from other people or to avoid encountering physicians, employers, and friends.

Behavioral Changes

Recently, the behavioral aspects of depression have been investigated by a number of researchers. Typically, the depressed patient's stooped posture and deliberate, slow movement reflect his "lack of energy," although the agitated patient will fidget and pace incessantly. Depressed patients tend to interact with a very limited number of people, and thus are extremely vulnerable emotionally when these relationships are disrupted. In several studies, Lewinsohn and his coworkers (1974) established that there is an overall reduction in depressed patients' activity levels. They are likely to be engaged in solitary activities of a passive nature, such as watching television or "sitting around and doing nothing." Lewinsohn notes that the inactivity may be partly caused by a lack of social skill or an inability to elicit positive reinforcement, such as signs of affection or approval, from significant others. Depressed patients tend to express dissatisfaction in their relationships with others and often report that they are anxious and ineffective in certain kinds of social interactions, especially those that require assertiveness.

Lazarus, recalling Skinner's definition of depression as a general weakening of the behavioral repertoire, suggests that depression might be defined further in terms of "a base rate of frequent weeping, decreased food intake, frequent statements of dejection and self-reproach, psychomotor retardation, difficulties with memory and concentration, insomnia or a fitful sleep pattern, and general apathy and withdrawal."

Changes in Physiological Function

Finally, there are common physical or vegetative symptoms. The depressed person often complains of headaches, fatigue, gastrointestinal distresses. Anorexia and libido loss are frequently observed. A large proportion of depressed patients experience difficulty in sleeping—they may wake earlier than usual, sleep lightly and restlessly, or have trouble falling asleep (see Chapter 6). Occasionally, depressed people find they are eating or sleeping more than usual.

Mania

Mania is seen in connection with some but not all depressive disorders, manic and depressive phases often occurring in a regular, cyclical pattern. In mania, the mood swings to elation, the feelings of inferiority to a sense of self-confidence and even grandiosity. While in a depressive phase, the patient may suffer from "paralysis of the will," when manic he may take on many projects and responsibilities, spend money recklessly and be ceaselessly active. He is gregarious and aggressive rather than passive and withdrawn, and obtains gratification from a wide range of experiences. He has an extremely favorable view of himself, overrating his abilities and attractiveness, and is highly optimistic—much more so than in a normal phase. Except for the sleep disturbance, which is common to both manic and depressive phases, the manic reactions appear to be the opposite of the depressive reactions. However, recent research suggests that there may be more underlying similarities between the two phases. This is discussed more fully in Chapter 14.

Diagnosis and Clinical Course

Depression has been called "the great masquerader." While its signs and symptoms may be readily observable to the clinician, depression may also be masked by a falsely hearty manner or present as a somatic illness whose psychiatric nature is revealed only through skillful questioning. It may be a hidden factor in marital difficulties, alcoholic behavior, sudden problems in doing schoolwork or maintaining employment. The failure to diagnose a serious depression can have tragic consequences, as the patient may attempt or commit suicide. It has been estimated that 15% of patients with primary affective disorder (patients who have had depressive or manic episodes but no previous psychiatric illness) ultimately kill themselves. Several researchers have found that a remarkably high proportion of suicides had consulted physicians within a few weeks prior to their deaths: this would seem to be evidence that serious depression and suicidal intent often go unrecognized even by professionals. Recently, a number of scales have become available which aid in the assessment of depression, among them the Hamilton Psychiatric Rating Scale, the Zung Self-Rating Depression Scale, and the Beck Depression Inventory.

Depressive episodes typically have a well-defined onset. They may or may not be precipitated by obvious traumatic events such as the failure of a love relationship, death of a spouse, loss of a job or income; the so-called "precipitating event" is often difficult to identify. Symptoms will generally become increasingly severe until the condition "bottoms out." From this point the patient improves steadily until he has recovered. Spontaneous recovery from a depressive episode is common, complete recovery occurring in 70–95% of cases; however, there is a definite tendency toward recurrence. In a patient with multiple episodes of depression, the attacks last about the same length of time (median duration is 6.3 months for inpatients and about 3 months for outpatients), but the symptom-free periods between episodes become shorter.

Of course, in treating any depression, the clinician must take into account the possibility of suicidal behavior. Certain variables may be valuable in assessing suicidal risk, e.g., if the patient has been recently divorced, has been charged with a crime, or has a history of previous suicidal behavior, the suicidal risk is increased.

The patient himself is an important source of information: he may be questioned directly about suicidal intent. An especially crucial period for suicide risk in the depressive is the first three to six months after the depressive episode has apparently been resolved, or following discharge from treatment or from the hospital. It should be noted that not all people who kill themselves have been depressed: one study found that only 10 to 40% of suicides had been diagnosed depressed by a psychiatrist. Current research suggests that the relationship between depression and suicidal behavior may be explained by the presence of hopelessness, which is common to both, and seems to be a better indicator of suicidal risk than depression itself.

Types of Depression

Students of depression are often confused by its semantics. The term "depression" may be used to designate the "blues"—normal, low moods which we all experience. Secondly, "depression" may signify a cluster of symptoms which is not a disease in itself, but a psycho-pathological dimension accompanying other disorders, such as schizophrenic reaction or organic brain disease. Finally, "depression" may refer to a definite disease having a specific kind of onset, course, and outcome. When the term is used in this way, a subcategory is frequently specified, such as "reactive" or "endogenous" depression.

The relationships between normal low moods and clinical depression, and among the various subcategories of depression, have been a subject of debate involving various differences in conceptualizing depression. The school of thought favoring the "unitary hypothesis" claims that there is a continuous series of reactions from normal unhappy moods through mild and moderate depressions and with psychotic depression (in which signs such as delusions and hallucinations are present) at the extreme. This group sees depression as an intensification of a normal state, and the difference between neurotic and psychotic depression as primarily a difference in severity. The "pluralistic" school views neurotic and psychotic depressions as separate disease entities, both qualitatively different from the "blues." The latter view may be traced to Emil Kraepelin (1856–1926), an influential German psychiatrist whose scheme for classifying the psychiatric disorders forms the basis for current efforts.

In practice, neurotic and psychotic depressions are usually identified respectively with the exogenous (reactive, or psychogenic) and endogenous (autonomous) depressions, although these terms imply etiological differences: endogenous depressions show little emotional response to environmental changes and are presumed to have a hereditary basis. Opinion is divided regarding the status of the "involutional melancholia" label, which designates depression occurring in later life.

The complexities and inconsistencies of available systems for classifying the affective disorders has posed serious difficulties for research. Currently, the establishment of diagnostic subgroups is considered an issue of central importance both to research and treatment, and additional classification systems have been suggested. Robins and Guze (1972) propose that the affective disorders should be divided into primary and secondary classes. The "primary affective disorders" are those occurring in patients who have histories of no psychiatric illness or previous histories of mania or depression only. "Secondary depression" occurs in patients who have had pre-existing psychiatric illness other than depression. Within the group of primary affective disorders, a distinction is made between unipolar and bipolar types; the bipolar types are those in which there is a history of a manic phase. The unipolar cases, which today constitute the overwhelming majority, are sometimes separated into early-onset and late-onset groups. The unipolar-bipolar distinction has led to the sorting of depressed patients on a variety of clinical, genetic, biochemical, and pharmacological grounds (see Chapters 5 and 14).

Winokur and his coworkers have divided depressive illness into "pure depression" and "depression spectrum disease" categories, chiefly on the basis of family studies which indicate that the latter group has family histories showing a greater prevalence of alcoholism, sociopathy, or depression than the "pure depressive" group. The "pure depressives" have less familial psychiatric disorder than the "depression spectrum disease" cases, but the psychiatric disorder that occurs is primarily depression.

As Andreasen (1975) writes in his review of this much-debated area, "the entire issue of subtyping, a critical one for sophisticated biochemical research, remains unresolved."

The Psychology of Depression

The nature and origin of depression have been the subject of much speculation; a number of explanatory models have been developed. It is likely that depression actually represents a heterogeneous mix of disorders. For an individual case, it may be necessary to understand the depressive picture in terms of a wide spectrum of influences: genetic and biochemical predisposition, early life experiences, psychodynamic, environmental, and sociological factors, etc. One of the recent approaches that appears to hold great promise for enhancing our understanding and treatment of depression involves the study of cognitive factors in this disorder. For this reason, a discussion of the cognitive approaches to depression will be presented in some detail. (In Chapter 10 the pharmacological approaches to depression are described.)

The depressed person's disturbances in affect are accompanied—and, in many cases, brought about—by a negative view of himself, the world, and the future. Despite the fact that his negative evaluation of himself may be wholly unjustified by objective criteria, the depressed person blames his own failures for his unpleasant situation. In acute cases, his sense of causality may be so egocentric that he blames himself for catastrophes in world affairs, natural disasters, etc. Apparent successes, such as in business or professional life, do not serve to contradict this view; he may feel they are unimportant or unsubstantial and he actually may feel worse when reminded of them, because he feels they have deceived others by concealing his true ineptitude or harmfulness. Frequently the attributes he had previously valued most highly—were they intelligence, artistic creativity, moral rectitude, or financial clout—are those which he now sees himself as lacking.

His outlook on the world is also persistently negative. He takes a gloomy view of interpersonal interactions which he is witness to, as well as broad political and economic trends. He may see in trivial events, such as a slight increase in the number of motor accidents in his neighborhood, portents of cosmic doom. And he sees all these problems as extending indefinitely into the future, with little chance of remittance: he believes there is nothing he can do himself to alleviate his misery, and that there is not likely to be help from outside sources.

While the depressed person's global perception of reality is extremely negative, it is constantly reinforced by logical errors which he makes when he appraises daily events which have personal relevance to him. For example, a lecturer notices that one or two people in his audience walked out of the hall while he was speaking. He arbitrarily infers that they had not enjoyed his lecture; he then overgeneralizes and thinks that no one else present liked it and that, in fact, he has always been a "loser" at public speaking; consequently, he is worthless as a person and his life has no meaning. A newly divorced woman, thinking over the history of her experiences with men, selectively abstracts the bad ones as characteristic and concludes that she will never have a satisfying relationship with a man. She may attribute her difficulties to innate and irremediable flaws in herself. This woman also magnifies the importance of certain events, such as her current boyfriend's calling to cancel a date or criticizing her for some minor fault, and minimizes positive experiences.

The cognitive distortions in depression provide an explanation for the emotional, motivational, and behavioral phenomena previously outlined. The depressed person's feelings of sadness and gloom stem from his perception of himself as inadequate or unable to cope, his belief that he is deprived of or lacking something of great value. From the idiosyncratic cognitive schema also follow his behavioral inhibition and motivational eccentricities: if I am unable to do any better, he thinks, there is no point in doing anything at all. Thus paralyzed by his own cognitions, he may interpret his failure to act as confirmation of his weakness and despicability.

This model for depression has been supported by experimental evidence, and has led to the development of a cognitive-behavioral method for treating depression. Recent research has indicated that the negative thinking of depressed patients may be rapidly reversed by a combination of cognitive and behavioral techniques. Outcome studies have demonstrated the efficacy of this kind of treatment in alleviating even longstanding depressions.

At present, further research is in progress to determine not only the appropriateness of this model and treatment mode, but their applicability to the various depressive subtypes.

Selected References

Andreasen, N.J.C.: Clinical research on depression: A review. *J. Nerv. Ment. Dis.* 161: 63-69, 1975.

Beck, A.T.: *Depression: Clinical, Experimental, and Theoretical Aspects.* Hoeber, New York, 1967.

Beck, A.T.: *Cognitive Therapy and the Emotional Disorders.* International Universities Press, New York, 1976.

Beck, A.T., Ward, C.H., Mendelson, M., Mock, J.E., and Erbaugh, J.K.: An inventory for measuring depression. *Arch. Gen. Psychiat.* 4:561-571, 1961.

Guze, S.B., and Robins, E.: Suicide and primary affective disorders. *Br. J. Psychiat.* 117:437-438, 1970.

Lewinsohn, P.M.: Clinical and theoretical aspects of depression. In *Innovative Treatment Methods in Psychopathology,* Chapter 3, K. Calhoun, H. Adams, and K. Mitchell, eds. Wiley, New York, 1974, pp. 63-120.

Pokorny, A.: Myths about suicide. In *Suicidal Behaviors: Diagnosis and Management,* H.L.P. Resnik, ed. Little Brown, Boston, 1968, pp. 57-72.

Robins, E., and Guze, S.B.: Classification of affective disorders: The primary-secondary, the endogenous-reactive, and the neurotic-psychotic concepts. In *Recent Advances in the Psychobiology of the Depressive Illnesses,* T.A. Williams, M.M. Katz, and J. Shield, Jr., eds. U.S. Government Printing Office, Washington, D.C., 1972, pp. 283-293.

Rush, A.J., Khatami, M., and Beck, A.T.: Cognitive and behavioral therapy in chronic depression. *Behav. Ther.* 6:398-404, 1975.

Winokur, G.: The types of affective disorder. *J. Nerv. Ment. Dis.* 156:82-96, 1973.

Chapter 14

Biological Aspects of Mania and Depression

Alan Frazer

The past decade has seen an unprecedented expansion of investigation into, and theorization about, the biological changes associated with, and perhaps responsible for, clinical depression and mania. The demonstration that some drugs can alleviate the symptoms of depression and mania while others induce symptoms suggestive of depression, together with increasing evidence that genetic factors play an important role in the development of some forms of affective illness, have constituted the major spurs to this line of inquiry.

This upsurge of interest does not exclude or even diminish the possibility that psychological, social or developmental factors play an important role in the genesis of affective illness. It is unlikely that there will be any *one* answer to the problem of depression, as it is a heterogeneous clinical state with a variety of manifestations, pathologies, etiologies and treatments. Furthermore, several different factors probably contribute to the etiology of each form of the illness. For example, a genetic predisposition may render an individual vulnerable to specific types of stress, especially if these occur at certain stages of life when hormonal or enzymatic alterations increase susceptibility or reduce the capacity to cope. This requires that investigators be alert both to the possibilities of an abnormality which may be specific to a subgroup of patients as well as to the importance of interactions between systems.

The discussion which follows summarizes some of our current knowledge of the biological changes associated with depression. While we are still at a somewhat preliminary stage of investigation, considerable information has been gathered in depressives on various aspects of biogenic amine function; neuroendocrine function, especially hypothalamic-pituitary-adrenal cortex activity;

electrolyte metabolism and cell-membrane function. In reviewing some of the findings, we will consider them individually. However, it is essential to remember that they all interact with each other and that changes in one probably lead to changes in others. It is possible that some alteration in the interrelationships or balance between these systems is more important to the etiology of depression than is any change in the activity of an isolated system.

Biogenic Amines

After the discovery by Walter Cannon in 1915 that animals exposed to rage- or fear-inducing situations secrete increased amounts of epinephrine (adrenaline), there has been considerable interest in the association between emotional behavior on the one hand and epinephrine and the other biogenic amines on the other. A further spur to such investigations was the finding that some patients with high blood pressure who were treated with the drug reserpine developed a syndrome thought by some to be similar to clinical depression. When reserpine was shown in the mid-1950's to produce depletion of brain norepinephrine, this caused several investigators to suggest that depression is due to deficient functioning of biogenic amine systems. Subsequent investigations into the pharmacological effects of tricyclic antidepressants and monoamine oxidase inhibitors (see Chapter 10) demonstrated their potent effects on biogenic amine systems. From these pharmacological data, the biogenic amine hypotheses of affective disorders were proposed, namely that *depression is associated with reduced activity of biogenic amine-containing neuronal systems at key sites in the brain. Mania, conversely, was stated to be associated with excess activity in these neuronal systems.* These hypotheses have provided a very important framework for subsequent investigations.

In the United States, much of the research has focused on the catecholamines, dopamine (DA) and norepinephrine (NE), whereas in Europe serotonin systems have received most of the attention. While an impressive body of data has been gathered that is consistent with these theories, an equally substantial corpus of information is available which does not support them. [Clearly, part of the confusion among the various studies arises from difficulties in proper patient diagnosis, and proper control of diet, locomotor activity, and psychotropic drug medication.] The discussion that follows will review briefly the strategies that have been employed by the clinical investigator and summarize the results obtained.

Fig. 1 gives a schematic representation of a noradrenergic synapse. Also indicated in the diagram are sites of action of various psychotropic drugs. This model is similar to that for serotonin and dopamine. Using this as a reference point, it is easy to visualize the types of strategies employed to explore these theories. Investigators have measured biogenic amine metabolite excretion in urine or metabolite levels in cerebrospinal fluid, in the hope that this will provide some measure of the level of activity of biogenic amine systems in depressed and in manic patients. In addition, the behavioral effects of drugs

Schematic Representation of a Noradrenergic Synapse

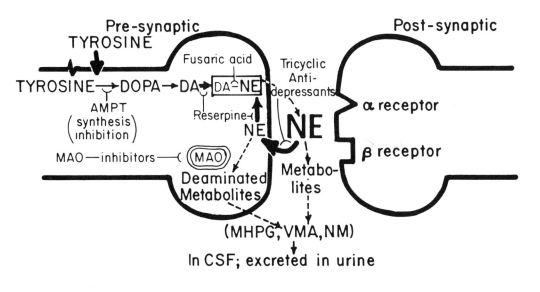

Fig. 1. Schematic representation of a noradrenergic synapse. Representative drugs inhibiting the synthesis (AMPT; fusaric acid), storage (reserpine), metabolism (MAOIs), and inactivation (tricyclic agents) of norepinephrine are indicated.

which should increase or decrease biogenic amine activity have been studied to see if the effects produced were consistent with the pharmacologically-derived biogenic amine theories.

Urinary Studies

One of the methods frequently used to explore the relationship between biogenic amines and affective illness has been the measurement of the concentration of amine metabolites in the urine of depressed and manic patients. Unfortunately, no more than 5% of most urinary amine metabolites comes from brain, which makes it difficult to infer much about brain function from these studies. One possible exception to this is 3, methoxy-4-hydroxyphenylgycol (MHPG). This compound is the main metabolite of brain norepinephrine and it has been reported that about 30% of urinary MHPG may originate in the central nervous system.

Robins and Hartman (1972) have summarized the findings from nine urinary studies of both depressed and manic patients in which catecholamines and their metabolites were measured. A result consistent with the catecholamine theory would be viewed as one in which the concentration of the amines or their metabolites was lower in the depressives as compared to a control population or was lower in patients when depressed as compared to when recovered from depression. The converse situation would be the case with regard to mania. They reported that the urinary findings were in general not consistent with the catecholamine hypothesis of depression, whereas the findings with manic patients were more consistent. The increased amine and metabolite excretion seen in manic patients could be secondary to the increased activity exhibited by such subjects.

Since a considerably higher percentage of the total MHPG in urine might come from the brain, when compared to other norepinephrine metabolites, attention has been focused on it. Several investigators have reported that the urinary output of MHPG in certain types of depressed patients is lower than that measured in either controls or other types of depressives.

This result highlights one of the problems associated with research into the biology of affective disorders, namely, that they are a heterogeneous group of diseases. In studying patients with the nonspecific general syndrome of depression, significant abnormalities in discreet subgroups of patients may be obscured by the larger group of those in whom this abnormality is absent. Thus, all depressed subjects do not have abnormal excretion of MHPG. Some do, and the question is whether such patients have other clinical or biochemical features in common which would provide a basis for a meaningful subgroup of depressives.

There have been many attempts to divide depressed patients into subgroups. In the main, these separations are based on concepts, such as endogenous, reactive, neurotic, psychotic, involutional, agitated, retarded and presenile. In general, patients grouped in these ways have not shown consistent differences in biochemical parameters or treatment response. More recently, Rob-

ins and Guze and their associates suggested a classification based on prior psychiatric history. A primary depressive would be a patient with an affective episode who has been either psychiatrically well or who has had no pre-existing diagnosable psychiatric illness other than depression or mania. In contrast, a secondary depressive would be a patient with an affective episode who has had another pre-existing diagnosable psychiatric illness. The key to this classification scheme, then, is chronology: the presence or absence of a pre-existing diagnosable psychiatric disorder.

The group of primary depressives can be subdivided further into either bipolar or unipolar depressives. Bipolar depression describes patients who have both depressive and manic episodes, while unipolar depression refers to patients with recurrent depressive episodes, without evidence of mania or hypomania. Some of the reported differences between bipolar and unipolar depressives are shown in Table 1. Several differences may be noted with regard to clinical and biochemical characteristics and with regard to treatment response to administration of lithium ion. The lesson to be remembered is to be on the alert for clusters of patients with a particular clinical course, treatment response, biochemical change or other distinctive features.

To return, then, to urinary MHPG excretion, it is the bipolar depressives who exhibit low excretion of this metabolite, whereas other depressives may not. Furthermore, three groups of investigators have followed several manic-depressive patients over time, and found reduced urinary MHPG during depressive phases as compared with periods of mania or normothymia. The results of these studies have been interpreted by some as being compatible with the hypothesis of reduced central noradrenergic activity in depression (reflected in the lower urinary MHPG concentration).

Recently, data has been reported

Table 1. Differences reported between bipolar and unipolar depressives

	Bipolar	Unipolar
History of mania	Positive	Negative
Family history of mania	Positive	Negative
Age of onset	Younger	Older
Sex distribution	Male = Female	Male < Female
Mania response to tricyclic drugs	Positive	Negative
Anti-depressant response to lithium ion	Positive	Negative
Platelet monoamine oxidase activity	Decreased	Normal
Urinary 17-hydroxy-corticosteroids	Decreased	Normal

which suggest another reason to be interested in urinary MHPG concentration: patients with low urinary MHPG prior to treatment respond to therapy with the tricyclic drug, imipramine, while those with normal or high excretion of MHPG respond to a different tricyclic antidepressant, amitriptyline. While this claim awaits further confirmation, it exemplifies an area in which the biological approach to mental disease can provide valuable assistance. Once drug therapy for depression is started, it is usually (in the absence of significant side effects) continued for at least two weeks and often longer before a clinical decision is made whether the patient is responding. For this reason, it is important to choose carefully the drug that will be used initially. Unfortunately, response to a drug is still quite often a hit or miss proposition when only clinical parameters are used as a guide to drug selection. For example, it is not uncommon for a depressive to respond well to the drug imipramine but not to amitryptyline. Another patient, with similar symptomatology will respond to amitryptyline but not to imipramine. We do not know why this is so. Biochemical parameters, then, may be important in subdividing patients into meaningful subgroups with regard to drug response. If low urinary MHPG does indeed predict response to imipramine, then it is an important parameter for the clinician to have measured. And this is so, regardless of what importance one attaches to MHPG with regard to the etiology of affective disorders. It is anticipated that other biochemical parameters will be found which will aid in drug selection for the individual patient.

Cerebrospinal Fluid Studies

Basal Concentrations — A number of investigators have measured the concentrations of biogenic amine metabolites in the cerebrospinal fluid of patients with affective illnesses. This strategy is based on the finding that the biogenic amine metabolites enter the cerebrospinal fluid from brain where they are produced. Since under most conditions these metabolites do not penetrate from blood into the cerebrospinal fluid, it is presumably brain (and spinal cord) metabolism that is being evaluated by measuring metabolites in cerebrospinal fluid. In man, cerebrospinal fluid is usually obtained at the lumbar level of the spinal cord. This poses a problem in that it is difficult to separate the contribution made by the spinal cord from that made by the brain to the concentration of metabolite measured.

Studies of lumbar spinal fluid homovanillic acid (HVA—the primary metabolite of dopamine) levels in depressed patients have yielded inconsistent results. There are reports of decreased concentrations in depressives which increase with clinical improvement, and other reports of no differences from levels found in control subjects. Studies with manic patients have been similarly inconsistent, with either low or normal HVA concentrations being observed.

The original report by Ashcroft and Sharman that depressed patients had significantly lower concentrations of the serotonin metabolite 5-hydroxyindoleacetic acid (5-HIAA) in lumbar spinal fluid than did neurological patients, has been confirmed by some, but not all, investigators. There are also reports of low lumbar fluid 5-HIAA in some schizophrenic patients. Of interest are the reports that some manic patients also have low 5-HIAA concentrations and that there may be little change in the low 5-HIAA values seen in some depressed and manic patients with treatment and clinical recovery. In other words, the abnormality in serotonin-containing neuron activity, inferred from the low lumbar spinal fluid 5-HIAA concentrations, may persist regardless of the clinical state of the patient. If this is so, it may represent some underlying defect that predisposes the individual to affective symptomatology.

MHPG concentrations in lumbar spinal fluid of depressives have been reported to be low by some, but not other investigators and may remain low after clinical recovery in some patients. Lumbar spinal fluid MHPG concentration has been reported to be either normal or elevated in both manic and acute schizophrenic patients.

Probenecid Studies — In an attempt to obtain more consistent and meaningful data about brain amine metabolism, several investigators have studied the accumulation of dopamine and serotonin metabolites in lumbar spinal fluid after the administration of probenecid. Probenecid blocks the active transport of organic acids, such as 5-HIAA and HVA, out of the cerebrospinal fluid. Over time, then, these substances continue to enter the cerebrospinal fluid from brain so that their concentration in this fluid increases. This is ultimately expressed as an increase in the concentration of these metabolites found in lumbar spinal fluid. The extent of the rise in metabolite concentration after probenecid seems to provide an index of the level of activity in biogenic amine neurons in the brain. This is shown in Fig. 2. When patients are given L-dihydroxyphenylalanine (L-DOPA) to increase dopamine synthesis, the extent of the probenecid-induced accumulation of the dopamine metabolite, homovanillic acid, is greatly enhanced. In contrast, α-methyl, ρ-tyrosine (AMPT), which inhibits dopamine biosynthesis, lowers the accumulation of HVA. Precursors of serotonin like tryptophan and inhibitors of serotonin synthesis like p-chlorophenylalanine (PCPA) alter the probenecid-induced accumulation of 5-hydroxyindoleacetic acid but not that of homovanillic acid.

There is no accumulation of MHPG after probenecid administration, so that this technique is not used to study norepinephrine metabolism in the central nervous system.

Results obtained using the probenecid technique are somewhat more consistent than those reported of basal metabolite concentrations. In most studies, decreased lumbar spinal fluid accumulations of both 5-HIAA and HVA have been reported in depressives in comparison with control subjects (usually, neurological patients). Quite interestingly, low accumulation of these metabolites has been observed in hypomanic patients as well.

Unfortunately, interpretation of these results is quite complicated. Originally, these data were offered as support of the amine theories of depression, in that the low metabolite accumulation was thought to reflect low activity of biogenic amine systems. Now, however, data are available which indicate that, under some circumstances, the extent of metabolite accumulation is *inversely* related to the level of amine activity. Thus, blockade of dopamine receptors, which reduces the effects produced by dopamine-containing neuronal systems, in-

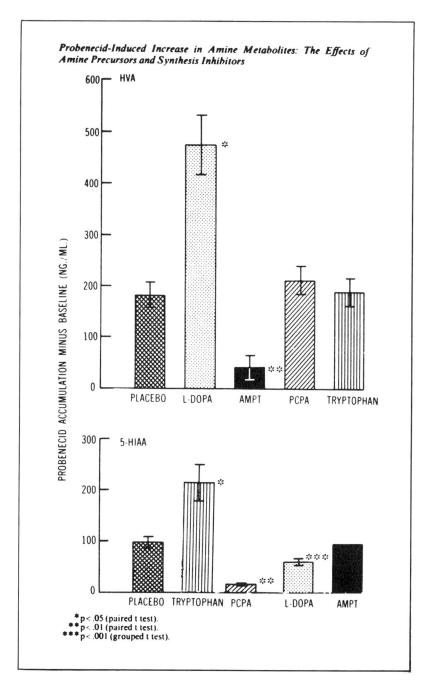

Probenecid-Induced Increase in Amine Metabolites: The Effects of Amine Precursors and Synthesis Inhibitors

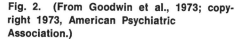

Fig. 2. (From Goodwin et al., 1973; copyright 1973, American Psychiatric Association.)

creases the probenecid-induced accumulation of homovanillic acid. This is presumably a reflection of the receptor blockade causing a compensatory increase in dopamine synthesis, release, and metabolism in the pre-synaptic neuron so as to overcome the post-synaptic receptor blockade. Also, treatment of depressives with tricyclic drugs further reduces the already low accumulation of 5-hydroxyindoleacetic acid seen in such patients. It is unclear, then, whether the low accumulation of amine metabolites seen in depressives after probenecid does reflect low activity of biogenic amine systems. Further research is needed to clarify this.

Furthermore, the significance of these results with regard to the etiology of the disease is unknown. Do these changes contribute toward the symptomatology of depression or predispose the individual to a depressive episode? Or rather, are they a consequence of the disease process or an associated abnormality, i.e., secondary changes? It is often difficult to determine whether the biological changes noted in depressives are primary (associated with the etiology and/or development of the condition) or secondary to either a primary biochemical change or to the illness itself. The secondary changes may actually obscure the primary manifestations. Many of the changes reported in depressives are not specific for the condition, but are secondary to the illness or some other factor. For example, depressives have elevated plasma catecholamine concentrations and this correlates with anxiety, which is almost always present together with depression, rather than depression *per se*. This indicates that the high plasma catecholamine concentrations seen in depressives are a secondary phenomenon due to the presence of concomitant anxiety.

In a similar manner, the abnormalities inferred in central biogenic amine containing neuronal systems in depressives may be secondary manifestations of the illness process.

Post Mortem Studies

Shaw and Pare and their associates have reported decreased serotonin concentrations in the hindbrains of suicide victims when compared to the hindbrains of persons who had died of other causes. Bourne et al. were unable to find any abnormality in brain serotonin levels but did report low concentrations of 5-HIAA. They also found no abnormality in hypothalamic and hindbrain norepinephrine or in dopamine concentrations in the caudate nucleus. In a study of discrete brain areas, Lloyd and his associates (1974) found that serotonin levels were reduced significantly in areas of the brain containing high concentrations of cell bodies for serotonin neurons, namely the raphe nuclei inferior (see Chapter 3). There are a large number of uncontrolled variables in any *post-mortem* study that make the results difficult to evaluate. Nevertheless, the approach used by Lloyd et al., with its emphasis on the study of discrete brain areas, may prove to be a useful strategy.

Amine Depletion Studies

The findings that some hypertensive patients treated with reserpine develop a syndrome resembling clinical depression and that a retarded behavioral state in rats similarly treated is associated with a depletion of brain biogenic amines played an important role in the formulation of the biogenic amine hypothesis of depression.

The multiple effects of reserpine on dopamine-, norepinephrine-, serotonin- and acetylcholine-containing neurons make it a poor drug for elucidating the role of particular amines in the development of depression. More specific depletion of catecholamines or of serotonin can be achieved by the administration of drugs which interfere with their biosynthesis. Thus, alpha-methylparatyrosine (AMPT) inhibits the synthesis of catecholamines (Fig. 1) and parachlorophenylalanine (PCPA) does the same to serotonin. The behavioral effects of these compounds in animals and in humans have been studied.

Lower animals treated with AMPT evidence sedation and decreased spontaneous motor activity but no behavioral changes suggestive of depression. In monkeys, Redmond et al. have reported that AMPT produces reduced motor activity, decreases in social initiatives and social interactions, and postural and facial changes suggestive of withdrawal. The monkeys continued to respond to the social initiatives of others, unlike most depressed patients, and did not show some of the characteristic biological signs and symptoms of depression, such as sleep disturbance, decreased appetite and loss of weight and libido.

Medical and schizophrenic patients treated with doses of AMPT sufficient to produce significant inhibition of peripheral, and presumably central, catecholamine synthesis showed evidence of sedation and, in some cases, anxiety, but did not become depressed. In another study, Brodie and colleagues found that AMPT produced improvement in the majority of manic patients treated with the drug. In the same study, three depressed patients were treated with AMPT and showed some aggravation of symptoms. The study of Brodie et al. offers some support for the catecholamine theory as the majority of manic patients improved when given AMPT and depressed patients had an exacerbation of symptomatology.

In another study, depressed patients who improved when treated with imipramine did not show any return of symptoms when given AMPT.

When AMPT is given, it depletes both dopamine and norepinephrine. In an attempt to focus more specifically on the role of norepinephrine in mania, Sack and Goodwin treated eight manic and hypomanic patients with fusaric acid, an inhibitor of the enzyme, dopamine-β-hydroxylase. This blocks the normal conversion of dopamine into norepinephrine (Fig. 1). Fusaric acid produced a 25% decrease in lumbar spinal fluid MHPG concentration (consistent with inhibition of dopamine-β-hydroxylase) and a significant increase in lumbar spinal fluid homovanillic acid in their patients. In contrast to the anticipated results, the more severe manic patients became *worse* with fusaric acid, while the milder hypomanics showed no change or improved slightly.

The behavioral effects of PCPA have also been assessed in animals and in human subjects. In animals, PCPA frequently causes insomnia, increases in sexual and aggressive behavior, and an irritability and hyperreactivity to the environment. If anything, these changes are more suggestive of mania than depression.

PCPA has been given to normal volunteers and patients with different medical illnesses, and produces a number of nonspecific effects, such as tiredness, restlessness, and anxiety, whereas at higher doses, confusion, agitation, and paranoid thinking have been noted. As with AMPT, depressive symptomatology is not a frequent occurrence.

In contrast to what was observed with AMPT, when depressed patients who had responded to imipramine were given PCPA, they all became depressed within 2 days despite continuation of the tricyclic drug. Upon withdrawal of PCPA, all the patients recovered from the depressive symptomatology. This is a very interesting strategy. It suggests, of course, some effect of serotonin depletion in susceptible individuals in the genesis of depressive features.

The available data, then, strongly suggest that the depletion of brain norepinephrine, dopamine, or serotonin is, *in itself*, not sufficient to account for the development of clinical depression. Such depletion, even if severe and accompanied by a major reduction in amine turnover, produces few *persistent* behavioral changes compatible with clinical depression. In fact, when one considers how much amine reduction is necessary to produce behavioral deficits in animals, it seems unlikely that such a severe depletion could occur in depressed patients and not be more readily detectable, unless it was sharply localized in one area of the brain. While these results do not rule out the possibility that biogenic amines play an important role in affect regulation, they do emphasize the need to consider other systems which may interact with changes in amine function.

Administration of Monoamine Precursors

In an attempt to increase biogenic amine containing neuron activity, a number of investigators have given precursors of the biogenic amines to depressed patients. The precursors penetrate into brain and are enzymatically converted there to the biogenic amines. The amines themselves (DA, NE, serotonin) cannot be given as they do not penetrate appreciably from the blood into the brain (see Chapter 3). Probably, much of the interest in this approach has stemmed from the successful use of the catecholamine precursor, L-DOPA, in the treatment of Parkinson's disease.

Depressed patients have been given large doses of L-DOPA, but there have been few reports of significant anti-depressant activity. There have been reports of the development of hypomanic-like activity without actual relief of the depressive mood.

The studies of the effects of serotonin precursors fall into two groups: 5-hydroxytryptophan (5-HTP), the immediate precursor of serotonin, and tryptophan, the precursor of 5-hydroxytryptophan (see Chapter 3).

The results with 5-hydroxytryptophan have been inconsistent, but in general suggest that it is not an effective antidepressant.

Several studies have been conducted testing the antidepressant efficacy of L-tryptophan. While Coppen and associates have suggested that L-tryptophan may be as effective as electro-convulsive therapy in the treatment of depression, most other investigators have not found tryptophan to be a useful antidepressant.

As with the amine depletion studies, the precursor load studies are not, in the main, supportive of the amine theories of depression. While partial improvement has been noted in some depressives with either L-DOPA or L-tryptophan, these compounds are not generally useful in the treatment of depression. Their efficacy certainly does not rival that of the tricyclic compounds or monoamine oxidase inhibitors.

Clearly, the amine theories of affective disorders must still be regarded as unproven. As with all good theories, though, their value is not dependent upon their being proven correct. Rather, their worth lies in the research they stimulated and the knowledge subsequently acquired. There is no doubt that these theories fostered important methodological advances by which our knowledge of brain function has been expanded considerably.

Acetylcholine

Relatively little research has been conducted into possible abnormalities of central cholinergic function in depression. In a recent study, Janowsky et al.

found that they could produce rapid, though temporary, remission of manic symptoms by the intravenous administration of physostigmine, a centrally active acetylcholinesterase inhibitor. They also reported that in some of these patients physostigmine produced feelings of hopelessness along with psychomotor retardation and other signs and symp-

toms of depression. They suggest that *affective state may be determined by a balance between cholinergic and noradrenergic activity, with mania being a condition of relative adrenergic preponderance.* Clearly, further research into the possible relationship between cholinergic function and mood is indicated.

Neuroendocrine Systems

There has been a long-standing interest in neuroendocrine function in affective disorders. It is known that lesions in the hypothalamus may be associated with mood disturbance in man; that hypothalamic stimulation will produce intense affective responses; and that the regulation of appetite, sexual activities, menstruation and aggression, all of which may be disturbed in depressed patients, are mediated through the hypothalamus.

Hypothalamic-Pituitary-Adrenal Cortical (HPA) Function

A number of studies employing different strategies point to increased HPA activity in many depressed patients. There are reports, for example, of elevations in plasma, urinary and cerebrospinal fluid (CSF) cortisol. The increased adreno-cortical activity is not due to an exaggerated response of the adrenal gland to corticotropin (ACTH) but rather seems to result from increased hypothalamic-pituitary activity. In most studies, the elevation in the corticosteroid parameter measured returned toward normal with clinical recovery.

Many of these biochemical findings seen in depressed patients are also found in patients with diencephalic Cushing's syndrome. In this disease, there is overproduction of corticosteroids from the adrenal cortex. In diencephalic Cushing's syndrome, the primary defect is not in the adrenal cortex, but rather is

centered in the brain so that there is reduced control of ACTH release. Many patients with diencephalic Cushing's syndrome exhibit euphoria and depression. Furthermore, therapeutic administration of corticosteroids may produce mood changes. As Butler and Besser reported, it is not always easy to distinguish between Cushing's syndrome and severe depression insofar as tests of HPA function are concerned.

The elegant experiments of Sachar and his associates (1973) have provided a clearer picture of the scope of the HPA abnormality seen in depressives. These investigators sampled venous blood frequently in depressed patients and in controls over a 24-hour period. As shown in Fig. 3, there is normally a circadian variation in plasma cortisol concentrations such that late evening and night time values are much lower than those obtained in the early morning. In addition, there is a spiking pattern to the plasma cortisol concentrations, presumably a reflection of the pulsatile release of ACTH.

In depressed patients, however, the picture is quite different (Fig. 4). Such patients have an increased number of secretory episodes of cortisol and increased total cortisol secretion. Furthermore, in depressives, cortisol secretion occurs during the late evening and early morning—a time during which such secretion is minimal in normal subjects. Some remnant of a circadian pattern of cortisol concentrations usually persists in

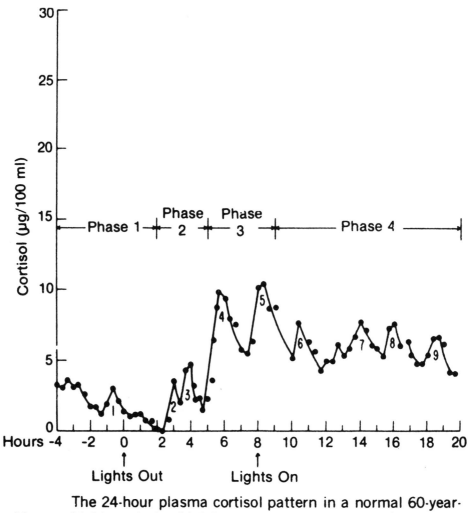

The 24-hour plasma cortisol pattern in a normal 60-year-old man. Lights out at midnight.

Fig. 3. (From Sachar et al., 1973.)

most depressives, though (Fig. 4).

Another strategy used by several investigators to test HPA function has been to administer the synthetic glucocorticoid, dexamethasone, to depressed patients. In normal subjects, this compound acts, as does cortisol itself, to suppress ACTH secretion, thereby lowering cortisol secretion and plasma cortisol concentrations. In many depressed patients, however, dexamethasone does not lower plasma cortisol concentrations. De-

pressed patients, then, are said to be "resistant" to suppression of plasma cortisol concentration induced by dexamethasone. In fact, what actually happens is that depressed patients initially suppress plasma cortisol concentrations in response to dexamethasone. The difference, though, is that this suppression does not last nearly as long in depressives as in nondepressed subjects. Doses of dexamethasone that suppress plasma cortisol concentrations for 24 hours in controls

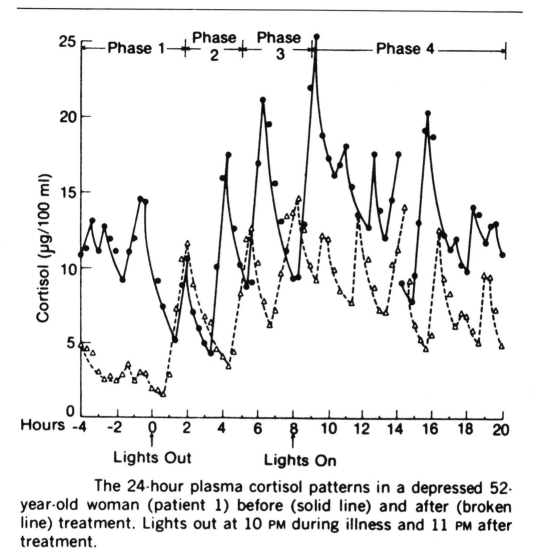

The 24-hour plasma cortisol patterns in a depressed 52-year-old woman (patient 1) before (solid line) and after (broken line) treatment. Lights out at 10 PM during illness and 11 PM after treatment.

Fig. 4. (From Sachar et al., 1973).

may only cause a two or three hour suppression in depressives. Thus, depressed patients "escape" early from the suppressive effect of dexamethasone. This abnormality is strongly related to the changes in circadian cortisol secretion described by Sachar and his colleagues (1973). Both are a manifestation of abnormal HPA regulation in depressives.

A question that has still not been adequately resolved is whether the elevations in the production rate of cortisol and its plasma concentration result in elevated exposure of tissues, especially brain tissue, to the steroid. Less than 10% of the total plasma cortisol circulates in a free form in plasma; most plasma cortisol circulates bound to plasma protein called either corticosteroid-binding globulin or transcortin. The effects of circulating glucocorticoids on tissues are presumed to be due to the small non-bound portion of circulating cortisol. Unfortunately, plasma free cortisol, which provide an index of tissue exposure, has not yet been measured in a sufficient number of depressives to make a definitive statement. When it has been measured, elevations in free cortisol have usually been observed.

Concentrations of cortisol in the CSF are closely related to plasma free cortisol levels and give an indication of the exposure of the central nervous system to cortisol. In the three studies measuring this parameter in depressives, values which were lower than in controls were reported in one study; in the second study, values similar to control levels were found; in the third investigation (in which the largest number of patients were studied), depressives were reported to have elevated concentration of cortisol in the CSF. The reason for this discrepancy is not readily apparent; further studies in depressives of this important parameter are needed.

Measurement of urinary free cortisol excretion provides another index of estimating tissue exposure to cortisol. Elevations in urinary free cortisol excretion have been noted in depressives. While it is not possible to make any definitive statement yet, a trend seems to be emerging from the different indirect measures that depressives do have increased tissue exposure to cortisol.

Direct examination of the question has been attempted by comparing the brain concentration of cortisol in patients dying by suicide with the concentration in brains of patients dying from other causes. In view of the results with the indirect measures, it is rather surprising that *low* cortisol levels have been found in the brains of subjects dying by suicide. Additional studies are needed to resolve this apparent paradox.

Several suggestions have been made as to the significance of the increased HPA activity seen in some depressed patients. While it may be the result of such nonspecific factors as the stress of the illness, concomitant anxiety, or hospitalization, this does not seem to provide an adequate explanation for several more recent findings. Thus, Carroll has reported that schizophrenic patients with psychosis ratings equivalent to depressives do not have any abnormality in dexamethasone suppression whereas the depressed patients do. Also, there is no consistent correlation between the elevated adrenocortical activity and manifest anxiety. Furthermore, administration of antianxiety drugs does not suppress the exaggerated adrenal cortical activity observed in these patients.

Another explanation for this phenomenon favors the idea of a deficiency in the functioning of monoamine-containing neurons in depressives, i.e., the biogenic amine theories of depression. Hypothalamic neurons containing biogenic amines are involved in the regulation of the release of corticotropin-releasing factor which, in turn, regulates ACTH release (see Chapter 4). Thus, the increased adrenocortical activity found in some depressed patients may be a reflection of a reduction in activity of amine-containing neurons which normally inhibit the release of corticotropin-releasing factor. The primary neuroendocrine lesion in depressives, according to this view, is a disinhibition of the HPA axis due to abnormal functioning of biogenic amine-containing neurons. This would result in increased ACTH release, with subsequent increased adrenocortical activity. While the exact mechanism responsible for the HPA abnormality in depressives remains to be established, it seems clear that it is not related to either psychosis or anxiety. Rather the abnormality seems peculiar to some depressives and, indeed, may represent an important component of the illness.

Sex Hormones

There is considerable evidence that factors associated with aspects of sex hormone functions may be of importance in our understanding of the development of depression. Thus, depression is more common in females than in males, especially among unipolar depressives (this may be due to genetic rather than to hormonal factors); depression is more likely to occur at times of endocrine change—premenstrually, *post-partum*, at the menopause, or in association with oral contraceptive administration.

It is unlikely that we are dealing with a simple increase or decrease in the level of a particular hormone but rather with a more complex action. For example, there may be sex-related differences in the activity of monoamine oxidase which could contribute to alterations in amine function. To date, little attention has been directed toward this issue, and there are a number of important lines of investigation which need to be developed.

Electrolyte Metabolism

Electrolytes play a central role in several critical aspects of neuronal function. This includes their involvement in maintaining the normal resting potential of nerves; the carrying of the current required for the action potential; in the synthesis, storage, release and inactivation of neurotransmitters; and in carrying the current responsible for depolarization of post-synaptic membranes. Depression and mania are presumably associated with an alteration in neuronal function, and it is, therefore, conceivable that an abnormality of electrolyte metabolism may be of importance in their development.

Perhaps the most consistent electrolyte finding in depressives involves sodium metabolism. Normally, the kidney regulates water and sodium excretion to maintain a balance between the amount ingested and the amount excreted. However, during periods of depression, this balance is disturbed so that not all the sodium taken in is excreted. In other words, several investigators have shown clinical depression to be associated with a retention of sodium. Upon clinical recovery, the excess sodium that was retained during depression is excreted in the urine.

The storage site for the excess sodium has not yet been established. Coppen and Shaw suggested that the sodium retained during clinical depression resulted in an increase in residual sodium —defined as the combination of intracellular sodium and bone sodium. Further investigation of this possibility is needed. It should be emphasized that we do not as yet know whether such changes in sodium metabolism represent some primary defect or are secondary to another, perhaps hormonal, defect.

Extensive studies of magnesium, potassium and calcium concentrations have not revealed any consistently significant findings to date.

Cell Membrane

Attention has been focused recently on the possibility that some depressed patients may have altered functioning of the processes responsible for the cation distribution across the cell membrane.

Mendels and Frazer (1974) suggest that there is a subgroup of depressed patients with a genetically determined abnormality in some aspect of cell membrane properties which regulate the movement of electrolytes across the plasma membrane. This subgroup of patients may partially overlap with patients diagnosed as bipolar depressives. The findings suggestive of an alteration in cell membrane activity come from a variety of sources. They include the following: (1) depressed patients who respond to lithium treatment distribute the cation differently across the erythrocyte membrane than do patients who do not respond to lithium; (2) the distribution of the lithium ion across the erythrocyte membrane seems to be under genetic control and to be dependent upon intrinsic properties of the erythrocyte membrane; (3) reduced transport of radioactive sodium from erythrocytes obtained from patients with bipolar depressive illness; (4) higher sodium activity and lower hydrogen ion activity in saliva of depressed patients than that measured in the saliva of controls suggesting reduced reabsorption of sodium and of bicarbonate (measured as pH) in the depressed patients; and (5) reduced rate of entry of radioactive sodium from plasma into lumbar spinal fluid.

Additional research into membrane transport properties of depressives would seem to be a promising area of investigation.

Interactions Between Biochemical Systems

Increasing attention is being directed to many ways in which the different systems discussed in this review interact with each other. For example, biological theories of affective disorders have arisen concerning the balance between serotonin and norepinephrine systems. Such an idea is not new; it was, perhaps, first formally stated some twenty years ago by Brodie and Shore, who suggested that NE and serotonin were transmitters for systems mediating opposing central nervous system effects. Recently, other investigators have expanded and refined such ideas. Thus, there is some evidence to support the view of reduced functioning of serotonin systems in both depression and in mania. When coupled with low activity of NE systems, the low serotonin activity leads to depression; if there is a high level of NE activity, mania ensues.

As noted previously, Janowsky et al. favor a balance between cholinergic and adrenergic systems—cholinergic predominance causing depression whereas adrenergic excess leading to mania. While such ideas remain speculative, they illustrate a refinement of previous thinking. It is no longer adequate to think of too little or too much activity in any one system. Now, the manner in which the system in question interacts with other components in the central nervous system must be researched and considered.

In addition to the interactions between different biogenic amine systems, electrolytes and steroid hormones can influence activity of amine-containing systems. Cations, such as sodium, calcium and magnesium play key roles in the synthesis, storage, release and re-uptake of monoamines. Similarly, steroid-hormone administration can alter both monoamine synthesis and monoamine-induced responses. It seems possible, then, that disturbances in electrolyte metabolism or steroid hormone regulation would modify monoamine function. Alterations in central monoamine activity may not only cause disturbances in other systems but may, in fact, be the result of such disturbances. If subsequent research supports this idea, it suggests that cycles may be established in patients with affective disorders due to consecutive disturbances in multiple systems.

Mania-Depression Relationship

Some of the prevalent biological theories of affective disorders are clearly based on the view that depression and mania are polar opposites—a view that is apparently supported by aspects of manifest symptomatology (see Chapter 13). However, a number of clinical, biochemical and neurophysiological observations suggest that mania and depression may have a number of biological changes in common.

For example it is not unusual to see patients with clinical features of both mania and depression simultaneously—a manic patient may start to cry when discussing his problems.

Other observations such as this one imply that the view that mania and depression are polar opposites is an oversimplification. There do seem to be certain biochemical alterations that are similar in depressed and in manic patients. As was mentioned previously, both manic and depressed patients showed decreased lumbar spinal fluid accumulation of HVA and 5-HIAA after probenecid administration. In addition, hypomanic and depressed patients have sleep disturbances which have many features in common. Lithium carbonate is not only effective in mania but may also have antidepressant properties in selected depressed patients. Furthermore, both manics and bipolar depressives demonstrate an increase in the amplitude of the average evoked response—a measure of the cortical potential produced by sensory stimulation—with increasing light intensity.

Results such as these have led to alternative ways of conceptualizing the relationship between the two affective states. According to these ideas, the states of mania and depression may have certain predisposing physiological and biochemical alterations in common. Other secondary factors would then determine the actual affect observed, which could be either "pure" depression or mania or some combination of the two states.

Biochemical and pharmacological data, then, have contributed toward a rethinking of the association between depression and mania. It is hoped that further investigation will contribute to our understanding of the cyclical nature of the illness and to the appearance of spontaneous remissions. Most current biological theories of affective disorders offer no explanation for these phenomena. The lithium ion, though, may offer assistance in this regard, as it is the first drug shown to affect the natural course of the illness. Investigation of the pharmacological effects of this cation may provide leads for understanding the biology underlying the cyclical nature of affective disorders. Perhaps the time is not too distant when we will understand how the biological factor involved in affective disorders expresses itself.

224   FRAZER

Selected References

Baldessarini, R.J.: The basis for amine hypotheses in affective disorders. A critical evaluation. *Arch. Gen. Psychiat.* 32:1087-1093, 1975.

Davies, B., Carroll, B.J., and Mowbray, R.M.: *Depressive Illness: Some Research Studies.* Charles C. Thomas, Springfield, Ill., 1972.

Durell, J.: Sodium and potassium metabolism. Lithium salts and affective disorders. In *Factors in Depression*, N.S. Kline, ed. Raven Press, New York, 1974, pp. 67-96.

Goodwin, F.K., Post, R.M., Dunner, D.L., and Gordon, E.K.: Cerebrospinal fluid amine metabolites in affective illness: The probenecid technique. *Am. J. Psychiat.* 130: 73-79, 1973.

Holzbauer, M., and Vogt, M.: Depression by reserpine of the noradrenaline concentration in the hypothalamus of the cat. *J. Neurochem.* 1:1-7, 1956.

Lloyd, K.G., Farley, I.J., Deck, J.H.N., and Horneykiewicz, O.: Serotonin and 5-hydroxyindoleacetic acid in discrete areas of the brainstems of suicide victims and control patients. *Adv. Biochem. Psychopharmacol.* 11:387-397, 1974.

Mendels, J. and Frazer, A.: Alterations in cell membrane activity in depression. *Am. J. Psychiat.* 131: 1240-1246, 1974.

Perris, C.: A Study of bipolar, (manic-depressive) and unipolar recurrent depressive psychoses. *Acta. Psychiat. Scand.* 42 (Suppl.): 194, 1966.

Pletscher, A., Shore, P.A., and Brodie, B.B.: Serotonin as a mediator of reserpine action in brain. *J. Pharmacol. Exp. Ther.* 116:84-89, 1956.

Robins, E., and Hartman, B.K.: Some chemical theories of mental disorders. In *Basic Neurochemistry*, R.W. Albers, G.J. Seigel, R. Katzman, et al., eds. Little, Brown and Co., Boston, 1972, pp. 607-644.

Sachar, E.J., Hellman, L., Roffwarg, H., Halpern, F., Fukushima, D., and Gallagher, T.: Disrupted 24 hour patterns of cortisol secretion in psychotic depression. *Arch. Gen. Psychiat.* 28:19-24, 1973.

Schildkraut, J.J.: *Neuropsychopharmacology and the Affective Disorders.* Little, Brown and Co., Boston, 1970.

Chapter 15

Opiate Dependence

T. Alan Ramsey

Introduction

The goal of this chapter is to present some theories about biological factors which are important in causing and maintaining drug dependence and some pharmacological approaches which are used to treat it. It is clear that biological factors are not the only ones which are important in drug dependence. Social and psychological factors are of great importance in this phenomenon, and non-pharmacological treatment approaches have been used on their own or in com-bination with pharmacological modali-ties. However, a detailed discussion of non-pharmacological and non-biological factors is not within the scope of this chapter.

Emphasis will be placed on opiate de-pendence because it can be considered a prototype of other types of drug de-pendence, and pharmacological treat-ment approaches have been developed to a much greater extent with opiate dependence than with any other form of drug dependence. Alcohol depen-dence, which is the most frequent kind of drug dependence in the United States, will be covered in a separate chapter, and the reader is referred there for a detailed discussion of this problem.

History

The historical origins of drug dependence are shrouded in antiquity. However, drug preparations with high dependence potential have been used by man since before the beginnings of recorded history. The use of opiate preparations was recorded prior to the birth of Christ. Cannabis preparations have been employed in the Middle East for hundreds of years, and the use of alcohol extends back into the past, perhaps to the beginnings of civilization itself.

Opiate preparations have been available in the United States since the early part of the 19th Century; however, the Civil War gave rise to the first large-scale problem of opiate dependence in this country. Morphine was widely used as an analgesic (painkiller) for wounded soldiers, and many of them became dependent. In fact, opiate dependence became known as "the soldiers' disease."

Initially, opium preparations were widely available in America without medical prescription. In 1914, the Federal Government took the first steps to limit the availability of opiates with the passage of the Harrison Narcotics Act. This Act limited the use of opiates to medical purposes only. Over the next few years, the enforcement of this law and the court interpretations of it effectively confined the medical use of opiates to analgesic, cough suppressant, and anti-diarrheal indications. Physicians were not permitted to prescribe opiates in order to maintain addicts. As a consequence, the use of opiates for nonmedical purposes became a crime, fostering the development of an illicit supply system.

The beginning of this century saw the first systematic efforts to treat opiate dependence in the United States. This period was characterized by the establishment of several institutions in different parts of the country to treat opiate dependence. In 1898, heroin was introduced for the treatment of opiate dependence, because it was found to suppress morphine abstinence symptoms. Modern techniques for assessing the dependence-producing potential of drugs were not available, and it was not until several years later that the addiction potential of heroin was recognized.

In 1935, the Federal Government established a hospital at Lexington, Kentucky, for the treatment of opiate dependence, and another at Fort Worth, Texas, in 1938. Federal prisoners with a history of narcotic dependence were sent to these hospitals, and voluntary admissions were also accepted. These institutions remained the mainstay of treatment efforts until the 1960's. Opiate detoxification was followed up with several months of work, vocational training, and in some cases individual and group psychotherapy. Despite the fact that a broad-based treatment approach was used, outcome studies revealed a very high rate of relapse to opiate dependence among addicts treated in these hospitals. This, plus the development of methadone maintenance in the 1960's, led to the decline and eventual phasing out of these hospitals as major treatment centers. Since the middle 1960's, there has been an emphasis on community-based treatment programs as the major approach to the treatment of opiate dependence. Because community-based programs are of recent vintage, evaluation of long-term outcome is ongoing. Initial assessment indicates that community-based treatment programs are of value in the rehabilitation of opiate addicts and are probably better than treatment by institutionalization. However, it is clear that attempts should continue to be made to improve the effectiveness of all treatment approaches to drug dependence.

Definitions and Terminology

A variety of terms have been used to describe the self-administration of drugs to produce subjective states. Drug abuse is a frequently used term which refers to drug-taking behavior which conflicts with *socially accepted* patterns of drug use.

For the purposes of this discussion, the term *drug dependence* will be used. A 1969 World Health Organization definition of drug dependence describes it as: "A state, psychic and sometimes physical, resulting from the interaction between a living organism and a drug, characterized by behavioral and other responses that always include a compulsion to take the drug on a continuous or periodic basis in order to experience its psychic effects, and sometimes to avoid the discomfort of its absence."

This definition refers to most of the important elements that characterize those states which are usually considered as drug dependence. A compulsion to take a drug, usually accompanied by a subjective craving for the drug, is a necessary component of drug dependence. When this compulsion occurs with drugs which do *not* produce physical dependence, it is considered to be a *psychological dependence*.

Reference to the interaction between the drug and the individual is made in the definition of drug dependence. This is of crucial importance to the consideration of drug dependence as a medical problem, since it is the nature of this interaction which constitutes the disorder. For drug dependence to warrant treatment as a medical illness, the interaction between the drug and the individual should produce adverse consequences for the individual. It often also results in adverse consequences for society as well. In addition to toxic physical effects and the dangers of overdose, the most common adverse individual consequence of drug dependence is the tendency for the involved person to begin to feel that the effects produced by the drug are necessary for his/her well-being, and to become increasingly preoccupied with its procurement and use, usually to the exclusion of many other useful behaviors.

In summary, the criteria for *a state of drug dependence which warrants treatment* should require both an element of compulsion and craving as well as evidence that adverse consequences accrue to the individual due to drug involvement. Drug-dependent individuals may also be said to be drug abusers, but this term includes many people who are casual users or drug experimenters, and in our society may be applied to almost all situations of non-medical use of psychoactive drugs.

Scope of the Problem

Determining the incidence and prevalence of drug dependence is a particularly difficult task because of the illegality of almost all non-medical drug use. Addicts may not cooperate with investigators for fear that it might expose them to legal authorities; therefore, indirect techniques are often used to estimate the extent of drug dependence. Different techniques have been used, such as records of Federal Bureau of Narcotics* arrests, or the Baden** Formula, but these techniques have serious deficiencies.

---

*Now the Drug Enforcement Administration.

**Dr. Michael Baden, Chief Medical Examiner of New York City. (Number of heroin deaths each year) $\times$ 200 = number of opiate addicts.

Beginning in the early 1960's, there was a rather rapid upswing in opiate and other drug use in this country. This rise was reflected in an increased number of deaths attributable to narcotic overdose and in a mounting number of narcotic-related arrests. This situation created considerable public alarm, and governments at the federal, state, and local levels began to establish treatment programs, and to strengthen law enforcement efforts against the illicit supply of drugs.

The Federal Government recognized a need for more accurate and up-to-date information on the illicit use of drugs to help in planning treatment, law enforcement, and research efforts—and the proper allocation of available resources to combat the problem. Out of this concern grew several government-supported efforts to create a system of monitoring illicit drug use which provides current information on incidence and prevalence, and identifies shifts in drug preference among users.

Among such systems is the Drug Abuse Warning Network (DAWN), a reporting system operated jointly by the National Institute on Drug Abuse (NIDA) and the Drug Enforcement Administration (DEA). This network consists of selected emergency rooms, medical examiners, inpatient treatment units, and crisis intervention centers across the country. These units report incidents of illicit drug use which come to their attention in daily operation. In addition to DAWN, information is also collected through the Drug Enforcement Administration's Narcotic Arrests Report and reports of the frequency and kinds of drug use in clients seeking treatment from government-sponsored treatment programs.

Also, nationwide surveys are sponsored by the National Institute on Drug Abuse, with interviewing of selected population samples to determine their beliefs, attitudes, and behavior with regard to a wide range of illegal drugs. Table 1 presents a summary of the findings of a relatively recent (August 1975) survey regarding non-medical drug use in the United States. Of particular interest in this report is the finding that marihuana is the most commonly used psychoactive drug* by both adults and youth, with one in every five adults and almost one in every four youths having tried marihuana at least once. Heroin and other opiates have been used by a small but substantial proportion of both adults and youths.

While these figures are of interest and provide information about general trends and patterns of drug use, it should be kept in mind that both the information provided by DAWN and the data about non-medical drug use refer to drug abuse rather than drug dependence. Recent estimates of the prevalence of *opiate dependence* in this country have ranged from 100,000 to 500,000 addicts, depending on the source of the estimate. Estimates of the cost of drug dependence to this country have ranged from $3-billion a year for the cost of heroin-related crime to $17-billion a year in total costs.

Biological Aspects

General Pharmacology

Opiate refers to any chemical compound which has a morphine-like profile of pharmacological action. Sometimes the term "opiate" is restricted to those drugs which are derived from the natural products of the opium poppy, while the term opioid is used to designate both natural and synthetic compounds which have morphine-like properties. In this chapter, opiate will refer to both natural and synthetic substances.

Opiates exert their main effects on

---

*Figures do not include alcohol use.

Drug	Ever Used		Past Month		Past Year Not Past Month		Not Past Year		Never Used	
	Youth*	Adult**	Youth	Adult	Youth	Adult	Youth	Adult	Youth	Adult
Psychotherapeutic drugs, non-medical use	10%	13%	3%	2%	3%	3%	4%	8%	88%	87%
Marihauana	23%	19%	12%	7%	7%	3%	4%	9%	77%	81%
Hashish	10%	9%	3%	2%	5%	3%	2%	4%	90%	91%
Glue and other inhalants	8.5%	2.8%	0.7%	0.1%	1.7%	0.2%	6.1%	2.5%	91.5%	97.1%
LSD and other hallucinogens	6.0%	4.5%	1.3%	0.6%	3.0%	0.9%	1.7%	3.0%	94%	95.6%
Cocaine	3.6%	3.4%	1.0%	0.7%	1.7%	1.3%	0.9%	1.4%	96.4%	96.7%
Heroin	1.0%	1.3%	- -	0.1%	0.4%	0.2%	0.6%	1.0%	98.9%	98.7%
Methadone	0.7%	0.8%	0.2%	0.1%	0.4%	0.2%	0.1%	0.5%	99.4%	99.2%
Other opiates	6.1%	3.3%	0.5%	0.2%	2.5%	1.0%	3.1%	2.1%	93.9%	96.7%

* Ages 12-17
** 18 or Older

the central nervous system (CNS) and the bowel. CNS effects include analgesia, sedation, and changes in mood. Opiates include the most effective analgesics known to man and are of great value in the modern practice of medicine. Of importance to their analgesic action is their capacity to alter mood states to decrease the unpleasant emotional reaction to pain. Mental distress, such as anxiety or depression which often accompany severe pain, is decreased. Analgesic effects of opiates may be due primarily to actions on the thalamus, though actions in other areas of the CNS also probably enhance these effects. In any case, the mood-altering properties of these drugs probably contribute substantially to their over-all analgesic action.

Other CNS effects of opiates include: an emetic (vomiting) effect, pupillary constriction, effects on the hypothalamus resulting in endocrinological changes, and suppression of the cough reflex. Pupillary constriction (pinpoint pupils) is a sign often used to detect opiate use.

At much higher doses than those which are required for most pharmacological actions, opiates produce excitatory effects and can cause convulsions. Most opiates cause death from respiratory depression long before doses high enough to produce convulsions are achieved.

After the CNS actions, the next most significant effects of opiates are those exerted on the gastrointestinal tract. Opiates decrease peristaltic contractions while increasing the tonicity, leading to spasm and reduced motility. They were used for centuries to treat diarrhea before their analgesic effects were discovered. Flushing and itching of the skin often accompany opiate administration. This effect is probably due to histamine release. The itching and flushing contribute to the overall "feeling" of the opiate rush and high when these drugs are self-administered intravenously by addicts.

The subjective feelings produced by intravenous injection of heroin or morphine are variable and influenced by such factors as the setting in which the drug is administered, the prior opiate experience of the individual taking the drug and his/her expectations of the drug effect. Most individuals have a pleasurable response, accompanied by a decrease in anxiety and a sense of well-being. Usually there is some mental clouding, and a person may lapse into a state of easily arousable somnolence ("nodding"). Non-tolerant individuals often become nauseated and vomit. Of particular interest is the sensation called a "rush" or "flash" which seems to be located in the abdomen and has been likened by many addicts to sexual orgasm. Once considerable tolerance has developed, the addict may no longer be able to achieve a "rush" when the drug is injected.

Upon cessation of chronic opiate administration, an abstinence syndrome occurs. The abstinence syndrome of opiates is characterized by CNS excitability. Is usually begins with evidence of autonomic overactivity, such as perspiration, yawning, tearing, and a runny nose. As the time after the last dose increases, the addict becomes restless, irritable, and develops dilated pupils, goose-flesh, nausea and vomiting, abdominal cramps, diarrhea, and muscle spasms. In addition to these physiological disturbances, the withdrawing individual exhibits drug-seeking behavior. This behavior may be relentless and sometimes involves imaginative manipulations on the part of the addict. The opiate withdrawal syndrome is very distressing but is rarely if ever fatal. Fluid and electrolyte imbalances may result from vomiting and diarrhea, but generally no permanent effects are produced by opiate withdrawal. The intensity of the abstinence syndrome depends on the potency of the drug, the dose taken, and the rate of elimination of the drug from the body. Potent drugs which have a short-lasting action, with rapid excretion and inactivation bring about abstinence syndromes which have a rapid onset and are more intense than

drugs which are more slowly excreted. The withdrawal syndrome of methadone comes on more slowly, lasts longer, and in equipotent doses is less intense than that produced by heroin.

An exception to the statement that the opiate withdrawal syndrome usually has no serious consequences may be abstinence which is precipitated by a narcotic antagonist (a drug which blocks the effects of opiates). When a narcotic antagonist is given to someone who is physically dependent on opiates, an abstinence syndrome is precipitated within minutes. The severity of the abstinence syndrome depends on the degree of physical dependence and the dosage of the narcotic antagonist. However, for a given level of dependence, precipitated abstinence is more intense than abstinence due to sudden drug withdrawal. This is probably caused by the sudden massive displacement of opiate molecules from receptor sites in the CNS by antagonist molecules. Some cases have been reported of methadone maintenance patients mistakenly taking a large dose of a narcotic antagonist believing that it was some type of opiate. These individuals had the onset of a very acute abstinence syndrome, with severe vomiting, diarrhea, and delirium. It is possible that death might occur from the precipitated abstinence syndrome.

Structure-Activity Relationships

A large number of compounds exhibit the opiate pharmacological profile. The structure-activity relationships of these drugs are interesting and have relevance to attempts to develop better pharmacological tools for therapy of drug dependence. While most of the currently used opiate agonists and antagonists are derived from six series of compounds, opiate activity has also been discovered in several other types of compounds as well.

Fig. 1 illustrates the basic structures of six common series of compounds. In

Structure	Series	Substituents	Compound
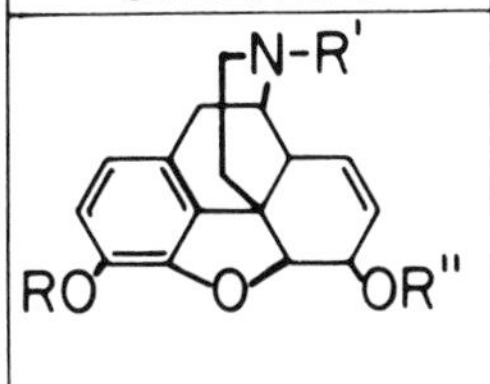 (N–R'; RO, OR")	Morphine	$R''{=}R{=}H; R'{=}CH_3$ $R''{=}R{=}H; R'{=}CH_2CH{=}CH_2$ $R''{=}R{=}CH_3C{=}O; R'{=}CH_3$ $R''{=}H; R{=}CH_3O, R'{=}CH_3$	Morphine Nalorphine Heroin Codeine
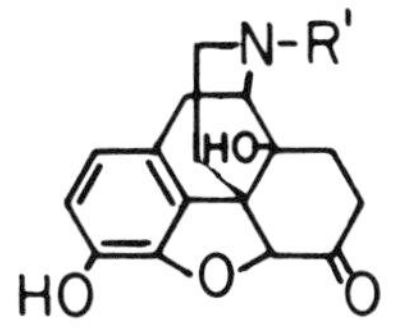 (N–R'; HO, HO, O)	Oxymorphone	$R'{=}CH_2CH{=}CH_2$ $R'{=}CH_2{-}\Delta$	Naloxone Naltrexone
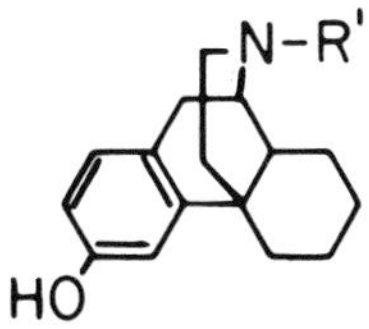 (N–R'; HO)	Morphinan	$R'{=}CH_3$ $R'{=}CH_2CH{=}CH_2$	Levorphanol Levallorphan
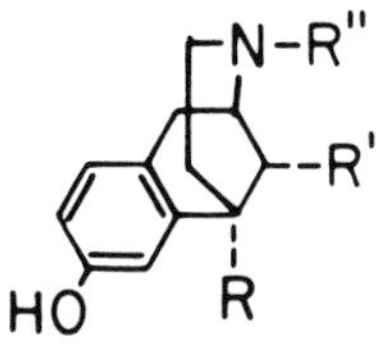 (N–R"; –R'; HO, R)	Benzomorphan	$R{=}R'{=}CH_3; R''{=}CH_2CH{=}C(CH_3)_2$ $R{=}R'{=}CH_3; R''{=}CH_2{-}\Delta$	Pentazocine Cyclazocine
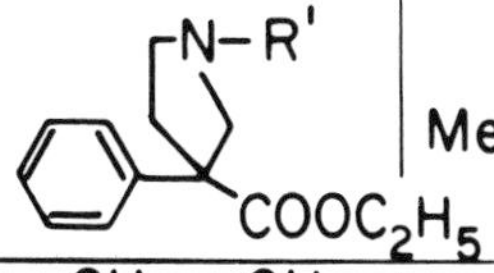 (N–R'; COOC₂H₅)	Meperidine	$R'{=}CH_2CH{=}CH_2$	N–allylnormeperidine
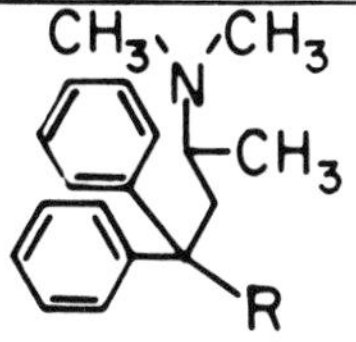 (CH₃, CH₃ N, –CH₃, R)	Diphenylpiperidine	$R{=}C_2H_5CO$ $R{=}CH_3COO$	Methadone Acetylmethadol

Fig. 1. Chemical structures of some compounds with opiate activity.

the morphine series, there are several important structural characteristics. First is the piperidine nitrogen with the R' substituent, the second is the five-ring structure, and the third is the phenolic hydroxyl group. These features are important because changes in these areas of the molecule have significant effects on pharmacologic activity. For instance, if the phenolic hydroxyl group is changed to a methoxy (CH_3CO) group, it becomes codeine, with considerable reduction in analgesic activity. If both hydroxyl groups are changed to acetyl (CH_3CO) groups, then it becomes heroin. From the standpoint of narcotic antagonists, the piperidine nitrogen is the most important structure. If the substituent on the piperidine nitrogen is a small moïety, such as a one-carbon methyl group, then usually there is opiate agonist (morphine-like) activity. If the size of this moiety is increased to 2, 3, or 4 carbon groups, then often antagonist activity occurs. The most common R' groups used to obtain antagonist activity are the 3-carbon allyl group and the 4-carbon cyclopropyl-methyl group.

One of the earliest strategies of molecular modification in the opiates was that of removing portions of the morphine molecule and seeing whether or not it retained its analgesic activity. In this manner, it was discovered that much of the molecule was not necessary for opiate effects and opened the way for the development of numerous synthetic analgesics, several of which are illustrated in Fig. 1.

Mechanisms of Action

The exact mechanism of action of the opiates in producing analgesia, tolerance, and physical dependence is as yet unknown. Since analgesic effects often closely parallel those of euphoria, the mechanism of action of analgesia may be of importance in understanding the production of drug dependence. Tolerance and physical dependence are also of great importance in the development of opiate dependence.

Tolerance is the property of a drug which results in increasing amounts of the drug being needed to attain the same pharmacological effect. *Physical dependence* is the characteristic of a drug which produces an abstinence syndrome characterized by physiological changes when the administration of the drug is discontinued. Tolerance and physical dependence often occur together; however, they can each occur separately. For example, tolerance develops relatively rapidly with repeated

administration of lysergic acid diethyla-mide (LSD), but this drug does not produce physical dependence. Opiate abstinence syndromes have been precipitated by narcotic antagonists after single doses of methadone when no tolerance was demonstrable.

Most models of physical dependence and tolerance postulate some adaptive change in the central nervous system in response to a narcotic drug, leading to a decrease in the effect of the drug, or tolerance. This adaptive change causes an excess of some CNS element producing an hyperexcitable state which is masked by the presence of the opiate. This hyperexcitable state represents physical dependence. When the opiate is withdrawn, this state is no longer masked and expresses itself as the abstinence syndrome.

Biochemical systems that have been postulated to be involved in tolerance and physical dependence are protein synthesis and RNA coding, immune mechanisms, and neurotransmitter mechanisms.

It has been shown that inhibitors of RNA or protein synthesis block or delay the development of tolerance to chronic opiate use. Administration of RNA precursors to animals has been shown to increase the rate of tolerance development to certain pharmacological effects of opiates. The exact role of RNA and protein synthesis in the production of tolerance is unknown, but several possibilities have been proposed. For example, there may be a requirement for protein and RNA synthesis in the formation of new receptors for transmitter substances or in increased synthesis of enzymes involved in transmitter metabolism.

Some investigators have proposed that immune mechanisms may be involved in the production of tolerance. It has been demonstrated that antibodies specific for opiates can be produced in certain animals. However, it remains to be demonstrated that the immune response plays a significant role in the development of opiate tolerance.

One theory of tolerance and physical dependence proposes that administration of an opiate inhibits an enzyme which is involved in the synthesis of a neurotransmitter. This leads to a compensatory increase in the synthesis of this enzyme. When the drug is withdrawn, the excess enzyme causes an increased synthesis of the neurotransmitter whose actions produce the abstinence syndrome.

Because biogenic amines play key roles as neurotransmitters in the CNS, the relation between brain biogenic amines and the pharmacological effects of opiates have received considerable attention. The possible role of norepinephrine in the acute effects of opiates and in the development of tolerance and physical dependence has been studied extensively. Alterations in the levels of CNS norepinephrine have been shown to affect opiate responses. Increases in these levels enhance acute effects of opiates, such as analgesia, while inhibition of the biosynthesis of norepinephrine decreases such acute effects. The development of tolerance in some animals has been shown to be blocked by the inhibition of norepinephrine synthesis and abstinence symptoms are decreased under these circumstances. It has also been found that acute administration of many opiates depletes CNS levels of both norepinephrine and dopamine, but this effect does not occur in tolerant animals.

While these findings strongly suggest that norepinephrine may play a role both in the acute effects of opiates as well as in tolerance and physical dependence, the exact nature of its role is as yet unclear.

Research on the possible role of dopamine in mediating opiate effects is more recent and not as extensive. However, a number of findings indicate that dopamine may be involved in the pharmacological actions of opiates. Haloperidol, a potent dopamine antagonist, has been shown to block opiate abstinence signs in a dose-dependent way. Dopamine agonists have been observed to antagonize acute effects of morphine and to exacerbate certain morphine withdrawal responses. Acute injections of morphine increase the synthesis of dopamine in rat brain; however, tolerance develops to this effect, paralleling the development of tolerance to other opiate effects. Opiate abstinence is accompanied by an increased rate of dopamine synthesis in the CNS.

Serotonin also may be involved in the production of narcotic effects. Inhibition of serotonin synthesis has been reported to antagonize both the acute effects of opiates as well as the development of tolerance and physical dependence. Serotonin turnover has been reported by some investigators to be elevated in the brains of tolerant animals, but others have not been able to confirm this finding.

Acetylcholine has been implicated in the mechanism of action of opiates. Morphine has long been known to inhibit acetylcholine release in the guinea pig ileum, and more recently evidence has been presented which indicates that acetylcholine release in the CNS is also inhibited by opiate administration.

While the preceding summarizes evidence that catecholamines, serotonin, and acetylcholine are involved in the mechanism of acute opiate actions and in the development of tolerance and physical dependence, no single neurotransmitter explains the multiple pharmacological effects of opiates. Also, other neurotransmitters which have not yet been adequately investigated, such as gamma-aminobutyric acid, may play a role in mediating opiate actions. In the future, the exact role of various neurotransmitters may be clarified. At present, one can only conclude that many different neurotransmitters are involved in some way in mediating the expression of opiate actions.

It has also been proposed that there

may be an alteration in the nature of receptors to produce tolerance and dependence. For example, it has been hypothesized that tolerance may result from an increase in the numbers of or sensitivity of receptors for a biogenic amine. The abstinence syndrome would result from the exposure of excess receptors or supersensitive receptors to a normal level of neural activity after administration of the opiate has been discontinued. In support of this are recent findings that morphine inhibits neurotransmitter-stimulated adenylate cyclase, the enzyme that might be the receptor for catecholamines (see Chapter 3). When morphine is withdrawn in tolerant animals, an exaggerated response of adenylate cyclase to catecholamines is observed.

A neurophysiological theory of tolerance and physical dependence proposes that exposure to opiates leads to the opening of redundant CNS pathways by blocking the normal pathways of impulses. When the drug is withdrawn, both the normal pathway and the redundant pathway are operative, leading to an excess of neural activity.

The structure-activity relationships of opiates and their stereo-specificity strongly imply the existence of specific opiate receptors in the CNS. The demonstration of opiate receptors in vertebrate CNS tissue has been reported. It was shown that a component of nerve membranes selectively bound opiate drugs at very low concentrations. This binding was stereospecific and closely paralleled the pharmacological potencies of the drugs. Investigations in a number of animal species have indicated that these receptors are not distributed homogeneously throughout the CNS, but are localized in certain areas, such as the caudate-putamen, locus coeruleus, amygdala, substantia nigra, medial thalamus, and periventricular and periaqueductal regions. Many of these areas have been shown to be involved in mediating the pharmacological actions of opiates.

In 1974, Goldstein suggested that there might be an endogenous opiate produced by the body which acted on these receptors. Several investigators have now isolated a substance which has morphine-like properties. This morphine-like factor appears to be a polypeptide and has been named *enkephalin*. It has been found in the brains of several animal species and in human cerebrospinal fluid. The physiological function of enkephalin and the opiate receptor are unclear; however, one interesting speculation is that the opiate receptor is a regulator of adenylate cyclase activity in opiate-sensitive neurons. Enkephalin may be an endogenous inhibitor of adenylate cyclase and part of a physiological regulatory mechanism for controlling its activity. In any case, these mechanisms provide a possible link through which the opiate-receptor interaction can affect neurotransmitter actions and thus, central nervous system function.

From the standpoint of drug dependence, the question of the exact nature of the opiate receptor and the mechanism of action of opiates is of some importance. A better understanding of these issues may make it possible to design analgesic drugs with little or no dependence potential. Thus, investigation of opiate receptors is likely to have important theoretical and practical implications.

Causes of Drug Dependence

It is not surprising that a disorder whose essence is the interaction between a drug and the individual has multiple, complex causal factors. Since the natural course of drug dependence is that of a chronic illness with periodic remissions and relapses, factors which contribute to relapse become as important as those which created the initial condition. In general, factors which contribute to cause or relapse can be divided into two categories: biological and social.

Biological Factors

Under this heading are grouped a variety of factors ranging from the pharmacological effects of drugs to personality and conditioning variables.

Pharmacological Effects — The single most important pharmacological factor motivating psychoactive drug use is the capacity of certain drugs to produce an altered subjective state called euphoria (an exaggerated sense of well-being). Little is known about the neurochemical and neurophysiological substrates of this state. It may involve changes in the amounts of certain biogenic amines at crucial CNS receptor sites. Probably, euphoria is not a unitary state, but a variety of subjective states which have in common a feeling of well-being on the part of the individual and the property of positive reinforcement to the individual for continued drug taking.

While the positive reinforcement properties of a drug are of great importance in motivating drug use, perhaps of equal importance in sustaining drug use are tolerance and physical dependence. The significance of tolerance in compulsive drug use comes from the fact that increasing doses of the drug are needed to achieve the sought-after euphoria. A physical abstinence syndrome has aversive properties that result in avoidance behavior, i.e., continued drug administration. Once an addict becomes tolerant to large doses of a drug, his continued use of the drug may be due more to his need to avoid abstinence symptoms than to continuing positive reinforcement from the drug. Often, when addicts become very tolerant, their drug habit becomes so large and expensive that further increase of drug intake is

impractical because of the large expense involved. At this point, the euphoria achieved from the drug diminishes, and the continued drug use is primarily sustained by the need to avoid the withdrawal syndrome.

Other pharmacological factors also are of importance in the addiction potential of drugs. For example, the absorption characteristics of a drug, the distribution, the rate of metabolism, and the route of metabolic breakdown all influence the intensity of effects and the duration of action. Also, the rapidity of onset and intensity of the abstinence syndrome is influenced by the duration of action of the drug and by the rapidity with which it is eliminated from the body. Thus, many of the pharmacological properties of a drug have a bearing on its dependence potential.

Genetic Factors — In recent years increasing attention has focused on genetic factors which are important in determining drug effects. Numerous genetic influences have been discovered which affect such things as the rate of drug metabolism, sensitivity to drug effects, etc. (see Chapter 5). However, there has been a paucity of investigations concerned with the role of genetics in predisposing individuals to drug dependence. Now a small number of such studies is underway in this area, and in the future they may begin to cast some light on this important problem.

Conditioning Factors — In a disorder which is characterized by compulsive behavior, e.g., drug use, it is not surprising that considerable interest has been focused on the role of conditioning in maintaining the behavior. In the discussion of pharmacological factors, two conditioning factors were mentioned: positive reinforcement and negative reinforcement. Behavior whose consequences result in either of these types of reinforcement is called operant behavior, and when responses are conditioned in this manner it is called operant conditioning.* The positive reinforcement from the euphoric effects of dependence-producing drugs undoubtedly results in some conditioning of drug-taking behavior. In addition, the aversiveness of withdrawal symptoms may negatively condition drug-taking as an avoidance behavior. The exact contribution of these conditioning factors in maintaining drug-taking behavior is difficult to assess; however, they are under intensive investigation at the present time.

In addition to operant conditioning in drug dependence, there is evidence that classical conditioning also plays a role. Wikler demonstrated in rats that certain signs of opiate abstinence could be conditioned to stimuli which had previously been contiguous with early withdrawal. For example, "wet dog" shakes, one sign of abstinence in the rat, could be conditioned to occur in the cage environment in which the animals had previously experienced the morphine abstinence syndrome. This phenomenon has been termed "conditioned abstinence." There are many anecdotal reports from addicts about suddenly experiencing withdrawal symptoms when returning to their old drug-taking haunts, even months after having been detoxified from drugs. Systematic investigation of this phenomenon in humans is underway and preliminary reports indicate that conditioning of abstinence symptoms may be possible in humans.

It is very important to establish this, for if conditioning factors play an important role in relapse to drug-taking behavior, then merely detoxifying the addict and maintaining him drug-free for a period of time is not likely to extinguish the conditioned responses. In the future, treatment programs may begin to incorporate the active and planned extinction of conditioned abstinence and of operantly reinforced drug-taking behavior.

Physiological Factors — The physiological derangements of the opiate abstinence syndrome are accompanied by a subjective craving for drugs which facilitates continued self-administration. While many people assume that the abstinence syndrome is over within a few days of drug termination, there is evidence that the physiological changes induced by physical dependence may last much longer than is generally assumed. In both rats and man, Martin and his associates have demonstrated a protracted abstinence syndrome lasting six months or longer. This consists of alterations in blood pressure, pulse rate, body temperature, and pupil diameter. Martin has suggested that these continuing changes cause the postaddict to be physiologically and psychologically more vulnerable to stress than normal people. Since relapse to drug use is most frequent during the first six months to a year after drug detoxification, it is possible that the protracted abstinence syndrome plays a significant role in relapse.

Personality — This is determined by both biological and social factors. Many studies have explored personality variables which make individuals more vulnerable to becoming addicts. Some investigators have suggested that sociopathic personality traits are frequently associated with drug dependence. While these individuals may tend to become involved in illicit drug use, drug dependence is not specific for any particular personality type. It may be found in individuals whose psychological state ranges from relatively normal to those with psychoses. However, individuals who are characterized by low tolerance for delayed gratification probably have a predisposition to drug dependence.

---

*Operating on the environment to avoid unpleasant or produce desired consequences.

Social Factors

Availability of drugs is a necessary but not sufficient cause of drug dependence. Probably, any drug which has dependence potential will result in a certain number of addicts if it is made easily available to a population. However, the extent of the dependence and the social and individual harm which results is contingent on numerous other factors.

Attitudes and values regarding the use of psychoactive drugs play an important role in the genesis of drug dependence. Strong social condemnation of psychoactive drug use may prevent many individuals in a society from experimenting with drugs, thus removing them from those at risk for drug dependence. However, social condemnation may stimulate others to try dependence-producing drugs, particularly if they identify with a group which opposes the dominant social values. Peer group pressures may be even more powerful than the values of society in determining drug-taking behavior. Epidemiological studies of the spread of drug use reveal that drugs spread through existing friendship groups in a manner that resembles the diffusion of a contagious disease. In the wake of this initial spread of drug experimentation, a number of chronic addicts are left.

Socio-economic factors, such as poverty, and social disorganization are often associated with a high incidence of drug dependence. In neighborhoods which are both economically deprived and have a breakdown in social organization, dominant social attitudes towards drug use are less potent in preventing experimentation. Also, the inaccessibility of traditional social reinforcers may predispose individuals to the immediate reinforcement which is available through the use of drugs or alcohol.

Treatment of Opiate Dependence

The majority of pharmacological approaches to the treatment of opiate dependence can be classified under the following categories:

Detoxification

This is the oldest pharmacological treatment of drug dependence and consists of administering gradually decreasing doses of an opiate until the individual is completely withdrawn from the drug. In this way, physical dependence on the drug is gradually decreased while the drug is tapered until only minimal dependence remains when administration of the drug is stopped. This procedure minimizes the discomfort and danger of the abstinence syndrome, though the individual usually does experience some signs and symptoms of withdrawal.

A variety of techniques have been used to withdraw addicts. Historically, morphine was used to withdraw addicts until the introduction of methadone after World War II. Almost all detoxification is now performed with methadone. Methadone is usually given orally and has the advantages of a long duration of action, necessitating one or two doses per 24-hour period during withdrawal. Experience has shown that a dose reduction of 20% per day is usually well tolerated during detoxification. Most addicts can be withdrawn in a week or less though low-grade symptoms may continue for a few days longer. The dose of methadone used must be determined empirically, since addicts' estimates of their level of dependence is often unreliable. Many physicians begin by observing the addict for a period without drugs. If significant abstinence signs appear, then 15–20 mg of methadone are given. Further dosages are determined according to the degree of suppression of withdrawal symptoms achieved by the initial dose.

Despite its long use, detoxification by itself is of limited value in the treatment of opiate dependence. Follow-up studies of addicts detoxified in the federal hospitals at Lexington and Fort Worth showed that the rate of relapse to drug taking was 90% or greater. Detoxification followed by treatment with a narcotic antagonist or in a therapeutic community may substantially increase its effectiveness. Although detoxification may do little to modify the tendency for drug-taking behavior, it may be useful for engaging an addict in a treatment alliance and is preferable to the abrupt termination of drug for medical and humanitarian reasons.

In recent years, there has been an upswing in multiple drug use. Therefore, there is always the possibility that the person undergoing withdrawal may be physically dependent on other drugs in addition to opiates. Of particular concern in this respect are the sedative-hypnotics whose abstinence syndrome can result in significant mortality if untreated. Any addict who continues to exhibit signs, such as insomnia, irritability, or tremulousness, despite what seems to be adequate doses of opiate should be suspected of sedative-hypnotic dependence.

Maintenance Therapy

In the early 1960's, a new conceptualization of the treatment of opiate dependence began to take shape in this country. Up to that time, almost all treatment approaches practiced in the United States had abstinence as the ultimate goal of treatment. However, in maintenance therapy the main goal is the psychological and social rehabilitation of the addict.

In New York City where the increase in opiate addiction was felt most acutely,

Dole and Nyswander (1965) began a program of opiate maintenance using methadone. This was based on the hypothesis that physical dependence on narcotics resulted in a long-standing metabolic alteration such that the addict had a biological drive to use opiates (however, the exact nature of this metabolic alteration was not known). To maintain the addict on methadone was to provide him with adequate medication to "normalize" this drive so that he could be freed from the abnormal feelings produced by the metabolic alteration. As a consequence, the addict would no longer need to engage in illicit activities to provide himself with heroin. In this way, with proper vocational counseling and training and other services, the addict could be rehabilitated and become a productive, working citizen in spite of his continuing drug dependence.

A second factor that was felt to be important in methadone maintenance was its ability to "block" the effects of heroin. In fact, this was not true pharmacological blocking as with narcotic antagonists, but due to cross-tolerance between methadone and heroin. Rather large doses of methadone were used for maintenance, and this, plus the relatively weak heroin available on the street, meant that small doses of heroin produced little euphoria. Obtaining enough heroin to get significant euphoria was very expensive, thus discouraging illicit opiate use by methadone patients.

This new model of treatment for opiate dependence represented a major change in direction from the approaches used in this country since the passage of the Harrison Narcotics Act. Thus, opiate dependence was viewed as a medical illness resulting from altered physiology. The illness was treated pharmacologically like other medical diseases, and this view tended to blunt the social stigma normally attached to opiate-taking.

Although maintenance therapy is relatively new in the United States, it has been a traditional approach in Great Britain for many years, though heroin was the most prevalent maintenance drug used there. There are both similarities and differences between methadone and heroin maintenance.

Methadone was originally synthesized in Germany during World War II because of a shortage of natural opiate alkaloids. It was used as a morphine substitute and is a potent analgesic. When given parenterally, its actions are similar to morphine; its duration of action is four to six hours, and it is approximately equipotent to morphine. When given intravenously, it produces substantial euphoria and has very high dependence-producing potential. Most importantly, it is effective orally, whereas heroin is not. Orally, methadone has a longer duration of action and does not produce the euphoric high that is characteristic of repeated intravenous administration of heroin. A single oral dose of methadone will prevent abstinence for at least 24 hours, thereby allowing single, daily administration of methadone in a clinic. The oral administration of methadone also eliminates frequent intravenous administration, which is the cause of many medical complications—such as hepatitis, thrombophlebitis and other infections—in heroin addicts. Therefore, the most important advantages of methadone over heroin maintenance result mainly from the different route of administration rather than any marked difference in the pharmacological profile of the drugs.

The efficacy of methadone maintenance in decreasing illicit drug use and in rehabilitating addicts to a more productive social role is now generally accepted, and this method represents the most common approach to treating opiate dependence at present. As practiced today, methadone maintenance includes more than just dispensing the drug. Although the specifics vary from program to program across the country, most of them provide psychological counseling

of some type, vocational counseling, and assistance with job finding. In addition, most programs check urine samples for the presence of illicit drugs.

Evaluation of patients who have been on long-term methadone maintenance indicate that there is little or no organ toxicity from long-term methadone administration and minimal side effects. The most common side effects reported are increased sweating, constipation, insomnia, decreased libido, difficulty in achieving orgasm, and daytime sedation.

There are certain problems and drawbacks of methadone maintenance. One of these is the illicit distribution of methadone. Most programs allow drug take-home privileges for selected patients, and this contributes to methadone diversion. Illicit methadone may be used by heroin addicts during periods when heroin is scarce in order to prevent going through withdrawal. Take-home methadone has also been a source of overdose deaths by children or others. Despite the cross-tolerance produced by large doses of methadone, drug-seeking behavior will continue to be seen in some patients.

When methadone maintenance was originally started by Dole and Nyswander, rather large maintenance doses were used—80 to 120 mg. As other programs got under way, the initial trend was to continue to employ these high doses of methadone partly out of belief that high dosages "blocked" use of other opiates which was an important component of the therapeutic effect of methadone. However, as more experience was gained with methadone maintenance, drawbacks of high doses of the drug became apparent. Because of the low potency of street heroin, many addicts were made much more physically dependent on opiates than they had been when taking heroin. Controlled studies which have compared the efficacy of high-dose versus low-dose methadone have failed to show appreciable differences in the use of illicit drugs by patients. Recently, the trend in methadone programs has been toward using lower dosages for maintenance.

Now that maintenance has been used for several years, many programs have a number of patients who have been successfully rehabilitated and who wish to be withdrawn from methadone. Some programs have detoxified these long-term maintenance patients with mixed success. Some of these detoxified subjects have relapsed to heroin dependence, suggesting that either these patients may have to be on opiate maintenance indefinitely or that a more effective therapeutic intervention will have to be devised in order to improve the results of terminating maintenance therapy.

Because of the problem of illicit diversion of methadone, interest has grown in developing a longer-acting opiate which might obviate the need for take-home medication. Most interest has centered on a diphenylpiperidine compound which resembles methadone, 1-α-acetylmethadol (levomethadyl, methadyl acetate). This drug is currently undergoing extensive testing. Early clinical trials have indicated that 80 mg of acetylmethadol administered three times weekly is equivalent to 100 mg of methadone administered daily with respect to side effects and abstinence suppression. Suppression of withdrawal symptoms for 48–72 hours by acetylmethadol reduces the frequency of maintenance clinic visits required and eliminates the need for weekend visits. In addition, longer-acting maintenance drugs may decrease the cost of maintenance programs.

Opiate agonists with other properties may contribute to the improvement of maintenance therapy. In the future, the clinician treating opiate dependence may have a choice of a variety of agonists available for maintenance therapy, so that the therapy can be tailored to the individual patient, depending on the specific characteristics of his drug-dependence problem.

Blocking Agents

Narcotic antagonists are drugs which block the actions of opiates by occupying opiate receptor sites and blocking the access of opiate molecules to these sites. A pure antagonist has no agonist (intrinsic morphine-like) actions of its own and therefore occupies the receptor site without acting on it. However, with the exception of the drug naloxone, most antagonists are actually mixed agonist-antagonists and have both agonist actions and the ability to block the actions of other opiates. These compounds present a continuum which ranges from drugs which are weak antagonists and strong agonists such as pentazocine (Talwin®) to compounds which are relatively pure antagonists, such as naloxone. Many of the mixed agonist-antagonists have an atypical profile of agonist actions, which is characterized by dysphoria and psychotomimetic effects. Nalorphine is the prototype of this group. Other mixed agonist-antagonists have morphine-like subjective effects. The nalorphine-like drugs also have many actions similar to those of morphine, such as analgesia, respiratory depression, and the production of physical dependence. Tolerance develops to the agonist actions of mixed drugs in the same way as it does with other opiates. This makes it possible to administer nalorphine-type drugs in slowly increasing doses to produce tolerance without incurring the unpleasant dysphoria which characterizes them.

The possibility of using narcotic antagonists in the treatment of opiate dependence was first advanced by Martin in 1965 and was stimulated by the observation that cyclazocine, a mixed agonist-antagonist of the benzomorphan series (Fig. 1), had a duration of action of 24 or more hours when given orally. This made it possible to administer an antagonist once daily in a maintenance clinic in much the same manner as methadone. Cyclazocine has been used in a small number of experimental programs, with promising enough results to warrant continued efforts to develop improved antagonists.

Antagonists may act therapeutically in two ways. If drug-taking behavior is maintained by operant conditioning through frequent positive reinforcement by the drug, then maintaining an addict on an antagonist may allow extinction of this behavior. If the addict takes an opiate while on an antagonist, he does not experience any effect. Theoretically, repeated experiences of this sort may lead to extinction of the operantly conditioned aspects of the drug-seeking behavior. Studies are now underway to experimentally evaluate the importance of this factor in sustaining drug-seeking behavior.

The second way in which antagonists may be effective is by preventing readdiction in those situations where an addict may temporarily succumb to temptation and take drugs while abstinent. Typically, this leads to increasing drug-taking until dependence is re-established. However, if the addict is taking an antagonist, then this chain may be broken by protecting the addict from experiencing opiate effects.

Experience to date with the use of antagonists indicates that the following drug characteristics are desirable for an antagonist which is to be used in a drug-treatment program: (1) high potency of opiate-blocking action, (2) little or no agonist actions, particularly unpleasant side effects, (3) absence of potential for physical or psychological dependence, (4) long duration of blocking activity, (5) oral effectiveness, and (6) relatively low-cost and synthesis from precursors that are readily available. Naloxone, which is the purest antagonist, has been tried in a very limited manner in the treatment of opiate dependence, but has numerous limitations which include relative ineffectiveness when given orally, short duration of action and compara-

tively high expense. Several other antagonists are being evaluated as potential agents for treating drug dependence. Naltrexone, the cyclopropylmethyl congener of naloxone (Fig. 1), appears to be the most promising of these at the present time. Naltrexone is a relatively pure antagonist, though it probably has some mild agonist properties. It is effective orally, and 50–100 mg produce blockade to substantial doses of heroin for 24 to 48 hours. It is being used in a small number of investigational programs across the country, and initial results appear promising.

Antagonists offer an alternative pharmacological approach to the use of methadone maintenance. They are likely to be more acceptable to those who feel the main emphasis of treatment should be drug abstinence rather than just improved social and personal functioning. However, the effectiveness of antagonist treatment will depend on the number of addicts who are motivated to accept it. It is not yet known how large this proportion will be. Previous clinical investigations with antagonists suggest that they may be useful in the following addict populations: (a) long-term successful methadone maintenance patients who are motivated to be drug-free, (b) heroin addicts who are highly motivated to be abstinent, and (c) addicts who are on parole or probation or who are under some form of legal compulsion to seek treatment for their drug dependence. Most experienced observers feel that the above categories comprise only 10 to 15% of the opiate addict population. Nevertheless, it adds an important tool to the pharmacological armamentarium and increases the options available to the clinician who is treating opiate dependence.

In contrast to methadone maintenance, the person on an antagonist, such as naltrexone, is not physically dependent and receives no positive reinforcement from the drug. Therefore, there may be a greater temptation to miss doses and occasionally "chip" doses of heroin. Currently, attempts are underway to create long-acting antagonist preparations which could be given parenterally and might be effective for weeks. Several approaches are being explored, including the incorporation of an antagonist into a biodegradable polymer from which it would be slowly released, the formation of fatty acid salts of antagonists, and the synthesis of relatively insoluble complexes of antagonists. Long-acting preparations of an antagonist would decrease the frequency with which the addict would have to return to the clinic and would give relatively long-lasting protection against the urge to return to opiate-taking.

Conclusion

This chapter has tried to present an overview of drug dependence and pharmacological approaches to its treatment. It is hoped that the reader has gained an appreciation of the multiple factors which play a role in the causation of drug dependence and an understanding of the complex nature of this phenomenon. A summary of the relevant pharmacology of these drugs was presented and its role in the causation and perpetuation of drug dependence was outlined. Various treatment strategies were described and some possible future directions in this area were mentioned. The treatment of drug dependence has advanced considerably over the past decade, and even more effective approaches are likely to be developed in the future. The investigation of the mechanism of action of opiates and their interactions with the opiate receptor is a rapidly expanding area and may stimulate the development of radically new modes of treatment.

Dependence on non-opiate drugs, such as sedative-hypnotics and stimulants, was not discussed, though they are certainly important problems in their own right. It is hoped that by gaining knowledge about one specific type of drug dependence, i.e., opiate dependence, the reader will obtain insight into the relevant variables, many of which apply to other types of drug dependence. The differences between opiate dependence and other types of drug dependence are determined chiefly by the pharmacological properties of the drugs involved and the social attitudes and conditions associated with them. Those interested in learning in greater detail about opiate dependence or other types of drug dependence are referred to the bibliography at the end of this chapter.

Selected References

Braude, M.C., Harris, L.S., May, E.L., Smith, J.P., and Villarreal, J.E. (Eds.): *Narcotic Antagonists.* Raven Press, New York, 1973.

Clouet, D.H., and Iwatsubo, K.: Mechanisms of tolerance and dependence on narcotic analgesic drugs. *Annu. Rev. Pharmacol.* 15:49-71, 1975.

Dole, V.P., and Nyswander, M.E.: A medical treatment for diacetylmorphine (heroin) addiction. *J. Am. Med. Assoc.* 193:646-650, 1965.

Ellinwood, E.H. (Ed.): *Current Concepts on Amphetamine Abuse.* Proceedings of a Workshop, National Institute of Mental Health, U.S. Government Printing Office, Washington, D.C., 1972.

Essig, C.F.: Chronic abuse of sedative-hypnotic drugs. In *Drug Abuse: Proceedings of the International Conference,* Zarafonetis, C.J.D., ed. Lea and Fibiger, Philadelphia, 1972.

Freedman, D.X., and Senay, E.C.: Methadone treatment of heroin addiction. *Annu. Rev. Med.* 24:153-164, 1973.

Goldstein, A. (Ed.): *The Opiate Narcotics: Neurochemical Mechanisms in Analgesia and Dependence.* Pergamon Press, Elmsford, New York, 1975.

Martin, W.R., Gorodetzky, C.W., and McClane, T.K.: A proposed method for ambulatory treatment of narcotic addicts, using a long-acting narcotic antagonist, cyclazocine. *Committee on Problem of Drug Dependence,* 27th Meeting, Houston, 1965.

Martin, W.R., and Jasinski, D.R.: Physiological parameters of morphine dependence in man—tolerance, early abstinence, and protracted abstinence. *J. Psychiat. Res.* 7:9-17, 1969.

Pert, C.B., and Snyder, S.H.: Opiate receptor: Demonstration in nervous tissue. *Science* 179:1011-1014, 1973.

Chapter 16

Alcoholism

James L. Stinnett

Introduction

Alcoholism is a chronic behavior disorder that affects nine to ten million Americans directly, and indirectly affects society in many diverse ways. The scope of the problem and its impact on society can be realized by considering some epidemiological facts on alcoholism. It is the third largest public health problem after heart disease and cancer. Thirteen thousand people a year die of cirrhosis of the liver, which is thought to be due primarily to alcoholism. The life span of the average alcoholic is shortened by twelve years. The cost in

terms of human suffering to the nine to ten million people directly afflicted with this disorder and the twenty to thirty million family members of alcoholics is impossible to quantify. The economic cost of the problem has been estimated at about 25 billion dollars annually, resulting from decreased economic productivity, health and medical costs, motor vehicle accidents, treatment expenses, and the cost to the criminal justice and social welfare systems. It is thought that alcohol is involved in twenty-eight thousand traffic fatalities a year, which is one-half of all the deaths caused by traffic accidents. Alcohol is involved in half of all crimes of violence (murder, rape, and assault). These facts present a compelling argument for clinicians and researchers to learn more about this disorder which will directly affect a large number of the patients that they treat and, indirectly, will have an impact on the society in which they live.

Conceptualization of Alcoholism

Alcoholism has been viewed in various ways throughout recent history. It is important to have an idea of how a particular disorder is conceptualized since this strongly affects the way in which clinicians approach the disorder, and it determines the type of research questions investigators ask. The concept of alcoholism has evolved through a number of developmental stages which can be described as the three "D's": *deviancy, disease,* and *disorder of behavior.* In the 19th and the early part of the 20th Century, the alcoholic was regarded as a social deviant, and his behavior viewed as a manifestation of moral weakness. This view was legitimized by legislation known popularly as prohibition. The alcoholic was seen as being the concern and responsibility of the criminal justice system. With the repeal of prohibition in 1933, people slowly began to look at alcoholism more as a disease, something over which the patient has little, if any, control. This change has introduced some beneficial effects in the treatment of the alcoholic. It made alcoholism and its medical sequelae the legitimate concern of physicians. One negative aspect, however, has been that it has occasionally caused some alcoholics to view their problem as an "illness" or "disease," something over which they could exert little or no control, nor could they be held responsible for it. This led certain alcoholics to blame the "disease" for their problem rather than their inability to control their drinking behavior, and, in some cases, resulted in the alcoholic relinquishing responsibility for controlling his behavior. The most recent approach to alcoholism is to see it as a behavioral disorder which is subject to the laws of learning theory and, to varying degrees, under voluntary control. This viewpoint considers abnormal drinking behavior as being caused and shaped by stimuli controlling the behavior, and by various rewards which tend to reinforce and perpetuate the behavior.

From a more holistic perspective, alcoholism is regarded as a multi-causal, behavioral phenomenon with biological, psychological, and social determinants producing primary, secondary, and tertiary effects at biological, psychological, and social levels of organization (Fig. 1). Consideration of all of these dimensions of alcoholism is beyond the scope of this chapter, so the focus will be on discussing those determinants and effects at the biological level of organization. A particular individual with this problem may have different weights attached to specific determinants; however, it is important to remember that all of these factors interact together to produce the group of behaviors known as alcoholism.

Description

Alcoholism is a term applied to a complex series of behaviors centered on the excessive use of alcoholic beverages. Alcoholism must be viewed in the context of a continuum of drinking behavior, at one end of which is total abstinence from all alcoholic beverages, progressing through moderate drinking, "heavy"

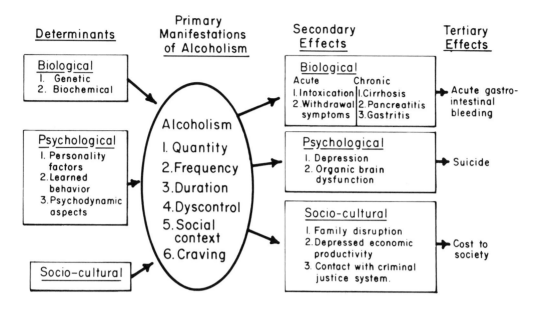

Fig. 1.   Schematic representation of determinants and effects of alcoholism.

drinking to—at the other end of the continuum—alcoholism. There are many definitions of alcoholism; however, most of these include excessive consumption of alcohol to the point of psychological or physiological dependence, which produces detrimental effects on the person's physical health and causes deterioration in social and economic functioning. It may lead to problems involving the criminal justice system. It is a matter of judgment, however, as to when a person actually crosses the line on the continuum from "heavy" drinking to drinking which could be characterized as "alcoholic drinking," just as it is difficult to look at a color spectrum and state where one color stops and another begins.

Alcoholism is a generic term that needs to be broken down into its constituent parts in order to understand what comprises the whole. These aspects of the problem are usually referred to as being the primary manifestations of the disorder, as opposed to the secondary manifestations which refer to the effects of drinking, such as cirrhosis of the liver, and social and economic deterioration.

Quantity

The amount of alcohol that a person consumes is an important parameter in determining whether a person is an alcoholic. Most, if not all, alcoholics drink large quantities of alcoholic beverages. What constitutes a "large quantity" may vary markedly from one culture to another and is dependent on certain social and cultural values. Amount alone does not determine whether a person can be legitimately classified as an alcoholic.

Frequency

How often a person drinks is an important dimension. A person drinking a pint of whiskey on just two days out of a month can hardly be classified as an alcoholic; however, if he drinks a pint of whiskey a day, every day out of the month, this obviously constitutes behavior of a much different magnitude and problem.

Duration

The length of time that a person has been drinking heavily is an important consideration. Long duration of frequent, heavy alcohol consumption usually connotes a more severe problem than does heavy drinking of a short duration.

The parameters of quantity, frequency, and duration, even though quantitative, are still relative since they refer to a subjective judgment or standard as to *how much* is *too much*. Other parameters of the primary manifestations of alcoholism are important to consider in the overall context of this disorder.

Dyscontrol

The inability to modulate or control the rate at which a person drinks during a particular episode of drinking is considered by many to be a critical factor in determining whether or not a person is an alcoholic. Dyscontrol refers to a person starting to drink and being unable to stop when he feels he should or when he wants to. In its most extreme form, dyscontrol is manifest by the person, who, once he starts to drink, continues to do so until he becomes so intoxicated that he is unable to drink anymore. Alcoholics do not manifest dyscontrol all the time when they are drinking.

Social Context

The social context in which drinking occurs is an important factor. There are certain specifically defined social occasions, depending greatly on the particular culture, in which drinking alcoholic beverages is not only acceptable but is considered to be normal social behavior. Examples of these situations are dinner parties, cocktail parties, business lunches, and various sporting events. Drinking in these situations is considered to be normal. If, however, a person were to drink in the morning before work, or drink during work, or at home alone, or have a few drinks before leaving to go to a party, or after coming home from a party, one might conclude that drinking in these situations is not occurring in the context of the usually acceptable social norms but is governed by an internal, psychological need.

Craving

The phenomenon of "craving" for alcohol usually denotes a pathological attitude toward it. Craving refers to the subjective sensation of internal, appetitive arousal which totally preoccupies the individual and is focused on one subject, alcohol. Craving is thought by some to be the psychological dimension of physiological dependence on alcohol, and is the subjective, emotional manifestation of the intense physiological state of arousal that occurs during the withdrawal and abstinent state.

All of these factors, amount, frequency, duration, dyscontrol, social context, and craving together comprise the primary manifestations of alcoholism. In addition to these primary manifestations, which are necessary though not sufficient for the diagnosis of alcoholism, one needs to look at the secondary effects that chronic alcohol ingestion has on a person's health or his social and economic functioning. Some authorities contend that a person may have all of the primary manifestations listed above but still not merit the diagnosis of alcoholism unless the excessive drinking has also had a significant impact on some aspect of his life.

Clinical Course of Alcoholism

Certain people develop alcoholism fairly early in their drinking career, and others become alcoholic later in life. Once the illness is manifest, the course varies considerably. Usually a person will alternate between "alcoholic" drinking and controlled drinking. Once treatment is begun, the course is marked by relapses and remissions. Treatment outcome depends on a number of factors, most importantly, the criteria for "cure." If total lifelong abstinence from alcohol is the criterion for cure, only a small percentage ever reach this goal. If moderate drinking with improved social and economic functioning are the criteria for "cure," then a larger number can be considered as having a successful treatment outcome.

Clinical Pharmacology of Alcoholism

The physiological and pharmacological mechanisms concerned with the absorption, distribution, metabolism, excretion, and acute behavioral effects of alcohol have been investigated and delineated in both normals and alcoholics. The pharmacology of alcohol in normals will be briefly reviewed here to serve as a conceptual foundation for a discussion later in this chapter of the mechanisms which are thought to be involved in the development of alcoholism.

Absorption

Alcohol is absorbed slowly and incompletely through the mucous membranes of the mouth and stomach and is absorbed rapidly in the small intestine. The intoxicating effect of alcohol depends on the concentration that reaches the brain, and the speed and intensity of that effect is mediated by a number of variables. Much depends on how quickly alcohol moves from the stomach to the small intestine. It is most rapid when the stomach is empty. Food in the stomach, especially fatty or oily foods, tends to slow the passage of alcohol from the stomach to the small intestine, thus delaying the absorption from the small intestine into the bloodstream. Some alcoholic beverages, such as beer, contain food substances which also decrease the rate of absorption.

The presence or lack of carbonation in the beverage has an effect on the rate of absorption. Carbon dioxide speeds the passage of alcohol through the lining of the intestine into the bloodstream.

In addition to the food in the stomach and the presence of carbon dioxide in the beverage, the effect of the pyloric valve in the stomach also plays a significant role in the regulation of absorption of alcohol. The pyloric valve is thought to control the rate at which gastric contents proceed from the stomach to the small intestine. When large amounts of alcohol are ingested, it occasionally causes a partial or complete closure of the pyloric valve which results in little or no alcohol leaving the stomach to go into the intestine. This tends to slow the rate of absorption of alcohol and, in certain people, produces nausea and vomiting. In those who tend to have this reaction, it constitutes a natural protection against dangerous or lethal amounts of alcohol being absorbed into the blood, which may happen if the alcohol were permitted to leave the stomach and go into the intestine.

Distribution

Alcohol is distributed equally throughout the body in the aquous phase. Blood is roughly 85% water, so that when alcohol is ingested and absorbed it is possible to measure the amount of alcohol in the blood and extrapolate from this to the amount of alcohol in the entire body.

Metabolism and Elimination

Ethanol (ethyl alcohol) or alcohol (as we will refer to it in this chapter) is removed from the body through metabolism by oxidation and elimination. Alcohol is eliminated by evaporation from the blood into the air of the alveoli of the lung and then exhaled. The concentration of alcohol in exhaled breath air is directly proportional to its amount in the blood passing through the lung at that time. This is the physiological basis of the "breathalyzer" test for blood alcohol concentration. Alcohol in the blood is also filtered by the glomerulus of the kidney into the urine and this, too, is a linear function of the concentration of alcohol in blood.

Only 10% of all the alcohol in the body is eliminated unchanged through either the kidney or the lungs. The remainder is metabolized by oxidation. The metabolic process of alcohol oxidation releases energy as with other food substances, such as fats, carbohydrates and proteins. In the case of alcohol, one gram of alcohol produces 7 calories of energy. For example, one ounce of 86 proof spirits yields about 75 calories, the same as 1½ pats of butter, a large slice of bread or 4½ teaspoons of sugar. The consumption of one pint of 86 proof spirits a day, which is not an unusual amount for many alcoholics, can generate around 1400 calories which represents roughly half the daily adult caloric requirement.

The process of oxidation of alcohol involves several steps schematically portrayed in Fig. 2. The first step is the oxidation of ethanol to acetaldehyde by the enzyme, alcohol dehydrogenase (ADH), which requires the co-factor nicotinamide adenine dinucleotide. This takes place primarily in the liver. Other enzyme systems, such as catalase and the microsomal ethanol oxidizing system, are also thought to be involved in the oxidation of alcohol. Acetaldehyde is pharmacologically active and quite toxic. It is rapidly oxidized by acetaldehyde dehydrogenase to acetate, carbon dioxide and water.

The rate at which alcohol is metabolized is dependent on the functional integrity of the liver and the characteristics of the various enzyme systems that oxidize ethanol. The fraction or proportion of the total body alcohol oxidized by the liver is constant and is the same for most people whose liver is functioning normally. Alcohol is oxidized and eliminated at the rate of approximately 15mg/100ml of blood (0.015%) per hour which is the equivalent of approximately ¾ of an ounce (½ jigger) of whiskey in a 150-lb man. A person could therefore ingest this amount slowly over a period of one hour without accumulating any measurable alcohol in his body. If, however, the same person ingested that same amount in a period of ten minutes, it would be absorbed more rapidly than it could be oxidized and eliminated, and would be detectable.

The behavioral effect of alcohol is

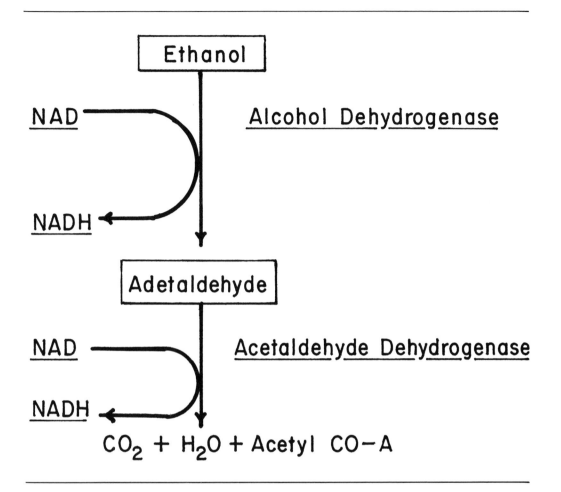

Fig. 2. Metabolism of alcoholism

determined by the concentration of alcohol in the blood that reaches the central nervous system. The concentration of alcohol in the blood at any one time is a function of three variables:

1. The rate of absorption of alcohol from the gut into the bloodstream.
2. The size of the person.
3. The constant rate of metabolism and elimination.

An analogy which more simply explains the interaction of these factors is to imagine the three variables as a tank of water with a spigot and a drain.

The amount of alcohol present in the tank will depend on the amount coming in the spigot (absorption) and the amount leaving the drain (metabolism and elimination). The steady state obtained will determine the amount. The size of the tank will determine the concentration which is the critical variable affecting the brain. An example of how these variables interact can be seen in the following illustrations: A 190-lb man who consumes two jiggers (3 ounces) of 86 proof whiskey (43% absolute ethanol) over a period of one hour will have a blood alcohol level of 50mg% or .050%. In the non-tolerant individual, this would cause a feeling of warmth, mental relaxation, less concern with minor irritations and restraints. If a 130-lb woman were to drink the same amount—two jiggers (3 ounces) of 86 proof whiskey over a period of an hour, it would produce a blood alcohol concentration of 73mg% or .073%. In the non-tolerant individual this usually causes a feeling of buoyancy, exaggerated emotion and behavior. The behavioral effect of the same amount of alcohol is dependent on its concentration in the blood and that, in turn, depends on the size and weight of the individual. It is important to remember that other factors, in addition to weight, will effect the concentration in the blood, such as the dilution of the alcohol in water or whether the person has eaten before or during the time alcohol is consumed.

The rate of metabolism is a constant 0.015% per hour. It will take the 190-lb man about three hours to metabolize this amount, whereas it will take the 130-lb woman about slightly more than four hours to metabolize the alcohol she has consumed.

Behavioral Pharmacology

When alcohol reaches the central nervous system, it begins to exert its behavioral effect. This effect is influenced by external factors, such as personality, past attitudes and expectations about drinking, mood at the time drinking occurs, and the social or "demand characteristics" of the particular social setting in which drinking takes place. Therefore, it is difficult to predict how a particular person may react behaviorally to alcohol ingested at a specific time. Within a wide range of variations, there are certain neuropsychological modes of expression of the way alcohol affects the central nervous system. Alcohol is a CNS depressant; however, different parts of the central nervous system react in different ways to increasing amounts of alcohol.

When low doses of alcohol are consumed, the higher cortical centers of the central nervous system are affected first. Alcohol appears to act on these brain areas by first causing depression of inhibitory centers which is manifest behaviorally as a "loosening of inhibitions" or a state of increased arousal and excitement. This is thought to account for the paradoxical effect of alcohol, a central nervous system depressant, causing a state of behavioral excitation. With increasing amounts of alcohol, the facilitative aspects of higher cortical functioning appear to be depressed. This results in decreased mental acuity, difficulty with abstract thinking and impairment of judgment. With increasing amounts of alcohol, the cerebellum is affected which results in cerebellar dysfunction, such as dysarthria (slurred speech), decrease in visual-motor coordination, and the well-known "alcoholic stagger" or ataxia. As more alcohol is consumed, it tends to depress the reticular activating system, resulting in a decreased level of consciousness and progressing through the stages of lethargy, stupor, and coma or unconsciousness. At very high levels of alcohol, the brain stem centers regulating respiration and cardiovascular control are affected, and this appears to be the mechanism by which extremely high amounts of alcohol cause death. One way to conceptualize the neuropsychological effect of alcohol on the central nervous system is to view the various brain areas (cortex, cerebellum, reticular activating system, and brain stem) as existing on a hierarchical continuum of tolerance to alcohol, which parallels the phylogenetic development of the mammalian nervous system. The area of the nervous system most sensitive to the effects of alcohol is the cortex which is the "newest" phylogenetically. Next is the cerebellum which is a little "older" phylogenetically, followed by the reticular activating system, down to the "old-est" part of the nervous system which is the brain stem. It is the brain stem that appears to be most resistant to impairment of function by alcohol.

Neuropharmacological Mechanisms in Alcoholism

In the sections above, we have outlined some of the descriptive aspects of alcoholism and the pharmacology of alcohol. In this section, we shall focus on the biological determinants of alcoholism and the effect of its prolonged, excessive consumption on the nervous system. It might help to view the relationship of these biological factors to alcoholism by assuming that the latter is the behavioral expression or final common pathway resulting from the interactions of multiple factors. These factors, in turn, can be divided into two subgroups: those that produce a vulnerability to manifest a certain disorder and those factors that precipitate or elicit the disorder. The biological factors we shall be discussing in this section are those that are presumed to contribute to the predisposition that a particular individual will develop alcoholism.

Genetic Determinants

It has been noted by many investigators that there is a high frequency of association of alcoholism in first degree relatives of alcoholic patients. This finding has raised the issue of the importance of hereditary factors in the etiology of alcoholism. A number of interesting research strategies have been employed to examine these hypotheses.

Family Studies — One approach has been to systematically investigate and document the prevalence of alcoholism among the relatives of alcoholics. In one series it was shown that 53% of alcoholics had fathers who were diagnosed as alcoholics and 6% had mothers who were

alcoholic. Almost without exception, every family study has shown higher rates of alcoholism among relatives of alcoholics than occur in the general population. It must be emphasized, however, that "familial" does not mean "hereditary" and it is incorrect to conclude from this data alone that alcoholism is genetically determined.

Twin Studies — A second strategy has been to carry out twin studies where the concordance rates of alcoholism among monozygotic twins are compared with the rates for dizygotic twins. One large study by Kaij showed a concordance rate for alcohol abuse in the monozygotic twin group of 54% compared to 28% in the dizygotic twin group. Even though this is a statistically significant difference, the data from this study does not present as compelling an argument in support of a genetic diathesis as do the data from twin studies with manic-depressive patients (see Chapter 5).

Adoption Studies — An interesting approach to this question is to perform adoption studies. This enables the investigator to attempt to separate genetic from environmental factors by studying individuals raised apart from their biological parents. In a recent report by Goodwin and his colleagues (1973) this general tactic was employed. These investigators compared two groups of adoptees. One group had one biological parent who had been hospitalized primarily for alcoholism. The other group consisted of controls, none of whose biological parents had ever had a hospital record of alcoholism. Both groups of adoptees had been separated from their biological parents prior to the age of 6 weeks and had been raised in foster homes that had been carefully screened for alcoholism and excluded if there were any indication of alcoholism in the adoptive parents. At the time of follow-up, both probands and controls were divided into four groups according to their drinking behavior: moderate drinkers, heavy drinkers, problem drinkers, and alcoholics. They found that there were four times as many *alcoholics* in the group of adoptees whose biological parents were positive for alcoholism than in the control group. On the other hand, there were more controls than probands in the problem drinking group. When these two groups (alcoholics and problem drinkers) were combined, there were still more probands than controls in the combined group; however, the difference was much less impressive. In interpreting these data, it must be kept in mind that it is often difficult to make the distinction between problem drinking and alcoholism. One tentative conclusion that can be drawn from this work is that alcoholism *per se* may not be genetically determined; however, the more severe forms of alcoholism may be partially determined or controlled by genetic factors.

Animal Alcohol Preference Studies — Another finding that adds indirect support to the notion of a genetic influence in alcoholism is that certain animals, such as mice and rats, can be selectively bred to prefer alcohol to other liquids. Experiments have suggested that preference for alcohol is influenced by hereditary factors. Rogers and McClearn (1962) cross-bred strains of rats with different levels of alcohol preference and found that the first generation fell nicely between the parental strains in their alcohol preference. They concluded that voluntary alcohol consumption may be "regulated by numerous genes."

At this stage of our understanding, the evidence that genetic factors play a significant role in the etiology of al-coholism is suggestive and intriguing rather than proven.

Biochemical Mechanisms

Genetic influences are usually expressed through complex biochemical mechanisms which, in turn, affect physiological reactions and psychological behavior. In this section, we shall examine some of the biochemical mechanisms that are hypothesized to be the biological substrate for alcoholism.

Endogenous Production of Alkaloids — A recent theory advanced by Davis and Walsh (1970) proposes a biochemical diathesis existing in alcoholics. This hypothesis states that, in alcoholics, acetaldehyde and the aldehyde derivatives of certain biogenic amines interact through a chemical process known as a Pictet-Spengler condensation to produce a class of compounds known as tetrahydroisoquinolines (THIQ). These compounds have a chemical structure which is very similar to highly addictive opiate alkaloids, such as heroin and morphine. It is speculated that the formation of THIQ *in vivo* may constitute the biochemical basis of alcohol addiction. An example of the mechanism of formation of one of these compounds, tetrahydropapaveroline, is shown schematically in Fig. 3. In this case, it is postulated that when a person consumes alcohol chronically, acetaldehyde generated in the liver by the metabolism of ethanol causes a relative competitive inhibition of the enzyme, aldehyde dehydrogenase, in brain. Aldehyde dehydrogenase catalyzes the conversion of the intermediate aldehyde derivatives of biogenic amines formed through the action of the enzyme monoamine oxidase. Inhibition of aldehyde dehydrogenase results in the accumulation of the intermediate aldehydes. One possibility is that the aldehyde may be diverted to a reductive pathway, with the formation of certain pharmacologically active al-

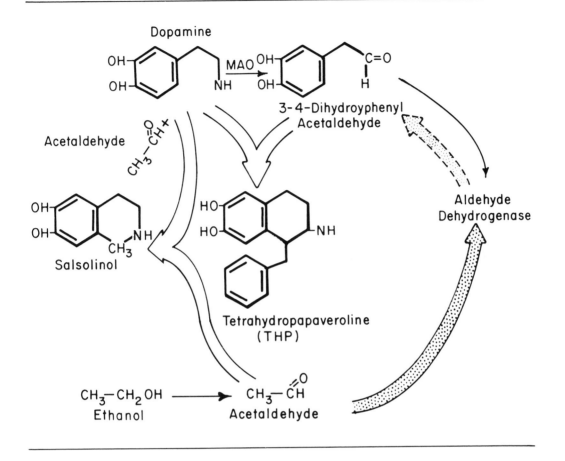

Fig. 3.   Formation of Tetrahydroisoquinolines
1. Dopamine and 3-4 Dihydroxyphenyl
Acetaldehyde → THP
2. Dopamine and Acetaldehyde→Salsolinol.

cohols, e.g., salsolinol. The other possibility is that at neutral pH the aldehyde (3-4-dihydroxyphenyl-acetaldehyde) is condensed with dopamine to form the compound tetrahydropapaveroline.

The tetrahydroisoquinolines have a number of interesting pharmacological properties. For instance, they are thought to compete for the same uptake and storage mechanisms as catecholamines in the brain. They also appear to be secreted in a manner similar to certain catecholamines, such as norepinephrine. Furthermore, they may act as "false"

transmitters and, under certain conditions, demonstrate properties similar to beta-adrenergic antagonists.

It is important to point out that, although there is some evidence that these compounds are formed *in vivo* under certain biological conditions, their relationship to the complex behavioral process of becoming addicted to alcohol is highly speculative. The theory is offered here to provide an example of current thinking in the area of possible biochemical determinants of the development of alcoholism.

Acetaldehyde — Another biochemical theory attempts to relate levels of acetaldehyde with an "aversion" to alcohol or, alternatively, lower levels of acetaldehyde permitting alcoholism to develop in certain individuals. Acetaldehyde is known to have a very marked psychophysiological effect. It is known that certain groups of individuals, especially some Orientals, develop an unpleasant reaction to the ingestion of even small amounts of alcohol. In those who exhibit this reaction with the ingestion of alcohol, it has been noted that, as a group, they have higher levels of acetaldehyde than do controls who do not demonstrate this idiosyncrasy. These findings have caused some to develop a "permissive" theory of the genesis of alcoholism, postulating that higher levels of acetaldehyde exert an aversive or protective effect against developing alcoholism, whereas lower levels of acetaldehyde remove this aversive inhibition to drinking alcohol, thereby "permitting" a person to drink more comfortably and, possibly, develop alcoholism. The evidence for this speculation is limited and inconclusive, and, once again, it is offered as an example of the type of questions that are being asked in an effort to relate certain biochemical changes to the development of alcoholism.

Pharmacological Tolerance and Dependence — Central to any concept of alcoholism is the process of addiction to the drug, alcohol. Although there are many definitions of addiction, most include the development of pharmacological tolerance and physiological dependence on alcohol. Tolerance develops in most people when they consume alcohol continually over a specific period of time. Tolerance is manifest as a decrease in the sensitivity to the effects of alcohol. An example of tolerance is to look at the effect of alcohol on a person's ability to do a specific behavioral task involving fine motor coordination. When a person takes alcohol, the ability to perform this task is impaired. With increasing amounts of alcohol consumed over a period of a few days to a week, the effect of alcohol is not as apparent on that particular task. A common everyday example of tolerance is shown by the person who is not used to drinking alcohol but has a few drinks and becomes noticeably intoxicated. In contrast, the person who may have been drinking moderately for quite some time can drink the same amount or more than the first person, yet show little, if any, effects of the alcohol.

Related to the concept of pharmacological tolerance is that of physiological dependence. This occurs in the person who has a pharmacological tolerance to a particular drug when that specific drug is abruptly discontinued. This results in a specific behavioral response which is opposite to the effects caused by the agent. This process is referred to as a "physiological withdrawal effect." In the case of alcohol, which depresses certain central nervous system functions, the withdrawal effect, seen when alcohol is discontinued, is just the opposite, i.e., a state of central nervous system excitability. The behavioral state of addiction occurs when a person finds it very hard to stop drinking because of the development of unpleasant withdrawal symptoms when drinking ceases. Usually the person learns that if he resumes drinking this will cause the withdrawal symptoms to abate.

The development of physiological dependence to alcohol and withdrawal has been explained on the basis of the ability of the central nervous system to compensate for the depressant effects of alcohol on brain cell function. In order to maintain an optimal level of brain cell function in the face of chronic alcohol administration, it is postulated that various compensatory mechanisms occur that increase the level of central nervous system stimulation to compensate for the depressant effect of alcohol. When alcohol is abruptly discontinued, there is a rebound effect produced by the central nervous system stimulation which is now no longer counteracted by the depressant effects of alcohol. New compensatory mechanisms are then brought into play that decrease the level of activation.

Biogenic Amines — Numerous attempts have been made to relate changes in biogenic amine metabolism to the development of addiction to alcohol, tolerance, and physiological dependence. The rationale for asking whether changes in biogenic amines may be relevant to alcoholism is based primarily on the finding that they are involved in so many other areas of normal and abnormal behavior, specifically in the affective disorders and schizophrenia. On a clinical level, there is evidence to suggest that there is a relationship between alcoholism and depression. On a neurophysiological level it has been shown that electrical stimulation of the lateral hypothalamus in rats facilitates the development of a permanent preference for ethanol over water. Other studies have indicated that these brain areas are richly supplied with noradrenergic nerve fibers, and it is thought, therefore, that norepinephrine and other biogenic amines may play a major role in the control of drinking.

Many of these studies have been performed in animals who have developed a "preference" for alcohol. One study demonstrated that intraventricular injection of minute quantities of serotonin precursors and metabolites altered the preference of monkeys for alcohol. In another experiment, rats who were selectively bred for alcohol preference had higher brain levels of serotonin before being exposed to ethanol and, after consumption of ethanol, the serotonin level increased even more.

A different approach is to see whether there is a relationship between changes in biogenic amine metabolism and the subjective effect of alcohol. One study approached this issue by looking at levels of dopamine beta-hydroxylase (DBH), the enzyme that catalyzes the conversion of dopamine to norepinephrine, in a group of normal subjects. These investigators found that those individuals who had low levels of DBH, when they drank alcohol, had fewer positive mood states in comparison to those with higher DBH levels who, after drinking, felt significantly better, less drunk and less sick. This study raises the intriguing hypothesis that some aspect of biogenic amine metabolism may be involved at the juncture of the interaction of alcohol and mood states which may constitute the critical factor in the genesis of alcoholism. This line of inquiry is supported by data from both human and animal experiments which show that alpha-methyl tyrosine, a drug that inhibits catecholamine synthesis, reduces alcohol-induced euphoria (in human) and decreased alcohol-induced locomotor stimulation (in rats and mice).

It appears that changes in biogenic amine metabolism are involved in alcoholism; however, the precise mechanisms operating in this relationship are not clear, and, as with other psychological states, there is the problem of whether changes in amine metabolism preceded the clinical state or whether they are the result of alcohol intake.

Alcohol Withdrawal Syndrome

The clinical manifestation of the withdrawal phenomenon in alcoholics when they stop drinking is known as the alcohol withdrawal syndrome (AWS). This occurs in the alcoholic who, after a long history of drinking, has achieved a state of pharmacological tolerance to alcohol. When he stops drinking or markedly decreases his intake of alcohol, a new group of symptoms, those of the abstinence or withdrawal syndrome become manifest. There are four major groups of abstinence symptoms which can be recognized: (1) a state characterized primarily by *tremulousness* and signs of mild autonomic nervous system hyperactivity such as increased perspiration, increased heart rate, mild increase in blood pressure, nausea and vomiting; (2) *Perceptual dysfunction*, manifest by the occurrence of either hallucinations or illusions; (3) *Seizures* which are usually grand-mal type; and (4) a state of *delirium* characterized by marked tremor, disorientation, hallucinations, rapid pulse rate, fever, diaphoresis and extreme psychomotor hyperactivity. We usually refer to this latter stage as "delerium tremens" or "DT's." The first three stages usually occur anywhere from 24 to 48 hours after cessation of drinking or marked decrease in alcohol intake. The stage of delirium usually sets in anywhere from 48 to 72 hours following the cessation of drinking. Each of the component subgroups may appear alone or in combination. Usually, they have a fairly predictable sequence, starting off with tremulousness, progressing to transient perceptual dysfunction and occasionally on to seizures. Signs and symptoms of the first three stages may appear to resolve only to be followed by the delirium later on. When seizures and delirium occur in the same patient, the seizures usually precede the delirium. It is thought that the intensity and severity of the withdrawal syndrome is correlated with the duration and amount of alcohol consumed. The very mildest manifestations of this syndrome is the well-known "hangover" which occurs after only one or two days of moderate to heavy drinking when, on awakening, the person experiences feelings of tremulousess, nausea, and hyperirritability. The more severe form of the abstinence syndrome, *viz.* hallucinations, seizures, and delirium, usually takes place when a person drinks at least a half to one quart of whiskey a day for a period of one to three months.

It is important to emphasize the clinical significance of the alcohol withdrawal syndrome. Not only is it an extremely uncomfortable and frightening experience for the patient to undergo, it also carries a small but significant mortality. In one series of patients, 5% went on to demonstrate signs and symptoms of delirium which is the most serious of the four stages of the withdrawal syndrome. Of more importance is the fact that 15% of those who developed delirium died.

There have been a number of attempts to delineate a biochemical or neurophysiological mechanism which underlies the alcohol withdrawal syndrome. One hypothesis proposes that low serum magnesium and elevation of pH in the blood are associated with the signs and symptoms of the alcohol withdrawal syndrome. Direct examination of patients who are undergoing this syndrome show a decrease in serum magnesium and an increase in blood pH which correlates with the initial phase of the alcohol withdrawal syndrome. Furthermore, the severity of the syndrome seems to bear a close relationship to the magnitude of change in these biochemical abnormalities. In addition to these direct observations, there is considerable indirect evidence to suggest that decreased serum magnesium and increase in blood pH are important in the causation of the withdrawal syndrome. Patients who have states of magnesium deficiency, not associated with alcohol, show signs of central and peripheral nervous system hyperirritability. In some cases, epileptic seizures have been known to occur when serum magnesium decreases. In man, magnesium deficiency states have been associated with tremor, twitching, visual and auditory hallucinations and other subjective symptoms similar to those occurring in the alcohol withdrawal syndrome. Most of these symptoms are quickly resolved with administration of magnesium. In addition, it has been shown that lowering the partial pressure of carbon dioxide (pCO_2), which occurs when there is hyperventilation, also tends to have an effect on neural excitability. Low pCO_2 may cause cerebral hypoxia by decreasing cerebral blood flow. The cerebral hypoxia may potentiate the direct effect of a low pCO_2 and increased pH on neural excitability.

The period from 10 to 48 hours following cessation of drinking, during which the signs and symptoms of the alcohol withdrawal syndrome are most severe, coincide with the period of great-est abnormality in arterial pH and serum magnesium. It is of interest that the patients who go on to develop the more severe form of the withdrawal syndrome, *delirium tremens*, seem to have the lowest levels of serum magnesium; however, their serum magnesium levels usually return to normal just at the time the delirium begins, so it is not possible to infer conclusively a direct causal relationship between low magnesium and the onset of delirium.

Treatment

Alcoholism is an extremely difficult disorder to treat. Measures of success depend greatly on criteria for cure and treatment outcome. Depending on the series studied, anywhere from 60% to 80% of all patients treated will relapse back to drinking at some stage in their treatment career; however, many of those who continue to drink have improved in other areas of their life, so that roughly one half to two thirds of those treated are improved in some fashion as a result of therapy. Most approaches to treatment utilize various aspects of group or individual psychotherapy. These span the spectrum of psychotherapeutic intervention from individual psychotherapy, counselling, psychoanalytic therapy, group counselling, alcoholics anonymous and, more recently, behavior therapy approaches. It is beyond the scope of this chapter to discuss these interventions in detail. In addition to these psychological therapies, there are biological methods, specifically pharmacological agents: disulfiram, antidepressants, and tranquilizers, which are used as adjuncts to psychological treatment modalities. Since our understanding of the specific biochemical mechanisms which underlie alcoholism are not as advanced as it is in depression and schizophrenia there is no specific biological treatment for alcoholism. Some of the drugs which have been useful in the over-all clinical management are discussed below. It is important to remember that pharmacotherapy is but one ingredient of a total treatment package that must be individually designed to fit the needs of each patient.

Disulfiram

Disulfiram is a drug which is used as an adjunct in the treatment of alcoholism. Disulfiram has a very specific metabolic effect which is thought to be the basis for its clinical usefulness in treating alcoholics. It inhibits the enzyme, acetaldehyde dehydrogenase. When a person who has taken disulfiram ingests alcohol, the alcohol is oxidized to acetaldehyde but the acetaldehyde cannot be metabolized further due to the competitive inhibition by disulfiram of the enzyme, acetaldehyde dehydrogenase. This results in an accumulation of acetaldehyde. As mentioned above, acetaldehyde is pharmacologically very active and quite toxic. The person who drinks alcohol while on disulfiram will experience a very intense and unpleasant psychophysiological reaction manifest by blushing, increased heart rate, dizziness, intense nausea, vomiting, and occasionally fainting.

Disulfiram is usually given to alcoholics who are in a state of remission and who have been abstinent from alcohol for a certain period of time. Its usefulness derives from the knowledge of the patient who is taking disulfiram that if he or she were to drink while taking disulfiram they would experience a very intense, unpleasant reaction. It is the realization of this that tends to strengthen the alcoholic's "willpower" to abstain from alcohol. Clearly the use of disulfiram is not a definitive treatment and it is also not useful for all alcoholics. Its effectiveness tends to be greatest in those alcoholics who are quite motivated to abstain from alcohol and who require something to help them resist the urge to drink.

Treatment of the Alcohol Withdrawal Syndrome

The major therapeutic thrust in the treatment of the alcohol withdrawal syndrome is to utilize a pharmacological agent that will counteract the state of increased central nervous system excitability and arousal which occurs in this syndrome. There has been a great deal of controversy as to the most effective psychotherapeutic drug to use in these situations and, over the years, a number of agents have been employed such as paraldehyde, phenothiazines, barbiturates and, most recently, minor tranquilizers, such as the benzodiazepines (chlordiazepoxide or diazepam). There are some definite factors which would tend to indicate that certain drugs are more useful and safer than others. Phenothiazines, for example, even though they have been widely used to treat this disorder, have one obvious major disadvantage: it is known that they tend to decrease the seizure threshold. Since seizures constitute one of the major undesirable sequelae of the abstinence syndrome, phenothiazines are theoretically contraindicated on this basis. Barbiturates also are contraindicated primarily

because, with the exception of phenobarbitol, most of them are metabolized by the liver. Most alcoholics have varying degrees of liver damage and may not be able to metabolize the barbiturate, thus causing a build-up of a drug which might produce a depression of vital central nervous system functions. A more important criticism of the use of barbiturates, however, is the fact that there is a high degree of cross-tolerance with alcohol, and this raises the problem of transferring an addiction from alcohol to barbiturates. Most clinicians prefer to use either chlordiazepoxide or paraldehyde. Paraldehyde has certain intrinsic disadvantages. It cannot be injected intravenously or intramuscularly safely because of the danger of tissue necrosis producing sterile abscesses. It also occasionally causes gastric irritation when given orally. In spite of the fact that patients who take paraldehyde often smell of the drug, only 5 to 10% of all paraldehyde is eliminated through the lungs. Most of it is oxidized by the liver. As mentioned above in the case of barbiturates, if there is some impairment in liver function, paraldehyde may accumulate, producing a state of metabolic acidosis. This compound presents still another problem in that it is a very labile substance which decomposes quite rapidly unless it is kept carefully stoppered in brown bottles. On the positive side is the fact that paraldehyde is an extremely effective drug to use in the treatment of the alcohol withdrawal syndrome. The minor tranquilizers, diazepam and chlordiazepoxide, have recently been widely employed because of their large margin of safety. They are easily tolerated both orally and parenterally, and do not cause, even in fairly high dosages, any untoward medical complications. In one study comparing the effectiveness of both paraldehyde and chlordiazepoxide, it was shown that chlordiazepoxide tended to decrease the duration of the abstinence syndrome; however, paraldehyde was slightly more effective in reducing the severity of the symptoms.

Conclusion

We have touched primarily on the biological variables thought to promote a disposition to developing alcoholism. It is important to remember that there are psychological and social variables which are critical in the development of this disorder. It is beyond the scope of this chapter to discuss these specific aspects in detail, and we will just briefly summarize them here. It is known that many alcoholics have certain personality variables in common, such as a tendency to indulge in impulsive behavior, difficulty in postponing gratification, or difficulty tolerating painful feelings for relatively long periods of time. Alcoholics describe subjective feelings of high levels of anxiety and tension which appear to persist over long periods of time. It is important to remember, however, that not all alcoholics have these characteristics and that these same traits are often found in a number of people who are not alcoholics.

There have been many psychodynamic profiles drawn of the typical alcoholic. He has often been characterized as a passive, dependent, and hostile person who finds it difficult to express his anger and hostility and, instead, turns his anger in upon himself. That is to say, he hurts others by hurting himself through drinking. This profile is not limited to alcoholics, and many alcoholics do not manifest this behavior.

There are social and cultural factors which play an important role in the development of alcohol abuse. The meaning of drinking in a particular culture is an important factor in the drinking practices of certain age groups. Adolescents and young adults are extremely susceptible to the notion that the mark of adult status in a particular society may be defined by whether a person can drink or how much he drinks. The effect of cultural attitudes can be seen by looking at epidemiological data on the incidence of alcoholism in various countries and in different nationalities. One example of this is the very high incidence of alcoholism in Scandinavian countries and France, as compared to Spain and Italy. Of interest is the fact that there is a low incidence of alcoholism in Jews and Chinese in the United States as contrasted with the high incidence in Irish-Americans.

In considering these various factors—biological, psychological, and sociological—it is important to realize that one cannot easily separate the biological from the psycho-social factors and give more weight to one than the other. In any particular patient who is afflicted with alcoholism it may very well be that one particular factor (biological, psychological, or sociological) may contribute more to the development of the problem than do other factors; however, all of these elements appear to be acting together to produce the behavioral end result which is alcoholism. The inappropriateness of separating the biological from the psycho-social dimensions of alcoholism is similar to attempting to determine how much the width of a field contributes to its area as opposed to the length.

The focus of this chapter has been on describing the clinical manifestations of alcoholism and its clinical course. We have tried to show how alcohol is absorbed, distributed, metabolized, and how it exerts its behavioral effect. Finally, we have tried to pinpoint certain biological factors which are thought to play a role in either the causes or perpetuation of alcoholism.

Selected References

Davis, V.E., and Walsh, M.J.: Alcohol, amines, and alkaloids: A possible biochemical basis for alcohol addiction. *Science* 167: 1005-1007, 1970.

Goodwin, D.W., et al.: Alcohol problems in adoptees raised apart from alcoholic biologic parents. *Arch. Gen. Psychiat.* 28:238-244, 1973.

Kaij., L.: *Studies on the Etiology and Sequels of Abuse of Alcohol.* Dept. of Psychiatry, University of Lund, Lund, 1960.

Keller, M. (Ed.): *Alcohol and Health.* Special Report to the U.S. Congress, U.S. Government Printing Office, Washington, D.C., 1974.

Kissin, B., and Begleiter, H. (Eds.): *The Biology of Alcoholism.* Plenum Press, New York, 1971. (Good review of metabolism of alcohol, neurochemistry of alcohol, and effects of alcohol on protein, carbohydrate, fat, and mineral metabolism.)

Rodgers, D.A., and McClearn, G.E.: Alcohol preferences in mice. In *Roots of Behavior,* E.L. Bliss, ed. Harper and Row, New York, 1962.

Siexas, F. (Ed.): Nature and nurture in alcoholism. *Ann. N.Y. Acad. Sci.* Vol. 197, 1972. (Collection of papers dealing with genetic and environmental factors in alcoholism).

Siexas, F. (Ed.): Alcohol and the central nervous system. *Ann. N.Y. Acad. Sci.* Vol. 215, 1973. (Collection of papers dealing with the action of alcohol on the brain, opiate alkaloid formation, alcohol preference in animals, tolerance, withdrawal states, and brain damage).

Index